GENDER AND HEALTH

Major Themes in Health and Social Welfare

Other titles in this series:

Medical Sociology
Edited and with a new introduction by Graham Scambler
4 volume set

Health Care Systems
Edited and with a new introduction by Jonathan Watson
4 volume set

Child Welfare
Edited and with a new introduction by Nick Frost
4 volume set

Death, Dying and Bereavement
Edited and with a new introduction by Kenneth J. Doka
4 volume set

Disability
Edited and with a new introduction by Nick Watson
4 volume set

Addiction
Edited and with a new introduction by Moira Plant and Martine Plant
4 volume set

Social Work
Edited and with a new introduction by Ann Buchanan
4 volume set

Mental Health
Edited and with a new introduction by Teresa L. Scheid
4 volume set

Health and Inequality
Edited and with a new introduction by Kate Pickett and Richard Wilkinson
4 volume set

Forthcoming

Social Issues of Aging
Edited and with a new introduction by Chris Phillipson
4 volume set

Caring for the Elderly
Edited and with a new introduction by Christina Victor
4 volume set

Suicide
Edited and with a new introduction by Keith Hawton and Rory O'Connor
4 volume set

GENDER AND HEALTH

Major Themes in Health and Social Welfare

Edited by
Kate Hunt and Ellen Annandale

Volume I
Theoretical and Methodological Developments

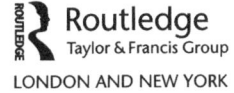

LONDON AND NEW YORK

First published 2012
by Routledge
2 Park Square, Milton Park, Abingdon, Oxon OX14 4RN

Simultaneously published in the USA and Canada
by Routledge
711 Third Avenue, New York, NY 10017

Routledge is an imprint of the Taylor & Francis Group, an informa business

© 2012 Kate Hunt and Ellen Annandale

All rights reserved. No part of this book may be reprinted or reproduced or utilised in any form or by any electronic, mechanical, or other means, now known or hereafter invented, including photocopying and recording, or in any information storage or retrieval system, without permission in writing from the publishers.

Trademark notice: Product or corporate names may be trademarks or registered trademarks, and are used only for identification and explanation without intent to infringe.

British Library Cataloguing in Publication Data
A catalogue record for this book is available from the British Library

Library of Congress Cataloging in Publication Data
Gender and health / edited by Kate Hunt and Ellen Annandale.
   p. ; cm. – (Major themes in health and social welfare)
   Includes bibliographical references and index.
   ISBN 978-0-415-56976-7 (set) – ISBN 978-0-415-56977-4 (v. 1) – ISBN 978-0-415-56978-1 (v. 2) – ISBN 978-0-415-56979-8 (v. 3) – ISBN 978-0-415-56980-4 (v. 4)   1. Health–Sex differences.
2. Women–Health and hygiene.   3. Men–Health and hygiene.
I. Hunt, Kate, 1959–   II. Annandale, Ellen.   III. Series: Major themes in health and social welfare.
   [DNLM: 1. Gender Identity–Collected Works.   2. Health Status Disparities–Collected Works.   3. Health Behavior–Collected Works.
4. Men's Health–Collected Works.   5. Sex Factors–Collected Works.
6. Women's Health–Collected Works.   WA 300.1]
   RA564.85.G45 2011
   613–dc23
                                                            2011007587

ISBN: 978-0-415-56976-7 (Set)
ISBN: 978-0-415-56977-4 (Volume I)

Typeset in 10/12pt Times NR MT
by Graphicraft Limited, Hong Kong

Publisher's Note
References within each chapter are as they appear in the original complete work

Printed and bound in Great Britain by the MPG Books Group

CONTENTS

Acknowledgements xv
Chronological table of reprinted articles and chapters xvii

General introduction 1

VOLUME I THEORETICAL AND METHODOLOGICAL DEVELOPMENTS

Introduction 5

PART 1
Making distinctions: sex and gender, the biological and the social 13

1 Sex and gender: the challenges for epidemiologists 15
LESLEY DOYAL

2 Genders, sexes, and health: what are the connections—and why does it matter? 26
NANCY KRIEGER

3 Shaping biology: feminism and the idea of 'the biological' 37
LYNDA BIRKE

4 The bare bones of sex: Part 1—sex and gender 51
ANNE FAUSTO-STERLING

5 Bodies, health, gender—bridging feminist theories and women's health 84
ELLEN KUHLMANN AND BIRGIT BABITSCH

CONTENTS

6 The egg and the sperm: how science has constructed a romance based on stereotypical male-female roles   101
EMILY MARTIN

PART 2
From women's health to gender and health: questioning binary thinking   117

7 Sexism, feminism and medicalism: a decade review of literature on gender and illness   119
JUANNE N. CLARKE

8 What is gender? Feminist theory and the sociology of human reproduction   139
ELLEN ANNANDALE AND JUDITH CLARK

9 Who is epidemiologically fathomable in the HIV/AIDS epidemic? Gender, sexuality, and intersectionality in public health   167
SHARI L. DWORKIN

10 Hegemonic masculinity: rethinking the concept   179
R. W. CONNELL AND JAMES W. MESSERSCHMIDT

11 The 'feminisation' of health   213
ELLIE LEE AND ELIZABETH FRAYN

PART 3
Capturing individual experience and gender contexts in research   235

12 Vaginal politics: tensions and possibilities in *The Vagina Monologues*   237
SUSAN E. BELL AND SUSAN M. REVERBY

13 Towards transnational feminisms: some reflections and concerns in relation to the globalization of reproductive technologies   260
JYOTSNA AGNIHOTRI GUPTA

14 Feminism meets the 'new' epidemiologies: toward an appraisal of antifeminist biases in epidemiological research on women's health   275
MARCIA C. INHORN AND K. LISA WHITTLE

15	Women's status and the health of women and men: a view from the States ICHIRO KAWACHI, BRUCE P. KENNEDY, VANITA GUPTA AND DEBORAH PROTHROW-STITH	302
16	Gender equity and socioeconomic inequality: a framework for the patterning of women's health NANCY E. MOSS	324
17	Healthy bodies, social bodies: men's and women's concepts and practices of health in everyday life ROBIN SALTONSTALL	348
18	Identity dilemmas of chronically ill men KATHY CHARMAZ	364

VOLUME II UNDERSTANDING THE PATTERNING OF HEALTH BY GENDER

	Acknowledgements	ix
	Introduction	1

PART 4
Early conceptualizations of the 'problem' of gender and health   9

19	Gender differences in mental and physical illness: the effects of fixed roles and nurturant roles WALTER R. GOVE	11
20	The future of sex mortality differentials in industrialized countries: a structural hypothesis CONSTANCE A. NATHANSON AND ALAN D. LOPEZ	29

PART 5
Gender patterning of mortality   45

21	Sex differences in mortality in Denmark during half a century, 1943–92 KARIN HELWEG-LARSEN AND KNUD JUEL	47

CONTENTS

22 Excess female mortality in rural Somalia: is inequality in the household a risk factor? 63
A. S. ADEN, M. M. OMAR, H. M. OMAR, U. HÖGBERG, L. Å. PERSSON AND S. WALL

23 Women's health status and gender inequality in China 76
MEI-YU YU AND ROSEMARY SARRI

PART 6
Gender patterning of morbidity: complicating the picture 101

24 Gender differences in health: are things really as simple as they seem? 103
SALLY MACINTYRE, KATE HUNT AND HELEN SWEETING

25 Sex difference in hospitalization due to asthma in relation to age 120
YUE CHEN, PAULA STEWART, HELEN JOHANSEN, LOUISE MCRAE AND GREGORY TAYLOR

26 Cross-national variation of gender differences in adolescent subjective health in Europe and North America 134
TORBJØRN TORSHEIM, ULRIKE RAVENS-SIEBERER, JORN HETLAND, RAILI VÄLIMAA, MIA DANIELSON AND MARY OVERPECK

27 Gender inequalities of health in the Third World 156
CHRISTIANA E. E. OKOJIE

28 Gender inequalities in US adult health: the interplay of race and ethnicity 179
JEN'NAN GHAZAL READ AND BRIDGET K. GORMAN

29 Gender differences in health: evidence from the Czech Republic 218
JOSEPH HRABA, FREDERICK LORENZ, GANG LEE AND ZDEŇKA PECHAČOVÁ

PART 7
Explanations for the gender patterning of health 235

30 Gender matters: an integrated model for understanding men's and women's health 237
CHLOE E. BIRD AND PATRICIA P. RIEKER

CONTENTS

31 Women, work, and well-being 1950–2000: a review and
    methodological critique   256
    PETRA L. KLUMB AND THOMAS LAMPERT

32 A two way view of gender bias in medicine   288
    M. TERESA RUIZ AND LOIS M. VERBRUGGE

33 Is patriarchy the source of men's higher mortality?   296
    D. STANISTREET, C. BAMBRA AND A. SCOTT-SAMUEL

PART 8
Gender and coronary heart disease   307

34 Sex matters: secular and geographical trends in sex differences
    in coronary heart disease mortality   309
    D. A. LAWLOR, S. EBRAHIM AND G. DAVEY SMITH

35 Decreased risk of death from coronary heart disease amongst men
    with higher 'femininity' scores: a general population cohort study   322
    KATE HUNT, HEATHER LEWARS, CAROL EMSLIE AND
    G. DAVID BATTY

36 Gender and images of heart disease in Scandinavian drug
    advertising   340
    ELIANNE RISKA AND THOMAS HEIKELL

37 Invisible women? The importance of gender in lay beliefs about
    heart problems   350
    CAROL EMSLIE, KATE HUNT AND GRAHAM WATT

PART 9
Gender and mental health   383

38 Gender, multiple roles, role meaning, and mental health   385
    ROBIN W. SIMON

39 Sex differences in distress: the impact of gender and work roles   406
    MARY CLARE LENNON

40 Gender differences in depression in 23 European countries:
    cross-national variation in the gender gap in depression   430
    SARAH VAN DE VELDE, PIET BRACKE AND
    KATIA LEVECQUE

CONTENTS

41 The social construction of gender and its influence on suicide: a review of the literature 452
SARAH PAYNE, VIREN SWAMI AND DEBBI L. STANISTREET

VOLUME III GENDER AND HEALTHCARE

Acknowledgements ix

Introduction 1

PART 10
Policy trends and health system change 9

42 Well women and medicine men: gendering the health policy agenda 11
ANNA COOTE AND LIZ KENDALL

43 Thinking about the production and consumption of long-term care in Britain: does gender still matter? 24
CLARE UNGERSON

44 Gender and equity in health sector reform programmes: a review 45
HILARY STANDING

45 Gender mainstreaming in health: looking back, looking forward 74
T. K. S. RAVINDRAN AND A. KELKAR-KHAMBETE

46 Reforming gendered health care: an assessment of change 99
MARY K. ZIMMERMAN AND SHIRLEY A. HILL

PART 11
The impact of gendered assumptions on health and healthcare 125

47 A funny thing happened on the way to the orifice: women in gynecology textbooks 127
DIANA SCULLY AND PAULINE BART

48 Doctor–patient negotiation of cultural assumptions 133
SUE FISHER AND STEPHEN B. GROCE

CONTENTS

49	Women as patients: a problem for sex differences research KATHY DAVIS	161
50	Sex differences and the new politics of women's health STEVEN EPSTEIN	174
51	Gender and the medicalization of healthcare SUSAN E. BELL AND ANNE E. FIGERT	202
52	Gendering the migraine market: do representations of illness matter? JOANNA KEMPNER	219
53	The influence of patient and doctor gender on diagnosing coronary heart disease ANN ADAMS, CHRISTOPHER D. BUCKINGHAM, ANTJE LINDENMEYER, JOHN B. McKINLAY, CAROL LINK, LISA MARCEAU AND SARA ARBER	239
54	Continuity and change in the gender segregation of the medical profession in Britian and France ROSEMARY CROMPTON AND NICKY LE FEUVRE	262
55	The feminization thesis: discourses on gender and medicine ELIANNE RISKA	280

PART 12
Accessing and experiencing healthcare   299

56	Help seeking for cardiac symptoms: beyond the masculine–feminine binary PAUL M. GALDAS, JOY L. JOHNSON, MYRA E. PERCY AND PAMELA A. RATNER	301
57	Gender and help-seeking: towards gender-comparative studies KATE HUNT, JOY ADAMSON AND PAUL GALDAS	318
58	Gender and access to HIV testing and antiretroviral treatments in Thailand: why do women have more and earlier access? SOPHIE LE CŒUR, INTIRA J. COLLINS, JULIE PANNETIER AND EVA LELIÈVRE	333
59	Gender, sexuality and embodiment: access to and experience of healthcare by same-sex attracted women in Australia JANE EDWARDS AND HELEN VAN ROEKEL	352

CONTENTS

60 Choosing Cesarean: feminism and the politics of childbirth in
the United States 370
KATHERINE BECKETT

61 Doing health, doing gender: teenagers, diabetes and asthma 396
CLARE WILLIAMS

VOLUME IV GENDER AND HEALTH BEHAVIOURS

Acknowledgements ix

Introduction 1

PART 13
Linking gender and health behaviours 9

62 Trends in gender differences in mortality: relationships to
changing gender differences in behaviour and other
causal factors 11
INGRID WALDRON

63 Constructions of masculinity and their influence on men's
well-being: a theory of gender and health 41
WILL H. COURTENAY

64 Healthy masculinities? How ostensibly healthy men talk about
lifestyle, health and gender 71
CLAIRE SLOAN, BRENDAN GOUGH AND MARK CONNER

65 Masculinity and perceived normative health behaviors as
predictors of men's health behaviors 96
JAMES R. MAHALIK, SHAUN M. BURNS AND
MATTHEW SYZDEK

66 'Real men don't diet': an analysis of contemporary newspaper
representations of men, food and health 112
BRENDAN GOUGH

CONTENTS

PART 14
Smoking and gender   133

67 Cigarette advertising policy and coverage of smoking and
    health in British women's magazines   135
    AMANDA AMOS, BOBBIE JACOBSON AND PATTI WHITE

68 Deadly targeting of women in promoting cigarettes   143
    ANNE MARIE O'KEEFE AND RICHARD W. POLLAY

69 Global patterns and determinants of sex differences in smoking   150
    FRED C. PAMPEL

70 Socioeconomic pattern of smoking in Japan: income inequality
    and gender and age differences   173
    YOSHIHARU FUKUDA, KEIKO NAKAMURA AND
    TAKEHITO TAKANO

71 Female ever-smoking, education, emancipation and economic
    development in 19 European countries   189
    MAARTJE M. SCHAAP, ANTON E. KUNST, MALL LEINSALU,
    ENRIQUE REGIDOR, ALBERT ESPELT, OLA EKHOLM,
    UWE HELMERT, JURATE KLUMBIENE AND
    JOHAN P. MACKENBACH

72 Loud, sad or bad: young people's perceptions of peer groups
    and smoking   206
    LYNN MICHELL

73 Women's smoking and family health   227
    HILARY GRAHAM

74 'If I don't smoke, I'm not a real man'—Indonesian teenage
    boys' views about smoking   249
    NAWI NG, L. WEINEHALL AND A. ÖHMAN

PART 15
Alcohol and gender   267

75 Alcohol and masculinity   269
    RUSSELL LEMLE AND MARC E. MISHKIND

76 Social roles and alcohol consumption: a study of
    10 industrialised countries   288
    SANDRA KUNTSCHE, RONALD A. KNIBBE AND GERHARD GMEL

CONTENTS

77 The specter of post-communism: women and alcohol in eight
post-Soviet states   308
BRIAN PHILIP HINOTE, WILLIAM C. COCKERHAM AND
PAMELA ABBOTT

78 The relationship between a less gender-stereotypical parenthood
and alcohol-related care and death: a registry study of
Swedish mothers and fathers   331
ANNA MÅNSDOTTER, MONA BACKHANS AND JOHAN HALLQVIST

79 Alcohol consumption and masculine identity among young men   353
RICHARD O. DE VISSER AND JONATHAN A. SMITH

80 Alcohol consumption, gender identities and women's changing
social positions   376
ANTONIA C. LYONS AND SARA A. WILLOTT

81 "Warning! Alcohol can seriously damage your feminine health":
a discourse analysis of recent British newspaper coverage of
women and drinking   411
KATY DAY, BRENDAN GOUGH AND MAJELLA McFADDEN

82 Childhood sexual abuse and adult binge drinking among
Kanak women in New Caledonia   433
CHRISTINE HAMELIN, CHRISTINE SALOMON, RÉMI SITTA,
ALICE GUEGUEN, DIANE CYR AND FRANCE LERT

Index   452

ACKNOWLEDGEMENTS

The publishers would like to thank the following for permission to reprint their material:

Baywood Publishing for permission to reprint Doyal, L. (2003) 'Sex and gender: the challenges for epidemiologists', *International Journal of Health Services*, 33, 3, 569–79.

Oxford University Press for permission to reprint Krieger, N. (2003) 'Genders, sexes, and health: what are the connections—and why does it matter?', *International Journal of Epidemiology*, 32: 652–7.

Routledge for permission to reprint Birke, L. (2003) 'Shaping biology: feminism and the idea of "the biological"', pp. 39–52 in S. Williams *et al.* (eds) *Debating Biology*, London: Routledge.

University of Chicago Press for permission to reprint Fausto-Sterling, A. (2005) 'The bare bones of sex: Part 1—sex and gender', *Signs*, 30, 21, 1491–527.

Elsevier for permission to reprint Kuhlmann, E. and Babitsch, B. (2002) 'Bodies, health, gender—bridging feminist theories and women's health', *Women's Studies International Forum*, 25, 4, 433–42.

University of Chicago Press for permission to reprint Martin, E. (1991) 'The egg and the sperm: how science as constructed a romance based on stereotypical male-female roles', *Signs*, 16, 3, 485–501.

Wiley for permission to reprint Clarke, J. N. (1983) 'Sexism, feminism and medicalism: a decade review of literature on gender and illness', *Sociology of Health and Illness*, 5, 1, 62–82.

Wiley for permission to reprint Annandale, E. and Clark, J. (1996) 'What is gender? Feminist theory and the sociology of human reproduction', *Sociology of Health and Illness*, 18, 1, 17–44.

Taylor & Francis for permission to reprint Dworkin, S. L. (2005) 'Who is epidemiologically fathomable in the HIV/AIDS epidemic? Gender, sexuality, and intersectionality in public health', *Culture, Health and Sexuality*, 7, 6, 615–23.

ACKNOWLEDGEMENTS

Sage for permission to reprint Connell, R. W. and Messerschmidt, J. W. (2005) 'Hegemonic masculinity: rethinking the concept', *Gender and Society*, 19, 6, 829–59.

Sage for permission to reprint Lee, E. and Frayn, E. (2008) 'The "feminisation" of health', pp. 115–33 in D. Wainwright (ed.) *A Sociology of Health*, London: Sage.

Elsevier for permission to reprint Bell, S. E. and Reverby, S. M. (2005) 'Vaginal politics: tensions and possibilities in *The Vagina Monologues*', *Women's Studies International Forum*, 28: 430–44.

Sage for permission to reprint Gupta, J. A. (2006) 'Towards transnational feminisms: some reflections and concerns in relation to the globalization of reproductive technologies', *European Journal of Women's Studies*, 13, 1, 23–38.

Elsevier for permission to reprint Inhorn, M. C. and Whittle, K. L. (2001) 'Feminism meets the "new" epidemiologies: toward an appraisal of antifeminist biases in epidemiological research on women's health', *Social Science & Medicine*, 53: 553–67.

Elsevier for permission to reprint Kawachi, I. *et al.* (1999) 'Women's status and the health of women and men: a view from the States', *Social Science & Medicine*, 48: 21–32.

Elsevier for permission to reprint Moss, N. E. (2002) 'Gender equity and socioeconomic inequality: a framework for the patterning of women's health', *Social Science & Medicine*, 54: 649–61.

Elsevier for permission to reprint Saltonstall, R. (1993) 'Healthy bodies, social bodies: men's and women's concepts and practices of health in everyday life', *Social Science & Medicine*, 36, 1, 7–14.

Wiley for permission to reprint Charmaz, K. (1994) 'Identity dilemmas of chronically ill men', *The Sociological Quarterly*, 35, 2, 269–88.

Disclaimer

The publishers have made every effort to contact authors/copyright holders of works reprinted in *Gender and Health (Major Themes in Health and Social Welfare)*. This has not been possible in every case, however, and we would welcome correspondence from those individuals/companies whom we have been unable to trace.

Chronological table of reprinted articles and chapters

Date	Author	Title	Source	Vol.	Chap.
1970	Diana Scully and Pauline Bart	A funny thing happened on the way to the orifice: women in gynecology textbooks	*American Journal of Sociology*, 78:4, 1045–51	III	47
1983	Juanne N. Clarke	Sexism, feminism and medicalism: a decade review of literature on gender and illness	*Sociology of Health and Illness*, 5:1, 62–82	I	7
1984	Kathy Davis	Women as patients: a problem for sex differences research	*Women's Studies International Forum*, 7:4, 211–17	III	49
1984	Walter R. Gove	Gender differences in mental and physical illness: the effects of fixed roles and nurturant roles	*Social Science & Medicine*, 19:2, 77–84	II	19
1985	Sue Fisher and Stephen B. Groce	Doctor–patient negotiation of cultural assumptions	*Sociology of Health and Illness*, 7:3, 342–74	III	48
1987	Hilary Graham	Women's smoking and family health	*Social Science & Medicine*, 25:1, 47–56	IV	73
1987	Mary Clare Lennon	Sex differences in distress: the impact of gender and work roles	*Journal of Health and Social Behavior*, 28, 290–305	II	39
1987	Constance A. Nathanson and Alan D. Lopez	The future of sex mortality differentials in industrialized countries: a structural hypothesis	*Population Research and Policy Review*, 6, 123–36	II	20
1989	Russell Lemle and Marc E. Mishkind	Alcohol and masculinity	*Journal of Substance Abuse Treatment*, 6, 213–22	IV	75
1991	Amanda Amos, Bobbie Jacobson and Patti White	Cigarette advertising policy and coverage of smoking and health in British women's magazines	*Lancet*, 3371, 93–6	IV	67
1991	Emily Martin	The egg and the sperm: how science has constructed a romance based on stereotypical male-female roles	*Signs*, 16:3, 485–501	I	6

Chronological table continued

Date	Author	Title	Source	Vol.	Chap.
1993	Robin Saltonstall	Healthy bodies, social bodies: men's and women's concepts and practices of health in everyday life	Social Science & Medicine, 36:1, 7–14	I	17
1994	Kathy Charmaz	Identity dilemmas of chronically ill men	The Sociological Quarterly, 35:2, 269–88	I	18
1994	Christiana E. E. Okojie	Gender inequalities of health in the Third World	Social Science & Medicine, 39, 1237–47	II	27
1995	Robin W. Simon	Gender, multiple roles, role meaning, and mental health	Journal of Health and Social Behavior, 36, 182–94	II	38
1996	Ellen Annandale and Judith Clark	What is gender? Feminist theory and the sociology of human reproduction	Sociology of Health and Illness, 18:1, 17–44	I	8
1996	Joseph Hraba, Frederick Lorenz, Gang Lee and Zdeňka Pechačová	Gender differences in health: evidence from the Czech Republic	Social Science & Medicine, 43, 1443–51	II	29
1996	Sally Macintyre, Kate Hunt and Helen Sweeting	Gender differences in health: are things really as simple as they seem?	Social Science & Medicine, 42, 617–24	II	24
1996	Anne Marie O'Keefe and Richard W. Pollay	Deadly targeting of women in promoting cigarettes	JAMWA, 51, 67–9	IV	68
1997	A. S. Aden, M. M. Omar, H. M. Omar, U. Högberg, L. Å. Persson and S. Wall	Excess female mortality in rural Somalia: is inequality in the household a risk factor?	Social Science & Medicine, 44, 709–15	II	22
1997	Lynn Michell	Loud, sad or bad: young people's perceptions of peer groups and smoking	Health Education Research Theory and Practice, 12:1, 1–14	IV	72

1997	M. Teresa Ruiz and Lois M. Verbrugge	A two way view of gender bias in medicine	*Journal of Epidemiology and Community Health*, 51, 106–9	II	32
1997	Hilary Standing	Gender and equity in health sector reform programmes: a review	*Health Policy and Planning*, 12:1, 1–18	III	44
1997	Mei-Yu Yu and Rosemary Sarri	Women's health status and gender inequality in China	*Social Science & Medicine*, 45:12, 1885–98	II	23
1999	Chloe E. Bird and Patricia P. Rieker	Gender matters: an integrated model for understanding men's and women's health	*Social Science & Medicine*, 48, 745–55	II	30
1999	Ichiro Kawachi, Bruce P. Kennedy, Vanita Gupta and Deborah Prothrow-Stith	Women's status and the health of women and men: a view from the States	*Social Science & Medicine*, 48, 21–32	I	15
2000	Anna Coote and Liz Kendall	Well women and medicine men: gendering the health policy agenda	A. Coote (ed.), *The New Gender Agenda*, London: IPPR, pp. 149–60	III	42
2000	Will H. Courtenay	Constructions of masculinity and their influence on men's well-being: a theory of gender and health	*Social Science & Medicine*, 50, 1385–401	IV	63
2000	Karin Helweg-Larsen and Knud Juel	Sex differences in mortality in Denmark during half a century, 1943–92	*Scandinavian Journal of Public Health*, 28, 214–21	II	21
2000	Clare Ungerson	Thinking about the production and consumption of long-term care in Britain: does gender still matter?	*Journal of Social Policy*, 29, 623–43	III	43
2000	Ingrid Waldron	Trends in gender differences in mortality: relationships to changing gender differences in behaviour and other causal factors	E. Annandale and K. Hunt (eds), *Gender Inequalities in Health*, Buckingham: Open University Press, pp. 150–81	IV	62
2000	Clare Williams	Doing health, doing gender: teenagers, diabetes and asthma	*Social Science & Medicine*, 50, 387–96	III	61
2000	Mary K. Zimmerman and Shirley A. Hill	Reforming gendered health care: an assessment of change	*International Journal of Health Services*, 30:4, 771–95	III	46

Chronological table continued

Date	Author	Title	Source	Vol.	Chap.
2001	Carol Emslie, Kate Hunt and Graham Watt	Invisible women? The importance of gender in lay beliefs about heart problems	*Sociology of Health and Illness*, 23:2, 203–33	II	37
2001	Marcia C. Inhorn and K. Lisa Whittle	Feminism meets the "new" epidemiologies: toward an appraisal of antifeminist biases in epidemiological research on women's health	*Social Science & Medicine*, 53, 553–67	I	14
2001	D. A. Lawlor, S. Ebrahim and G. Davey Smith	Sex matters: secular and geographical trends in sex differences in coronary heart disease mortality	*British Medical Journal*, 323, 541–5	II	34
2002	Ellen Kuhlmann and Birgit Babitsch	Bodies, health, gender—bridging feminist theories and women's health	*Women's Studies International Forum*, 25:4, 433–42	I	5
2002	Nancy E. Moss	Gender equity and socioeconomic inequality: a framework for the patterning of women's health	*Social Science & Medicine*, 54, 649–61	I	16
2003	Lynda Birke	Shaping biology: feminism and the idea of 'the biological'	S. Williams *et al.* (eds), *Debating Biology*, London: Routledge, pp. 39–52	I	3
2003	Yue Chen, Paula Stewart, Helen Johansen, Louise McRae and Gregory Taylor	Sex difference in hospitalization due to asthma in relation to age	*Journal of Clinical Epidemiology*, 56, 180–7	II	25
2003	Rosemary Crompton and Nicky Le Feuvre	Continuity and change in the gender segregation of the medical profession in Britain and France	*International Journal of Sociology and Social Policy*, 23:4, 36–58	III	54
2003	Lesley Doyal	Sex and gender: the challenges for epidemiologists	*International Journal of Health Services*, 33:3, 569–79	I	1

2003	Nancy Krieger	Genders, sexes, and health: what are the connections—and why does it matter?	*International Journal of Epidemiology*, 32, 652–7	I	2
2004	Katy Day, Brendan Gough and Majella McFadden	"Warning! Alcohol can seriously damage your feminine health": a discourse analysis of recent British newspaper coverage of women and drinking	*Feminist Media Studies*, 4, 165–83	IV	81
2004	Petra L. Klumb and Thomas Lampert	Women, work, and well-being 1950–2000: a review and methodological critique	*Social Science & Medicine*, 58, 1007–24	II	31
2005	Susan E. Bell and Susan M. Reverby	Vaginal politics: tensions and possibilities in *The Vagina Monologues*	*Women's Studies International Forum*, 28, 430–44	I	12
2005	R. W. Connell and James W. Messerschmidt	Hegemonic masculinity: rethinking the concept	*Gender and Society*, 19:6, 829–59	I	10
2005	Shari L. Dworkin	Who is epidemiologically fathomable in the HIV/AIDS epidemic? Gender, sexuality, and intersectionality in public health	*Culture, Health and Sexuality*, 7:6, 615–23	I	9
2005	Anne Fausto-Sterling	The bare bones of sex: Part 1—sex and gender	*Signs*, 30:21, 1491–527	I	4
2005	Yoshiharu Fukuda, Keiko Nakamura and Takehito Takano	Socioeconomic pattern of smoking in Japan: income inequality and gender and age differences	*Annals of Epidemiology*, 15:5, 365–72	IV	70
2005	D. Stanistreet, C. Bambra and A. Scott-Samuel	Is patriarchy the source of men's higher mortality?	*Journal of Epidemiology and Community Health*, 59, 873–6	II	33
2006	Katherine Beckett	Choosing Cesarean: feminism and the politics of childbirth in the United States	*Feminist Theory*, 6:3, 251–75	III	60
2006	Jyotsna Agnihotri Gupta	Towards transnational feminisms: some reflections and concerns in relation to the globalization of reproductive technologies	*European Journal of Women's Studies*, 13:1, 23–38	I	13

Chronological table continued

Date	Author	Title	Source	Vol.	Chap.
2006	Joanna Kempner	Gendering the migraine market: do representations of illness matter?	*Social Science & Medicine*, 63, 1986–97	III	52
2006	Fred C. Pampel	Global patterns and determinants of sex differences in smoking	*International Journal of Comparative Sociology*, 47, 466–87	IV	69
2006	Jen'nan Ghazal Read and Bridget K. Gorman	Gender inequalities in US adult health: the interplay of race and ethnicity	*Social Science & Medicine*, 62:5, 1045–65	II	28
2006	Torbjørn Torsheim, Ulrike Ravens-Sieberer, Jorn Hetland, Raili Välimaa, Mia Danielson and Mary Overpeck	Cross-national variation of gender differences in adolescent subjective health in Europe and North America	*Social Science & Medicine*, 62, 815–27	II	26
2007	Brendan Gough	'Real men don't diet': an analysis of contemporary newspaper representations of men, food and health	*Social Science & Medicine*, 64, 326–37	IV	66
2007	Kate Hunt, Heather Lewars, Carol Emslie and G. David Batty	Decreased risk of death from coronary heart disease amongst men with higher 'femininity' scores: a general population cohort study	*International Journal of Epidemiology*, 36, 612–20	II	35
2007	James R. Mahalik, Shaun M. Burns and Matthew Syzdek	Masculinity and perceived normative health behaviors as predictors of men's health behaviors	*Social Science & Medicine*, 64, 2201–9	IV	65
2007	Nawi Ng, L. Weinehall and A. Öhman	'If I don't smoke, I'm not a real man'—Indonesian teenage boys' views about smoking	*Health Education Research*, 22:6, 794–804	IV	74
2007	Elianne Riska and Thomas Heikell	Gender and images of heart disease in Scandinavian drug advertising	*Scandinavian Journal of Public Health*, 35:6, 585–90	II	36
2007	Richard O. de Visser and Jonathan A. Smith	Alcohol consumption and masculine identity among young men	*Psychology and Health*, 22:5, 595–614	IV	79

2008	Ann Adams, Christopher D. Buckingham, Antje Lindenmeyer, John B. McKinlay, Carol Link, Lisa Marceau and Sara Arber	The influence of patient and doctor gender on diagnosing coronary heart disease	*Sociology of Health and Illness*, 30, 1–18	III	53
2008	Steven Epstein	Sex differences and the new politics of women's health	S. Epstein, *Inclusion: The Politics of Difference in Medical Research*, Chicago: Chicago University Press, pp. 233–57	III	50
2008	Ellie Lee and Elizabeth Frayn	The 'feminisation' of health	D. Wainwright (ed.), *A Sociology of Health*, London: Sage, pp. 115–33	I	11
2008	Antonia C. Lyons and Sara A. Willott	Alcohol consumption, gender identities and women's changing social positions	*Sex Roles*, 59, 694–712	IV	80
2008	Anna Månsdotter, Mona Backhans and Johan Hallqvist	The relationship between a less gender-stereotypical parenthood and alcohol-related care and death: a registry study of Swedish mothers and fathers	*BMC Public Health*, 8, 312	IV	78
2008	Sarah Payne, Viren Swami and Debbi L. Stanistreet	The social construction of gender and its influence on suicide: a review of the literature	*Journal of Men's Health*, 5:1, 23–35	II	41
2008	T. K. S. Ravindran and A. Kelkar-Khambete	Gender mainstreaming in health: looking back, looking forward	*Global Public Health*, 3:S1, 121–42	III	45
2008	Elianne Riska	The feminization thesis: discourses on gender and medicine	*NORA—Nordic Journal of Feminist and Gender Research*, 16:1, 3–18	III	55
2009	Jane Edwards and Helen van Roekel	Gender, sexuality and embodiment: access to and experience of healthcare by same-sex attracted women in Australia	*Current Sociology*, 57:2, 193–210	III	59

Chronological table continued

Date	Author	Title	Source	Vol.	Chap.
2009	Christine Hamelin, Christine Salomon, Rémi Sitta, Alice Gueguen, Diane Cyr and France Lert	Childhood sexual abuse and adult binge drinking among Kanak women in New Caledonia	*Social Science & Medicine*, 68, 1247–53	IV	82
2009	Brian Philip Hinote, William C. Cockerham and Pamela Abbott	The specter of post-communism: women and alcohol in eight post-Soviet states	*Social Science & Medicine*, 68, 1254–62	IV	77
2009	Sandra Kuntsche, Ronald A. Knibbe and Gerhard Gmel	Social roles and alcohol consumption: a study of 10 industrialised countries	*Social Science & Medicine*, 68, 1263–70	IV	76
2009	Sophie Le Cœur, Intira J. Collins, Julie Pannetier and Eva Lelièvre	Gender and access to HIV testing and antiretroviral treatments in Thailand: why do women have more and earlier access?	*Social Science & Medicine*, 69, 846–53	III	58
2009	Maartje M. Schaap, Anton E. Kunst, Mall Leinsalu, Enrique Regidor, Albert Espelt, Ola Ekholm, Uwe Helmert, Jurate Klumbiene and Johan P. Mackenbach	Female ever-smoking, education, emancipation and economic development in 19 European countries	*Social Science & Medicine*, 68, 1271–8	IV	71

2009	Claire Sloan, Brendan Gough and Mark Conner	Healthy masculinities? How ostensibly healthy men talk about lifestyle, health and gender	*Psychology and Health*, i-First, 1–21	IV	64
2010	Susan E. Bell and Anne E. Figert	Gender and the medicalization of healthcare	E. Kuhlmann and E. Annandale (eds), *The Palgrave Handbook of Gender and Healthcare*, London: Palgrave, pp. 107–22	III	51
2010	Paul M. Galdas, Joy L. Johnson, Myra E. Percy and Pamela A. Ratner	Help seeking for cardiac symptoms: beyond the masculine–feminine binary	*Social Science & Medicine*, 71, 18–24	III	56
2010	Kate Hunt, Joy Adamson and Paul Galdas	Gender and help-seeking: towards gender-comparative studies	E. Kuhlmann and E. Annandale (eds), *The Palgrave Handbook of Gender and Healthcare*, London: Palgrave, pp. 207–21	III	57
2010	Sarah Van de Velde, Piet Bracke and Katia Levecque	Gender differences in depression in 23 European countries: cross-national variation in the gender gap in depression	*Social Science & Medicine*, 71, 305–13	II	40

GENERAL INTRODUCTION

Kate Hunt and Ellen Annandale

Research in gender and health has inspired considerable interest over the last four decades or so. The papers appearing in this four-volume collection are the fruits of our attempt to provide a good overview of how theoretical conceptualisations of gender have developed over this time and how they have been applied in empirical studies of the impact of gender on various aspects of health. Limiting our choices to the 80 or so papers which are reproduced in these volumes has been a fascinating and challenging task. Our choices have not only been constrained by limitations of space, but also by our efforts to produce a representation of different approaches to understanding the complex interlinking between gender and health. For example, we have tried to provide a balance between theoretical papers, empirical studies and reviews; we have tried to include papers from different parts of the globe and some with a clearly historical perspective to illustrate how the meaning of being male or female (and its implications for health) changes over time and space; and we have included empirical papers utilizing a range of methodological perspectives reflecting different disciplinary or ontological standpoints.

Inevitably, we have had to make some extremely difficult choices, leaving out some excellent scholarship to maintain this balance, but we hope that the resulting collection provides a stimulating resource for anyone interested in gender and health. We believe that the collection illustrates: how theoretical conceptualisations of gender have changed; the very different consequences of being a woman (or man) in one historical and geographical context rather than another (e.g. Somalia as compared with Europe or the USA); how the thorny issue of being able to integrate biological and more social understandings of gender is yet to be resolved; how health care systems and health behaviours can produce, reproduce and reinforce societal understandings of gender inequalities; and how good research conducted within epidemiology, sociology, psychology, biology, medicine and other disciplines all contribute to our growing understanding of gender and health. In making our selections for this collection we have had a wide readership in mind, from students from a broad range of social science and biological backgrounds, to those training to be health care providers (doctors, nurses, and other allied health professionals), and researchers and policy-makers with a primary interest in either gender, health or both.

Because most cultures draw binary distinctions between men and women, male and female, and use these to structure life chances and opportunities, research on gender and health is a fascinating lens on how social systems, social processes and social environments become written into/onto the body. Gender is a fundamental social distinction that persists throughout our lives; irrespective of how much as individuals we may resist gender categories. These accumulated differences in life chances by gender become 'written' on/in the body and one way in which they manifest themselves is in gender differences in health. This can be illustrated using life expectancy at birth. In many ways, gender presents a paradox in relation to health. A huge body of research on inequalities in health demonstrates how social advantage confers health benefits, including longer life expectancy and longer healthy life expectancy. However, despite the greater social advantages and opportunities which are conferred on men rather than women of otherwise similar social backgrounds historically and cross-culturally, it is *women* who fare better in terms of mortality. Over the last decade at least there have been very few countries in which the life expectancy of women does *not* exceed that of men, even though life expectancy varies hugely around the world. Figures from the World Health Organisation for 2008 show a more than twofold difference between life expectancy at birth between the countries with the longest and the shortest life expectancies at birth. For males, life expectancy at birth was shortest at just 40 years in Afghanistan, and only reached or exceeded 80 years in Iceland (80 years), Switzerland (80 years) and San Marino (81 years) (World Health Organisation, 2010). For females, Zimbabwe had the shortest life expectancy at birth in 2008 at 42 years, and Japan had the longest (86 years), but life expectancy was 80 years or more in 37 countries spanning a range of cultures in western Europe (e.g. Austria (83 years), Belgium (82 years), France (85 years)), central and eastern Europe (e.g. Czech Republic (80 years), Poland (80 years)), north, south and central American (e.g. Canada (83 years), USA (81 years), Costa Rica (81 years)), and the Western Pacific Region (Australia (84 years), New Zealand (83 years), Republic of Korea (83 years), Singapore (83 years) and Japan (86 years)). Life expectancy is higher for women than men in almost every country, leading the World Health Organisation to suggest that 'their innate constitution' gives women 'an advantage over men'. In 2008 male life expectancy exceeded female life expectancy in just two WHO member states (Tonga, male life expectancy 71 years, female life expectancy 70 years; Central African Republic, male life expectancy 49 years, female life expectancy 48 years), and males and females had the same life expectancy at birth in Cameroon (53 years), Mozambique (51 years), Nigeria (49 years), Qatar (76 years), Swaziland (48 years), and Zimbabwe (42 years). However, this differential is far greater in some countries (e.g. Japan) than others (e.g. Qatar, Botswana) and rapid changes in the sex differential in life expectancy (e.g. as seen in the ex-Soviet Union in the 1980s–1990s) can only be explained by social factors. Statistics of course only tell part of the story. It is equally important for research to reveal the intricate lived reality of gender. Research on health can thus demonstrate the ways that different societies (historically and cross-culturally) create differential life chances and opportunities for men and women, boys and girls, and a window to understand how the social world 'gets under the skin' and how human health can be improved.

This four-volume collection draws together key papers spanning theoretical developments and empirical research which uses a range of qualitative and quantitative methods in the dynamic and challenging field of gender and health. Each of the volumes provides its own introduction to the particular selection of papers that it includes. Here we provide an overview of why we think it is important to continue to research the links between gender and health, and the overarching considerations that helped to determine the themes for each of the four volumes. The selected papers focus on all stages of the life course, including youth and adolescence, middle age, and older age. The choice of papers aims to illustrate the progress of research in this field and to highlight challenges for future research. Throughout we hope that the choice of papers demonstrates the central issues, substantively, methodologically and theoretically, for current and future research on gender and health.

Volume I: Theoretical and Methodological Developments includes articles on sociological, anthropological, biological, psychological, epidemiological and feminist conceptualisations of gender. It considers the influence of second-wave feminism on research on gender, and gender and health. It also addresses the conceptual shift from 'gender' as a status that affects women's lives (an implicit assumption of much earlier research) to new ways of thinking about gender as enacted or performed, as well as the increasing focus on men as gendered too with the rise of studies on masculinities.

Volume II: Understanding the Patterning of Health by Gender focuses on the patterning of health status by gender in various parts of the world, and to a lesser extent on how assumptions about gender and health have led to the gendering of some aspects of ill-health (including coronary heart disease and mental ill-health). The papers challenge the outdated assumption that gender differences in health can be universally summarised by the apparent paradox that 'women get sicker, but men die quicker' which dominated early research in this area in the 1970s and 1980s.

Volume III: Gender and Health Care includes papers on: the medicalisation of gender, initially of women's health and more recently of aspects of men's health; gender equity/gender bias and health care use and provision; gender differences and similarities in help-seeking and in health care usage; and the attitudes of health providers towards patients and their influence on the way that care is provided.

Volume IV: Gender and Health Behaviours examines patterns of key health-related behaviours (with a particular focus on smoking and detrimental patterns of alcohol consumption) and their contribution to differences in morbidity and mortality between men and women. It also picks up the theme of 'doing' gender through 'doing' health, examining how the adoption of particular behaviours can be linked to different 'performances' of gender.

Reference

World Health Organisation (2010) *World Health Statistics 2010*. http://www.who.int/whosis/whostat/EN_WHS10_Full.pdf

INTRODUCTION

Kate Hunt and Ellen Annandale

The theoretical approaches taken towards 'gender and health' steer us in the direction of particular research questions and towards specific ways of researching them. The relationship between theory and method is symbiotic: new theoretical agendas often require new methods and in turn new methods can stimulate new ways of conceptualising research problems. The articles and book chapters reprinted in this volume have been chosen to highlight the various theoretical and methodological matters that have influenced gender and health research since the latter part of the twentieth century. They are grouped into three overlapping themes: 'making distinctions: sex and gender, the biological and the social'; 'from women's health to gender and health: questioning binary thinking'; and 'capturing individual experience and gender contexts in research'.

Part 1 Making distinctions: sex and gender, the biological and the social

The distinction between biological sex and social gender has been an organising principle of gender research since the 1970s (Stoller 1968; Oakley 1972). It was particularly important for early feminist-inspired health research since it helped to make the argument that women's ill-health results from the organisation of societies along patriarchal lines rather than from their 'defective biology'. More recently, this line of argument has been extended to the study of men's health. However, although sex and gender have been vital conceptual tools they have proved difficult to employ in actual research.

In the first article in the volume, Lesley Doyal (**1**) argues that we 'need to differentiate very clearly between the biological and the social if we are to achieve a rigorous understanding of complex health problems and to develop appropriate interventions for solving them'. She addresses five challenges to the effective integration of sex and gender into research. These are: (i) to deal with the conceptual confusion that surrounds the concepts; (ii) to broaden our understanding of the links between biological sex and health; (iii) to develop a more comprehensive understanding of how the health of women and men is shaped by social gender; (iv) to make sure that research designs are 'sex and gender sensitive'; and (v) to create ways of including sex and gender into wider gender-equality agendas. Nancy Krieger (**2**) advises us to think about sex and gender in the plural as 'new constructions of sexes and genders are entering the scientific domain' such as transgender, transsexual, intersexual. As she points out, these 'blur boundaries not only *between* but also *within* the gender/sex dichotomy' (emphasis in original). She also stresses that 'we do not live as a "gendered" person one day and a "sexed" person the next; we are both, simultaneously'. With these and other theoretical matters in mind, Krieger explores the empirical question of whether and how 'diverse permutations of sex and gender matter – or are irrelevant' to health in twelve case examples for women and men, boys and girls.

Although the sex/gender distinction has been a fruitful basis for research, it has not been without difficulties, as these articles demonstrate. One taxing problem has been the tendency to focus on the social, to the exclusion of the biological. Although this was politically important in the early days of feminist research since it helped to challenge patriarchal ascriptions of women's illness as biologically given and fixed (**2**), it also led to the exclusion of biology and the embodied nature of illness from many explanatory frameworks. Feminist biologist Lynda Birke (**3**) explores moves to '"bring back" the biological', but raises a crucial question for feminists: 'what *kind* of biology do we want to bring back in'? (our emphasis). More often than not 'the "body" that is at the centre of discussions of health remains quite passive, seeming to be acted upon by . . . various external agents'. Birke urges us to think differently. She conceptualises the body 'as *process(es)* rather than fixed', as an organism which develops in engagement with the world in which it lives, both changing and being changed by it (emphasis in original).

The articles by Anne Fausto-Sterling (**4**) and Emily Martin (**6**) draw attention to the arrantly political nature of sex and gender research. Martin shows how cultural metaphors and gender stereotypes shape the way biologists think about the body. In an exploration of medical texts she reveals how a story is constructed of 'the egg and the sperm', menstruation and spermatogenesis. She finds that medical texts 'have an almost dogged insistence on casting female processes in a negative light' (**6**) while extolling the virtues of the male reproductive body. The sperm is portrayed as active, even aggressive, while the egg sits passive or, in more recent accounts at the time of writing, rather aggressively 'captures' the sperm. Fausto-Sterling uses the evocative notion of the 'spreading oil spill of sex' (**4**) to describe the current movement to 'bring sex back in', but in highly deterministic ways (see also **53** on the implications of this for health care). Through the example of bone disease she shows how medical problems like osteoporosis cannot be understood by parsing them into biological (or genetic, hormonal) in opposition to cultural and social factors. Fausto-Sterling argues that 'bones are eloquent' and tell of lives lived in certain ways. The gender regimens that have operated in different times and places have steered men and women to different kinds of activity that influence bone density. She advocates a lifecourse systems approach which stresses that 'cells, nervous systems, and whole organisms develop through a process of self-organisation rather than according to a preformed set of instructions' as they are embedded within particular gender and cultural regimes (**4**).

The 'second wave' women's movement of the 1960s onwards made health a focal concern and the feminist approaches of sociologists, biologists, anthropologists and others have been vital to the development of gender and health research. However as Ellen Kuhlmann and Birgit Babitsch (**5**) observe, rather deep 'fault lines' have emerged between the work of feminist theorists and what they term 'women's health research'. They argue that recent feminist theories such as Judith Butler's 'performative bodies', Donna Haraway's 'cyborg bodies', and Elisabeth Grosz's 'volatile bodies' are disassociated from the material body in health and illness (Haraway 1991; Grosz 1994; Butler 1993). In its turn, the more empirical field of 'women's health research' has provided a thoroughgoing criticism of biomedical practices and drawn attention to the socially produced nature of illness but has failed to engage fully with theoretical debates about the materiality of the body.

Part 2 From women's health to gender and health: questioning binary thinking

In an agenda-setting article of the early 1980s, Juanne Clarke (**7**) contends that our (in)ability to make sense of the supposed differences in the health status of men and women, is in good part due to theoretical and methodological limitations in the way both illness and gender have been conceptualised. She critiques the adoption of biomedical definitions of health and illness in gender and health research and draws attention to the highly problematic consequences of the conflation of sex and gender in medical practice and social science research. She also cautions against the tendency of researchers, which is still widespread today, to approach the study of health status in terms of 'sex differences' and to explain these differences in terms of social roles extracted from the their 'social, political and economic surroundings' (**7**).

Continuing some of these concerns, Ellen Annandale and Judith Clark (**8**) explore the problems that can arise when researchers engage unproblematically with binary thinking about men/women, male/female, sex/gender, and social/biological. They argue that research which begins from a biologically or a socially essentialist position that men and women are different biological and/or social groups can be more enslaving than liberating. They maintain that a consequence of treating women as a group *a priori* distinct from men as a group is that 'women's health is constructed as "poor" against an implicit assumption that that male health is "good" ... in such a view women "cannot" be well and ... men "cannot" be ill: they are "needed" to be well to construe women as sick' (**8**). They consider how far a deconstructive approach (drawing on feminist post-structuralism) can help dislodge the oppositions that spawn these problems and help to move research forward, paying particular attention to the potential of new reproductive technologies (of the time) to deconstruct politically problematic binaries.

Shari Dworkin also reflects critically on conceptual hierarchies to show how women become visible in HIV/Aids debates and research through the 'tropes of heterosexuality and vulnerability' (**9**). She argues that the conflation of sex and gender construes women as biologically and socially vulnerable and men as biologically and socially powerful in HIV/Aids literature. The result is an inappropriate 'passive emphasised femininity' and 'aggressive hegemonic masculinity' (**9**) which passivises women and omits male vulnerability. More adequate theories, she proposes, need to take greater account of intersecting identities and experiences in surveillance categories and in current models of risk hierarchicalisation.

The work of Raewyn Connell and colleagues has been the catalyst for much research and theorising on gender and health in general and on men's health specifically (see for example, Connell 1995, 2009). Connell and Messerschmidt (**10**) trace the development of the concept of 'hegemonic masculinity'. From their in-depth review, the authors conclude that the concept should be reshaped to take better account of: gender hierarchies; of the global geography of masculine configurations; of embodiment as a social process; and of masculinities as configurations of practice that are profoundly dynamic. These are fertile theoretical propositions for the analysis of men's health.

The comparatively late recognition that men's health is also 'gendered' is associated with the longstanding and largely tacit assumption that patriarchal privileges in society confer only health advantages upon men. One consequence has been to render the potential associations between masculinity and health invisible until quite recently. However, patriarchy is now recognised to be as much a danger to men's health as to women's health (**1**). As well as being important in its own right, the more recent attention to men's health has also made it possible for research to be more gender comparative (Annandale and Hunt 2000). Ellie Lee and Elizabeth Frayn (**11**) highlight how discourses of health and illness prevention have shifted away from the feminist insistence on women's health disadvantage to a heavy focus on the health perils facing men. The 'male outlook on life', they argue, is increasingly equated with ill-health as we have come to believe that masculinity is 'bad' for health and femininity is 'good' (**11**). Thus researchers often see men as the 'forgotten victims' of various health problems from postnatal depression to reproductive cancers and mental illnesses. The upshot is that both women and men are encouraged to adopt 'illness identities' as increasingly they come to see themselves as vulnerable help-seekers (see Volume III for articles on gender and help-seeking).

INTRODUCTION

Part 3 Capturing individual experience and gender contexts in research

Health and illness can strike at the core of social and personal identity, including what it means to be a man or woman, boy or girl. In various ways the articles in this section underscore that the individual experience of health and illness can only be understood fully when it is contextualised within the social, cultural and political orders of wider society.

Susan Bell and Susan Reverby (**12**) reflect on the health and gender politics of performing Eve Ensler's (2001) *The Vagina Monologues*. The play is used by the authors as a vehicle to examine how the body, and particularly the vagina, has been politicised in the different feminist eras of the 1970s–1980s and the 2000s. They deliberate on whether the focus on the speakers' individual experiences of the body – personally liberating though it may be – ultimately misses the connection between our bodies and the body politic. They also ask *whose* personal life does the play make political, and worry just how far its messages can travel successfully beyond the USA specifically and the West generally.

As Lesley Doyal (**1**) points out, we need to be aware that sex and gender do not stand alone. Consequently we should be alert to how they interplay with other characteristics which also are related to health, such as social class, age, sexuality and ethnicity in different parts of the world. The concept of 'intersectionality', which was coined by Kimberlé Crenshaw in 1989, has recently become an important lens for research on gender and health (see e.g. Iyer *et al.* 2009). Jyotsna Agnihotri Gupta (**13**) takes up the issue of intersectionality in her consideration of new reproductive technologies (NRTs) and transactions in body parts and the 'challenges and dilemmas' they pose for 'feminist solidarity worldwide'. From the perspective that there are divisions between those women who profit from NRTs and those who are exploited by them, she questions whether there can be 'common gender interests'. In particular she explores whether the relatively new concept of 'transnational feminisms' has added value over the older concept of 'global sisterhood' which, it has been argued, failed to pay heed to differences amongst women.

Writing from an avowedly feminist perspective, Marcia Inhorn and Lisa Whittle (**14**) argue for a strong 'socio-cultural and political-economic contextualization' to understand why particular diseases affect particular individuals in particular times and places. They critique mainstream epidemiology for its 'arid and politically unsophisticated' approach to disease causation and its 'antifeminist bias'. They call for methodological approaches which show how gender oppression (and, importantly, not just the variable 'gender') shapes women's health outcomes and well-being. They argue that connections need to be made between women's lived experiences of health and illness and 'the various forms of oppression they encounter to larger social, economic and political forces' (**14**). Bringing us back to the theme of intersectionality, they also stress the need to take account of 'multiple, interlocking, and simultaneous forms of oppression based on gender, race, class, and nation'.

While commentators may generally agree that individual and structural factors both need to be brought into analysis, this has been hard to achieve in practice because methodological innovation often lags behind theory. Ichiro Kawachi and colleagues' paper (**15**) is an early attempt to capture the gendered macro context and the influence of place on health by exploring women's health status as an 'ecological characteristic'. In a cross-sectional analysis using multivariate regression models they found some correlations between four composite indices of women's status in the 50 US states – political participation, economic autonomy, employment and economic earnings, and reproductive rights – and female mortality rates, female cause-specific mortality rates, and activity limitations. Interestingly, they also found associations between these factors and some aspects of men's health, leading them to suggest that 'patriarchy and unequal status for women might spill over into worse health for men . . . [and that] a society that tolerates gender inequalities is also likely to be a more unhealthy place to live for both men and women, compared to a more egalitarian one' (**15**).

Nancy Moss (**16**) argues that contextualising gender and health research in terms of geopolitical frameworks is the next 'big step' for developing an integrated approach to women's health. She draws gender equity and socioeconomic inequality together in a unified and multi-level model that 'takes into account the historical, geographical, legal, and political frameworks that provide the overarching context in which men and women live'.

Robin Saltonstall's article (**17**) illustrates the capacity of qualitative research to tease out the connections between 'doing gender' and 'doing health' in everyday life, drawing on interviews with middle-class 'white' men and women in the USA to explore the embodied experience of health and illness. She utilises West and Zimmerman's (1987) insight that doing health is a form of doing gender to argue that 'the interplay between health, self, body and gender at the individual level is linked to the creation of a sense of healthiness in the social body, the body politic of society'. She found that while men and women in her study held broadly similar ideas about what constitutes health, this broke down into gender-specific aspects when they spoke about everyday actions in relation to their health and their own and others' health practices.

As noted earlier, men's health only became a significant research focus in its own right from around the mid-1990s. In her chapter from a collection of papers edited by Donald Sabo and David Gordon (1995) which was influential in stimulating this new field, Kathy Charmaz (**18**) explores how chronic illness can be a threat to masculine identity. This has become a dominant theme in research on men's health. Reminding us of Saltonstall's

(**17**) emphasis on health and 'doing gender' and the significance of hegemonic masculinity (**10**), Charmaz argues that men with chronic illness can find themselves marginalised within the wider gender order, and draws on interview data to examine how they endeavour to preserve and recapture their sense of self.

The articles and chapters reprinted in this volume demonstrate many of the complex theoretical and methodological challenges that have concerned gender and health researchers over the years. Further light is thrown on many of these concerns in the articles in the other volumes in this Major Works collection – on the patterning of heath by gender (Volume II), gender and healthcare (Volume III), and gender and health behaviours (Volume IV).

References

Annandale, E. and Hunt, K. (2000) 'Gender inequalities in health: research at the crossroads', pp. 1–35 in E. Annandale and K. Hunt (eds) *Gender Inequalities in Health.* Buckingham: Open University Press.

Butler, J. (1993) *Bodies that Matter.* London: Routledge.

Connell, R. (1995) *Masculinities.* Cambridge: Polity Press.

Connell, R. (2009) *Gender*, 2nd edn. Cambridge: Polity.

Crenshaw, K. (1989) 'Demarginalizing the intersection of race and sex: a black feminist critique of antidiscrimination doctrine, feminist theory and antiracist politics', *University of Chicago Legal Forum*: 139–67.

Ensler, E. (2001) *The Vagina Monologues: The V-Day edition.* New York: Villard.

Grosz, E. (1994) *Volatile Bodies.* Bloomington: Indiana University Press.

Haraway, D. (1991) *Simians, Cyborgs, and Women.* London: Routledge.

Iyer, A., Sen, G. and Östlin, P. (2009) 'Inequalities and intersections in health: A review of the evidence', pp. 70–95 in D. Sen and P. Ostlin (eds) *Gender Equity in Health: The shifting frontiers of evidence and action.* New York: Routledge.

Oakley, A. (1972) *Sex, Gender and Society*, London: Temple Smith.

Sabo, D. and Gordon, D. F. (1995) (eds) *Men's Health and Illness.* London: Sage.

Stacey, J. and Thorne, B. (1985) 'The missing feminist revolution in sociology', *Social Problems* 32 (4): 301–16.

Stoller, R. (1968) *Sex and Gender.* New York: Science House.

West, C. and Zimmerman, P. (1987) 'Doing gender', *Gender and Society* 1: 125–51.

Part 1

MAKING DISTINCTIONS: SEX AND GENDER, THE BIOLOGICAL AND THE SOCIAL

1
SEX AND GENDER
The challenges for epidemiologists

Lesley Doyal

Source: *International Journal of Health Services*, 33:3 (2003), 569–79.

> Gender issues are now receiving more attention on global and national health agendas. However, the evidence base for policy and practice in this area remains limited and conceptual confusion is still common. This article reviews the challenges facing epidemiologists and other researchers who aim to make their work more "gender sensitive." It begins by exploring the concepts of biological "sex" and social "gender" and assesses their implications for the health of both women and men. It then reviews a range of strategies for mainstreaming sex and gender into health research. The article concludes with brief comments on the links between gender equity and wider equality concerns.

What I want to do here is explore the challenges posed by sex and gender for epidemiologists. You may find this a strange topic because you all know about the differences between men and women, and presumably you believe that you take them into account in your work. But I want to argue that our thinking about these issues has changed dramatically over the past few years. It is clear that these matters are more complex than we had previously understood. And there is a growing acceptance that this has major implications for the work we do. I want to argue that three interrelated processes have caused this growing interest in the relationship between sex, gender, and health.

First, there has been a significant shift in social values. Gender inequalities in general and gender inequalities in health in particular are now being given much greater priority in both national and global debates. Indeed, the last decade has seen both the World Health Organization and the World Bank calling for much greater attention to be paid to these issues. Second, as a result of these changing priorities, policy makers and practitioners have been expected to reshape the services they deliver. But it has often been very unclear what these new "gender-sensitive services" should look like. As they try to develop these new approaches, health care providers have begun to ask new questions about the different patterns of health and illness experienced by women and men. Third, in response to these questions, researchers (including epidemiologists) have generated new knowledge about men, women, health, and health care. This has been extremely valuable and I will be referring to some of it later on. But one of the most important messages to emerge from this research is that there are no simple answers. In particular it has highlighted the need to include both biological sex *and* social gender as key variables in understanding how human health and illness are shaped. And it is here that the challenges for epidemiologists begin to emerge.

What I want to do in this presentation is to highlight five challenges facing epidemiologists as they try to integrate sex and gender concerns into their work in more appropriate and effective ways. The first challenge is one of conceptual clarification. Considerable confusion still seems to surround the use of the terms "sex" and "gender" themselves. The second challenge is to develop a broader understanding of the links between biological sex and health. The third is to create a more comprehensive understanding of the ways in which social gender shapes the health of both women and men. The fourth is to ensure that all research designs are both sex and gender sensitive. And the final challenge is to forge a strategy for integrating findings on both sex and gender into wider equality agendas. I want to look at each of these challenges in turn. And I will argue that epidemiology that fails to take them seriously is not only inequitable but quite simply bad science.

What are "sex" and "gender"?

The first challenge, then, is one of clarifying the concepts. What do we mean by sex and gender, and how do they relate to health? I know that this is an especially difficult task for Spanish speakers, since in Spanish as in many other languages these are not two separate words. But it is important that we are clear about what they mean in English since they represent two distinct aspects of reality, which are often confused.

The two words are not interchangeable, as is often assumed. Rather, the term "sex" should be used to describe the biological differences between women and men, while the term "gender" refers to the social differences between them. Thus sex differences are relatively unchangeable while gender differences are socially constructed and vary over time and place. Both these factors have a major influence on the health of individual men and women as well as shaping male and female patterns of health and illness at the population level.

Consider a very simple example from the epidemiology of cancer. Sex differences in biology mean that only women are at risk of developing cancer of the cervix and only men are at risk from cancer of the prostate. However, biology *cannot* be used to explain why men are currently much more likely than women to develop lung cancer. Instead we have to use the social concept of gender. Men have traditionally been much more likely than women to smoke in just about every country in the world. And the reasons for this are to be found not in their genes but in the different cultural expectations of male and female behavior. Biological risk factors are clearly unchangeable, but those related to gender are not. Indeed, Spain provides an excellent example of this. As women's lives have changed, rates of female smoking have increased, as have their rates of lung cancer—a trend repeated in many other countries, including the United Kingdom.

Both biological sex and social gender are therefore important in shaping the epidemiology of cancer and of other diseases. However, it is clear that these two variables operate through very different mechanisms. Hence we need to be very clear when we are talking about one and when we are talking about the other. We need to differentiate very carefully between the biological and the social if we are to achieve a rigorous scientific understanding of complex health problems and to develop appropriate interventions for solving them.

To take another simple example: if a study on the epidemiology of tuberculosis in a particular region shows that the prevalence is apparently lower among women than among men, then we need to know whether this is due to sex differences in susceptibility to the bacillus or whether it reflects social or gender differences in patterns of exposure to infection or in access to health care. Very often, of course, the answer lies in some combination of these factors. However, we will not be able to develop a scientific understanding of how this combination works until the different elements of sex and gender are clearly identified in research design and analysis.

Unless these different strands of causality are spelled out, it will not be possible to develop the most effective strategies for prevention and treatment. Yet reviews of existing studies in this and other areas indicate that there continues to be a disturbing level of confusion. If these confusions are to be avoided in the future, we will need to develop much greater clarity about what we mean by biological sex and what we mean by social gender and how each affects health. So let us move on to our second challenge, which is the development of a clearer understanding of the links between biological sex and human health.

How are sex and health related?

It is not surprising that biomedical scientists (including epidemiologists) have usually focused on male and female reproductive biology in explaining the differences in patterns of health and illness between the sexes. In particular, they have acknowledged the significance of women's reproductive potential in determining their health and have recognized the need to provide them with appropriate health care that meets their sex-specific needs.

For those of us living in the developed countries, it is easy to forget the significance of reproductive health needs. But maternal morbidity and mortality still remain unacceptably high in the developing world. In many countries in sub-Saharan Africa, a woman still has a one in seven chance of dying in childbirth at some stage of her life, and the figure for women in Afghanistan is very similar. So epidemiologists (and others) working in this part of the world still have an important role to play in measuring this huge burden of reproductive death and disability and identifying its immediate causes.

But the last few years have seen a major shift in thinking about the impact of biology on health. As is increasingly recognized, variations in reproductive capacity provide an important starting point, but we need to look far beyond them if we are to properly understand the biological differences between the two sexes. Of course, it has long been recognized that hormonal differences are part of the explanation for the higher rates of premature deaths among men from coronary heart disease. But a growing number of studies have identified other hormonal, metabolic, and genetic differences that have a major influence on male and female patterns of health and illness.

As has long been known, for example, women are more likely than men to suffer from a variety of autoimmune diseases such as multiple sclerosis, systemic lupus, and rheumatoid arthritis. At the same time they also seem to be more resistant than men to a range of infectious diseases, including TB and malaria. Recent research indicates that these differences in the incidence and effects of particular diseases reflect underlying differences in male and female immune systems. Thus women may be biologically better equipped than men to resist some diseases at the price of being more vulnerable to others. The potential value of such findings for the development of new therapies is obviously very considerable, but the mechanisms underlying the differences are not yet clear.

The exploration of sex differences in biology is now a major growth area, especially in the United States. However, many more studies are still needed. Just to give some illustrations of puzzles in need of explanations: we need to understand why women who smoke are significantly more likely to develop lung cancer than men who smoke the same amount, why some pain medications are far more effective in relieving pain in women than in men, why some common drugs such as antihistamines and antibiotics can cause different reactions in male and female patients, and why women are much more likely than men to suffer a second heart attack within a year of their first one. Epidemiologists clearly have an important part to play in moving beyond reproduction to explore this exciting new area of biological difference across a range of different health and disease processes.

But biology or sex is only part of the story. As we have seen, social or gender differences also have a major influence on health, but they have traditionally received much less attention from epidemiologists. So we need to turn to our third challenge of enhancing our understanding of the impact of gender on health.

How are gender and health related?

What do we mean by gender differences between women and men, and how do they influence health? All societies are based on gender divisions. That is to say, whatever their age, race, or social class, individuals defined as "female" are usually treated very differently from those defined as "male." Women and men, girls and boys, are expected to behave in very different ways. They are given different duties and responsibilities and different levels of resources in order to carry them out. In most settings these are not merely differences but inequalities. As a recent U.N. Development Program report pointed out, there are no societies in which women are treated equally with men, and this inevitably affects their health as well as their access to health care.

There is now a very large literature exploring the links between gender divisions in daily life and female morbidity and mortality. In most countries women have the major responsibility for household work. And in many parts of the world they now have to combine this with waged work. Especially in poor countries, this double burden can be very heavy, and this is clearly reflected in patterns of health and illness.

To give just a few examples: around the world women are between two and three times more likely than men to report depression and anxiety, and this has been linked to their low status in the household, to the responsibility they carry for family survival, and to their unequal access to income, wealth, time, and other resources. Depression has also been identified as just one of the consequences of the violence that so many women experience as part of their daily lives. A recent study from the World Bank has estimated that about 5 percent of the total disease burden experienced by women in developing countries can be related to gender violence, while the comparable figure for developed countries is as high as 19 percent. These are extremely dramatic figures, especially when we realize that this is potentially *avoidable* death and disability.

More specific effects of the impact of the gender division of labor on women's health are evident from studies in a number of different areas.

Research has shown, for example, that women experience very high levels of some respiratory diseases in those countries where cooking is done inside with polluting fuels. Similarly, links can be drawn between women's work and schistosomiasis (bilharzia). We know that incidence of the disease is either equal in both sexes or higher among males up to the age of about 11. But afterwards the pattern is reversed. This has been attributed to gender differences in the use of water. Both boys and girls play in the water until puberty, when boys begin to take up other activities. Girls, on the other hand, remain in frequent contact with water through their domestic work and are therefore exposed more frequently than boys to the snails that carry the disease.

So the impact of gender on the health of females has been well documented. But what about males? Until recently, very little attention had been paid to the impact of gender on men's health. However, this is now changing as the links between masculinity and well-being start to emerge. At first glance it might seem that being a man would be positive for health, given men's relatively privileged access to a range of resources including income, wealth, and social status. And in many ways this is an accurate observation, since most men do have more of these valuable assets than women in the same social groups as themselves. However, closer examination reveals a more complex picture.

Being a male in a gender-divided society may have its own hazards. This is because the development and maintenance of a male identity usually requires the taking of risks that can be damaging to health. The most obvious examples of such risks come from the world of waged work. In most societies the traditional role of family provider has put men at greater risk than women of dying prematurely from occupational injuries. Though global forces are now reshaping the labor force, with more women now working outside the home, it is still men from the poorest communities who do most of the very dangerous jobs. So gender expectations mean that men may be put at risk by their external responsibilities just as women may be damaged by their domestic labor.

Alongside these risks in the workplace, many men also feel they must be involved in risk-taking behavior to "prove" their masculinity. As a result they are more likely than women to be murdered, or to die in a car accident or as a result of dangerous sports. In most societies they are also more likely than women to drink to excess and to smoke, as well as being more likely to desire unsafe sex. Again, much of this risky behavior is likely to be more common among men from the poorest communities. So it is clear that gender is not, as is often assumed, of relevance only to women. Gender divisions shape the lives of both men and women, and as a result they are a major influence on their health.

Similar arguments can be made about the relationship between gender and health care. Studies from the developing world in particular have shown that women are likely to face more obstacles than men in accessing appropriate and effective health care. There is also evidence of gender inequalities in the treatment received by individuals within health care systems. Studies from both developed and developing countries have shown that women's experiences of health care are often negative because of the discriminatory attitudes of service providers. Even more important perhaps is the growing volume of evidence of inequalities in technical aspects of care. Examples of this from the United States and the United Kingdom include women receiving fewer investigations than a man with the same symptoms of coronary heart disease and being less likely than a man with the same prognosis to be given a kidney transplant.

So gender divisions mean that women may be at a disadvantage compared with men in their access to health care and also in the quality of care they receive. But gender may also have a negative effect on men's use of services. In many cultures the process of male socialization—of bringing boys up to be "proper" men—can make it difficult for men to admit weakness. This may prevent them from taking health promotion messages seriously and from consulting a doctor when problems arise. So, many men face their own obstacles in trying to make the best use of services, and these are again related to their gender.

Epidemiologists therefore need to include gender as well as sex in their studies of both health and health care if they are to capture all the determinants of morbidity and mortality among women and among men. But how is this to be done? This takes us on to our fourth challenge, which is how to integrate sex and gender issues into epidemiological research.

Creating sex- and gender-sensitive research

As I am sure many of you are aware, debate about these issues has been increasing in recent years. In the United States in particular, the arguments have become increasingly sophisticated, and this has led to significant changes in policy. Although the main focus has been on clinical trials, epidemiological studies have also come under critical review. In this section I want to summarize some of these debates and explore the related policy issues. In particular I want to identify some of the major strategies that have been adopted to "mainstream" sex and gender issues in medical research.

Many of the arguments about sex and gender sensitivity in research have begun with relatively simple arguments about the numbers of women and men included as subjects in particular studies. Some of the earliest papers on this topic in the United States, in Canada, and in the United Kingdom highlighted the very clear male bias in the selection of subjects for many epidemiological studies on heart disease. In some famous cases, such as the "Mr. Fit" study of the relationship between heart disease, cholesterol, and lifestyle, the sample included no female subjects at all. As critics pointed out, this reflected a mistaken perception that heart disease is only a "men's problem" when it is also the major killer of women over the age of 55. The main thrust of these early arguments was that this approach to research was inequitable. It was based on the experiences of only half the population, but the results were then applied to the other half without any consideration of possible differences. The knowledge base for the treatment of women was therefore inferior to that available for the treatment of men. This was said to reflect a fundamental and unacceptable bias built into much of medical science.

In response to such criticisms, the United States developed a number of policies for achieving a more appropriate gender (and also race) distribution among research subjects. The most important of these was the passing of a law that prevented scientists from receiving federal funding for their work unless they could demonstrate that the proposed study took sex and gender issues seriously. Of course, a study of prostate cancer would need only male subjects, just as a study of cervical cancer would be all female. But in most studies an appropriate sample would be expected to include both male and female groups of sufficient size to ensure that statistically significant differences between them could be easily detected. This law had a major impact on patterns of research in the United States. The inclusion of sex and gender sensitivity in the criteria for funding meant that many scientists had to think about these issues for the first time. The effects of the legislation were complex, and it created a number of both methodological and ethical problems that have not been easy to resolve. However, it has certainly led medical scientists (including epidemiologists) to pay more attention to issues of sex and gender in the early stages of planning their research.

But greater equality of male and female subjects in a study will not be enough in itself to ensure that differences between men and women are taken seriously. It will also be important to ensure that any methodological tools used in the study are not themselves subject to gender bias. The potential importance of this problem is evident if we look at some of the problems that have been encountered in the increasing use of the disability-adjusted life year, or DALY, as a tool in epidemiology and public health research.

As you are all aware, the DALY is increasingly the preferred tool for measuring the burden of disease in a given population. It is also being promoted by both the WHO and the World Bank as an instrument to be used in making decisions about the allocation of scarce resources. However, a number of commentators have pointed out that there is evidence of considerable gender bias in the way this indicator is constructed. Though separate DALYs have been calculated for women and for men, it is clear that the underlying assumptions of the model are not neutral with regard to sex and gender.

The first problem is that what is measured by DALYs systematically underestimates the burden of disease borne by women. This is because most of the data are based on the recorded incidence of specific diseases, but the health problems of women are often much harder than those of men to fit into standard disease categories. For example, many gynecological problems are excluded altogether, as is the practice of female genital mutilation. This definitional problem is exacerbated by the use of incidence rather than prevalence data, since this prioritizes acute problems rather than the chronic ones that are more common among women. Finally, the summation of individual diseases covers up the interconnectedness of many women's health problems. In many parts of the world it is common for a woman to be pregnant, to be anemic, and also to be suffering from malaria. Yet this cumulative complexity is not reflected in the ways that DALYs are calculated.

In addition to these definitional problems, critics have also pointed out that overall there is less information available on women's health problems than on those of men. This reflects in part the sensitive nature of some of these problems. Information on gender violence, for example, and on termination of pregnancy is notoriously difficult to collect. More generally, because of the obstacles many women face in accessing health care, they are less likely than men to have their problems diagnosed and recorded. This of course will be especially true in the poorest countries, where we know that the official figures for women suffering from diseases such as HIV/AIDS, TB, leprosy, and malaria are significant underestimates. So it is clear that as well as choosing an appropriate sample, researchers also need to be aware of any bias in measuring tools.

But again, this is not enough. When they reach the stage of analyzing their findings, epidemiologists need to treat sex and gender as key variables and not just as optional extras. That is to say, they need to ensure that the possibility of variations between men and women is always investigated even if such differences are eventually found not to exist. Where such differences are found, it is of course essential that they are properly reported. Too often, the results of studies are presented in a way that obscures differences between women and men because they are not deemed to be important. It is for this reason that those concerned to mainstream sex and gender into medical research have argued so forcefully for the routine presentation of sex-disaggregated data.

So research *can* be made more sensitive to sex and gender differences at all stages in the collection and analysis of data. But the finding (and reporting) of empirical differences between men and women is of course only the beginning of a much longer process. These differences also need to be explained, and it is here that epidemiologists face some of their most difficult challenges. Are observed variations due to biology, to gender, or (more likely) to a combination of the two? Careful exploration will be required to unpick the underlying causal factors in each case, and the difficulties involved in making this kind of judgement are well illustrated in many studies of HIV/AIDS.

We know that there has been a massive shift in the epidemiology of HIV/AIDS as the pandemic has developed. Instead of affecting mainly gay men in the developed countries, it is now a disease of poor women. In the year 2000 more than 1.3 million women died from AIDS, and there are now more than 16 million living with the disease. As more and more researchers have explored the changing patterns of the disease, the complex relationships between the biological and the social have become ever more apparent.

On the one hand, as has now been (belatedly) recognized, there are major biological differences between women and men in their responses to the disease. We know for example that during unprotected sex with an infected partner, a woman's chance of contracting the disease is up to ten times greater than that of a man. But at the same time it is also clear that *gender* inequalities exert an enormous influence on women's capacity to protect themselves from exposure to the virus. In a situation where they have few opportunities for supporting themselves, women may feel compelled to stay with a male partner even when this is putting their life at risk. These relationships are often ones of profound inequality in which women feel they have no right to express their own needs and desires. Under these circumstances the avoidance of unsafe sex may be very low on a woman's list of priorities. But unless these social and psychological factors are properly understood, it may be very difficult to make sense of the findings from individual studies.

So the case of HIV/AIDS illustrates some of the challenges to be faced in using the concepts of sex and gender to solve particular empirical puzzles. We can see the way the epidemic is changing and this can be mapped in many different settings. But understanding the complex interplay of the biological and the social will require flexible and creative thinking. Epidemiologists are increasingly being required to think in this way, as the infectious diseases of the past are joined by new health hazards associated with globalization. Yet many are finding that their capacity to solve these problems in an integrated way is constrained by their disciplinary background.

A biomedical training is a preparation for exploring the biological. But as we have seen, the concept of gender is derived from the social sciences. Moreover the social reality of gender is much less amenable to the statistical methods usually used to explain the biological. The different dimensions of gender can certainly be subjected to empirical analysis through methods as rigorous as those applied to the biology of sex. But epidemiologists will need to think openly and creatively about both concepts and methods if they are to play their part in bringing these two dimensions of human health together.

In the coming decades, some of the most exciting work in health research will be interdisciplinary in approach, and epidemiologists are especially well placed to contribute to these developments. The growing interest in the links between the biological and the social offers unique opportunities for epidemiologists to work with colleagues across those disciplinary boundaries. With their history of using biomedical techniques in a social context, I believe they can play a central role in mainstreaming sex and gender in health research. Looking toward the future, then, I want to conclude by referring very briefly to our fifth challenge, which is the integration of sex and gender issues into the broader agenda of epidemiology.

A broader agenda

In this presentation I have focused on the biological and social differences between men and women and the implications of these differences for their health. I hope I have demonstrated that studies that fail to take both these factors into account can be neither equitable nor properly scientific. But of course this should not be taken to mean that I see sex and gender as the *only* structural determinants of health—or even necessarily as the most important.

As epidemiologists, you are only too aware that factors such as class or socioeconomic status, race/ethnicity, and age are also essential determinants of health and well-being. None of these operate independently of each other, yet there remains a great deal of confusion about their modes of interaction. If global inequalities are to be properly tackled, we need to understand much more about the ways in which biological sex and social gender interact with these other determinants of health. I think that epidemiologists have a vital role to play in developing that understanding, and I hope I have helped to identify some of the key aspects of what will be a continuing debate.

Note

This article is adapted from a paper presented at the Congress of the Spanish Society of Epidemiology, Barcelona, September 12, 2002.

Further reading

Doyal, L. Gender equity in health: Debates and dilemmas. *Soc. Sci. Med.* 51(6): 931–939, 2000.

Doyal, L. Sex, gender and health: The need for a new approach. *BMJ* 7320: 1061–1063, 2001.

Hanson, K. Measuring Up: Gender, Burden of Disease and Priority Setting Techniques in the Health Sector. 1999. www.harvard.edu/grhf/HUpapers/gender/hanson.html

Krieger, N. Epidemiology and social sciences: Towards a critical reengagement in the 21st century. *Epidemiol. Rev.* 11: 155–163, 2000.

Payne, S. "Smoke like a man die like a man"? A review of the relationship between gender, sex and lung cancer. *Soc. Sci. Med.* 53(8): 1067–1080, 2001.

Sundby, J. Are women disfavoured in the estimation of Disability Adjusted Life Years and the Global Burden of Disease? *Scand. J. Public Health* 27: 279–285, 1999.

Wizemann, T., and Pardue, M. *Exploring the Biological Contribution to Human Health: Does Sex Matter?* National Academy Press, Washington, D.C., 2001.

2
GENDERS, SEXES, AND HEALTH
What are the connections—and why does it matter?

Nancy Krieger

Source: *International Journal of Epidemiology*, 32 (2003), 652–7.

Open up any biomedical or public health journal prior to the 1970s, and one term will be glaringly absent: *gender*. Open up any recent biomedical or public health journal, and two terms will be used either: (1) interchangeably, or (2) as distinct constructs: *gender* and *sex*. Why the change? Why the confusion?— and why does it matter? After briefly reviewing conceptual debates leading to distinctions between 'sex' and 'gender' as biological and social constructs, respectively, the paper draws on ecosocial theory to present 12 case examples in which gender relations and sex-linked biology are singly, neither, or both relevant as independent or synergistic determinants of the selected outcomes. Spanning from birth defects to mortality, these outcomes include: chromosomal disorders, infectious and non-infectious disease, occupational and environmental disease, trauma, pregnancy, menopause, and access to health services. As these examples highlight, not only can gender relations influence expression—and interpretation—of biological traits, but also sex-linked biological characteristics can, in some cases, contribute to or amplify gender differentials in health. Because our science will only be as clear and error-free as our thinking, greater precision about whether and when gender relations, sex-linked biology, both, or neither matter for health is warranted.

Open up any biomedical or public health journal prior to the 1970s, and one term will be glaringly absent: *gender*. Open up any recent biomedical or public health journal, and two terms will be used either: (1) interchangeably, or (2) as distinct constructs: *gender* and *sex*. Why the change? Why the confusion?—and why does it matter?

As elegantly argued by Raymond Williams, vocabulary involves not only 'the available and developing meaning of known words' but also 'particular formations of meaning—ways not only of discussing but at another level seeing many of our central experiences' (ref. 1, p. 15). Language in this sense embodies 'important social and historical processes', in which new terms are introduced or old terms take on new meanings, and often 'earlier and later senses coexist, or become actual alternatives in which problems of contemporary belief and affiliation are contested' (ref. 1, p. 22).

So it is with 'gender' and 'sex'.[2,3] The introduction of 'gender' in English in the 1970s as an alternative to 'sex' was expressly to counter an implicit and often explicit biological determinism pervading scientific and lay language.[2-8] The new term was deployed to aid clarity of thought, in a period when academics and activists alike, as part of and in response to that era's resurgent women's movement, engaged in debates over whether observed differences in social roles, performance, and non-reproductive health status of women and men—and girls and boys—was due to allegedly innate biological differences ('sex') or to culture-bound conventions about norms for—and relationships between—women, men, girls, and boys ('gender') (Table 1). For language to express the ideas and issues at stake, one all-encompassing term—'sex'—would no longer suffice. Thus, the meaning of 'gender' (derived from the Latin term 'generare', to beget) expanded from being a technical grammatical term (referring to whether nouns in Latin and related languages were 'masculine' or 'feminine') to a term of social analysis (ref. 1, p. 285; ref. 4, p. 2; ref. 5, pp. 136–37). By contrast, the meaning of 'sex' (derived from the Latin term *secus* or *sexus*, referring to 'the male or female *section of humanity*' [rel. 1, p. 283]) contracted. Specifically, it went from a term describing distinctions between, and the relative status of, women and men (e.g. Simone DeBeauvoir's *The Second Sex*[9]) to a biological term, referring to groups defined by the biology of sexual reproduction (or, in the meaning of 'having sex', to interactions involving sexual biology) (ref. 1, p. 285; ref. 4, p. 2; ref. 5, pp. 136–37).

As the term 'gender' began to percolate into everyday use, however, it also began to enter the scientific literature,[3-8, 10] sometimes with its newly intended meaning, other times as a seemingly trendy substitute for 'sex'—with some articles[11] even including both terms, interchangeably, within their titles! Other studies, by contrast, have adhered to a strict gender/sex division, typically investigating the influence of only one or the other on particular health outcomes.[3-8, 10] A new strand of health research, in turn, is expanding these terms from singular to plural by beginning to grapple with new constructs of genders and sexes now entering the scientific domain, e.g., 'transgender', 'transsexual', 'intersexual', which blur boundaries not only <u>between</u> but also <u>within</u> the gender/sex dichotomy (Table 1).[8] The net result

Table 1 Definitions of 'sex' and 'gender'. From *A Glossary for Social Epidemiology*.[2]

Term	Definition
Gender, sexism, & sex	**Gender** refers to a social construct regarding culture-bound conventions, roles, and behaviors for, as well as relations between and among, women and men and boys and girls. Gender roles vary across a continuum and both gender relations and **biologic expressions of gender** vary within and across societies, typically in relation to social divisions premised on power and authority (e.g., class, race/ethnicity, nationality, religion). **Sexism**, in turn, involves inequitable gender relations and refers to institutional and interpersonal practices whereby members of dominant gender groups (typically men) accrue privileges by subordinating other gender groups (typically women) and justify these practices via ideologies of innate superiority, difference, or deviance. Lastly, **sex** is a biological construct premised upon biological characteristics enabling sexual reproduction. Among people, biological sex is variously assigned in relation to secondary sex-characteristics, gonads, or sex chromosomes; sexual categories include: male, female, intersexual (persons born with both male and female sexual characteristics), and transsexual (persons who undergo surgical and/or hormonal interventions to reassign their sex). Sex-linked biological characteristics (e.g., presence or absence of ovaries, testes, vagina, penis; various hormone levels; pregnancy, etc.) can, in some cases, contribute to gender differentials in health but can also be construed as **gendered expressions of biology and** erroneously invoked to explain **biologic expressions of gender**. For example, associations between parity and incidence of melanoma among women are typically attributed to pregnancy-related hormonal changes; new research indicating comparable associations between parity and incidence of melanoma among men, however, suggests that social conditions linked to parity, and not necessarily—or solely—the biology of pregnancy, may be aetiologically relevant.
Sexualities & heterosexism	**Sexuality** refers to culture-bound conventions, roles, and behaviors involving expressions of sexual desire, power, and diverse emotions, mediated by gender and other aspects of social position (e.g., class, race/ethnicity, etc.). Distinct components of sexuality include: sexual identity, sexual behavior, and sexual desire. Contemporary 'Western' categories by which people self-identify or can be labeled include: heterosexual, homosexual, lesbian, gay, bisexual, 'queer', transgendered, transsexual, and asexual. **Heterosexism**, the type of discrimination related to sexuality, constitutes one form of abrogation of sexual rights and refers to institutional and interpersonal practices whereby heterosexuals accrue privileges (e.g., legal right to marry and to have sexual partners of the 'other' sex) and discriminate against people who have or desire same-sex sexual partners, and justify these practices via ideologies of innate superiority, difference, or deviance. Lived experiences of sexuality accordingly can affect health by pathways involving not only sexual contact (e.g., spread of sexually-transmitted disease) but also discrimination and material conditions of family and household life.

is that although lucid analyses have been written on why it is important to distinguish between 'gender' and 'sex',[4-8] epidemiological and other health research has been hampered by a lack of clear conceptual models for considering <u>both</u>, simultaneously, to determine their relevance—or not—to the outcome(s) being researched.

Yet, we do not live as a 'gendered' person one day and a 'sexed' organism the next; we are both, simultaneously, and for any given health outcome, it is an empirical question, not a philosophical principle, as to whether diverse permutations of gender and sex matter—or are irrelevant. Illustrating the importance of asking this question, conceptually and analytically, Table 1 employs an ecosocial epidemiological perspective[2,12] to delineate 12 examples,[13-24] across a range of exposure—outcome associations, in which gender relations and sex-linked biology are singly, neither, or both relevant as independent or synergistic determinants.[25] These examples were chosen for two reasons. First, underscoring the salience of considering these permutations for any and all outcomes, the examples range from birth defects to mortality, and include: chromosomal disorders, infectious and non-infectious disease, occupational and environmental disease, trauma, pregnancy, menopause, and access to health services. Second, they systematically present diverse scenarios across possible combinations of gender relations and sex-linked biology, as singly or jointly pertinent or irrelevant. In these examples, expressions of gender relations include: gender segregation of the workforce and gender discrimination in wages, gender norms about hygiene, gender expectations about sexual conduct and pregnancy, gendered presentation of and responses to symptoms of illness, and gender-based violence. Examples of sex-linked biology include: chromosomal sex, menstruation, genital secretions, secondary sex characteristics, sex-steroid-sensitive physiology of non-reproductive tissues, pregnancy, and menopause.

As examination of the 12 case examples makes clear, not only can gender relations influence expression—and interpretation—of biological traits, but also sex-linked biological characteristics can, in some cases, contribute to or amplify gender differentials in health. For example, as shown by case No. 9, not recognizing that parity is a social as well as biological phenomenon, with meaning for men as well as women, means important clues about why parity might be associated with a given outcome might be missed. Similarly, as shown by case No. 11, recognition of social inequalities among women (including as related to gender disparities between women and men) can enhance understanding of expressions of sex-linked biology, e.g. age at perimenopause. Because our science will only be as clear and error-free as our thinking, greater precision about whether gender relations, sex-linked biology, both, or neither matter for health is warranted.

Table 2 Selected examples of differential roles of gender relations and sex-linked biology on health outcomes: only gender, only sex-linked biology, neither, and both.

Case	Diagrammed illustration	Exposure—outcome association	Relevance of: Gender relations	Relevance of: Sex-linked biology	Explication
1	gender relations ↓ exposure ——→ health outcome sex-linked biology	Greater prevalence of HIV/AIDS due to needle-stick injury among female compared with male health care workers providing patient care[13]	Yes: for exposure	No	• Gender relations: determinant of risk of exposure (needle stick injury), via gender segregation of the workforce (e.g. greater likelihood of women being nurses) • Sex-linked biology: not a determinant of risk of exposure • Risk of outcome, given exposure: risk of seroconversion same among women and men
2	gender relations ↓ exposure ——→ health outcome sex-linked biology	Greater prevalence of contact lens microbial keratitis among male compared with female contact lens wearers[14]	Yes	No	• Gender relations: determinant—among those wearing contact lenses—of risk of exposure to improperly cleaned contact lenses (men less likely to properly clean them than women) • Sex-linked biology: not a determinant of exposure • Risk of outcome, given exposure: risk of contact lens microbial keratitis same among women and men, once exposed to improperly cleaned contact lenses
3	gender relations ↓ exposure ——→ health outcome sex-linked biology	Greater prevalence of short stature and gonadal dysgenesis among women with Turner's syndrome compared with unaffected women[15]	No	Yes: for exposure	• Gender relations: not a determinant of exposure (X-monosomy, total or mosaic, or non-functional X chromosome) • Sex-linked biology: determinant of exposure • Risk of outcome, given exposure: not influenced by gender relations

4	gender relations ↘ sex-linked biology ↓ exposure ⟶ health outcome	Both similar and different adverse health outcomes among women and men due to ubiquitous exposure to cooking oil contaminated by polychlorinated biphenyls (PCB) ('Yusho' disease)[16]	No	Yes: once exposed	• Gender relations: not a determinant of risk of exposure (ubiquitous exposure to the contaminated cooking oil, in staple foods) • Sex-linked biology: not a determinant of risk of exposure • Risk of outcome, given exposure: partly influenced by sex-linked biology, in that although both women and men experienced chloracne and other dermal and ocular lesions, only women experienced menstrual irregularities
5	gender relations ↘ sex-linked biology ↓ exposure ⟶ health outcome	Higher risk of stroke among both women and men in the US 'stroke belt' in several Southern states, compared with women and men in other regions of the US (as distinct from differences in risk for women and men within a given region)[17]	No	No	• Gender relations: not a determinant of risk of exposure (living in the US 'stroke belt') • Sex-linked biology: not a determinant of risk of exposure • Risk of outcome, given exposure: neither gender relations nor sex-linked biology determine regional variation in stroke rates among men and among women (even as both may contribute to within-region higher risks among men compared with women)
6	gender relations ↘ sex-linked biology ↓ exposure ⟶ health outcome	Higher risk of hypospadias among male infants born to women exposed to potential endocrine-disrupting agents at work[18]	Yes: for exposure	Yes: once exposed	• Gender relations: a determinant of risk of exposure, via gender segregation of the workforce (e.g. high level of phthalate exposure among hairdressers, who are mainly women) • Sex-linked biology: not a determinant of risk of exposure • Risk of outcome, given exposure: different for women and men, and for female and male fetus, as only women can be pregnant, and adverse exposure can lead to hypospadias only among fetuses with a penis

Table 2 (cont'd)

Case	Diagrammed illustration	Exposure—outcome association	Relevance of: Gender relations	Relevance of: Sex-linked biology	Explication
7	gender relations → exposure; sex-linked biology → health outcome; exposure → health outcome	Geographical variation in women's rates of unintended pregnancy as linked to variation in state policies re family planning[19]	Yes: for exposure and once exposed	Yes: once exposed	• Gender relations: a determinant, at societal level, of risk of exposure, i.e. state policies and spending for family planning • Sex-linked biology: not a determinant, at individual level of the girl or woman at risk of pregnancy, of state policies and spending for family planning • Risk of outcome, given exposure: gender relations, at the individual level, influence women's access to—and ability to act on information obtained from—family planning programs, and sex-linked biology is a determinant of who can get pregnant
8	gender relations → exposure; sex-linked biology → health outcome; exposure → health outcome	Earlier age of human immunodeficiency virus infection among women compared with heterosexual men (in the US)[20]	Yes: for exposure	Yes: for exposure and once exposed	• Gender relations: a determinant of age of sexual partner and risk of unprotected sex (e.g. gender power imbalance resulting in sex between older men and younger women, the latter having a lesser ability to negotiate condom use) • Sex-linked biology: a determinant of exposure, via genital secretions • Risk of outcome, given exposure: sex-linked biology a determinant of greater biological efficiency of male-to-female, compared with female-to-male, transmission

#	Diagram	Example			Notes
9	gender relations → sex-linked biology → health outcome; exposure (a) → ; exposure (b) →	Parity among both women and men associated with increased risk of melanoma[21]	Yes: for exposures	Yes: for exposure	• Gender relations: a determinant of parity (via expectations of who has children, at what age) • Sex-linked biology: a determinant of who can become pregnant and pregnancy-linked hormonal levels • Risk of outcome, given exposure: decreased risk of melanoma among nulliparous women and men indicates that non-reproductive factors linked to parity may affect risk among both women and men, even as pregnancy-related hormonal factors may also affect women's risk
10	gender relations → sex-linked biology → health outcome; exposure → (with feedback)	Greater referral of men compared with women for interventions for acute coronary syndromes[22]	Yes: for exposure and once exposed	Yes: for exposure	• Gender relations: a determinant of how people present and physicians interpret symptoms of acute coronary syndromes • Sex-linked biology a determinant of age at presentation (men are more likely to have acute infarction at younger ages) and possibly type of symptoms • Risk of outcome, given exposure: gender relations are a determinant of physician likelihood of referral for diagnostic and therapeutic interventions (women less likely to be referred, especially at younger ages)
11	gender relations → sex-linked biology ↔ health outcome; exposure →	Earlier age at onset of perimenopause among women experiencing greater cumulative economic deprivation over the life course[23]	Yes: for exposure	Yes: as outcome	• Gender relations: a determinant of poverty, across the life course, among women (via the gender gap in earnings and wealth) • Sex-linked biology: a determinant of who can experience perimenopause • Risk of outcome, given exposure: risk of earlier age at perimenopause among women subjected to greater economic deprivation across the life course, including non-smokers, may reflect impact of poverty on oocyte depletion

Table 2 (cont'd)

Case	Diagrammed illustration	Exposure–outcome association	Relevance of:		Explication
			Gender relations	Sex-linked biology	
12	gender relations → exposure, sex-linked biology → health outcome, exposure → health outcome (with feedback from health outcome to exposure)	Greater rate of mortality among women compared with men due to intimate partner violence[24]	Yes: for exposure	Yes: for exposure and once exposed	• Gender relations: a determinant of likelihood of men versus women using physical violence against intimate partners, plus being encouraged to and having access to resources to increase physical strength • Sex-linked biology: a determinant of muscle strength and stamina, at a given level of training and exertion, and also body size • Risk of outcome, given exposure: risk of lethal assault related to on-average greater physical strength and size of men, and gender-related skills and training in inflicting and warding off physical attack

Key messages

- Gender, a social construct, and sex, a biological construct, are distinct, not interchangeable, terms; the two nevertheless are often confused and used interchangeably in contemporary scientific literature.
- The relevance of gender relations and sex-linked biology to a given health outcome is an empirical question, not a philosophical principle; depending on the health outcome under study, both, neither, one, or the other may be relevant—as sole, independent, or synergistic determinants.
- Clarity of concepts, and attention to both gender relations and sex-linked biology, is critical for valid scientific research on population health.

Acknowledgements

Thanks to Sofia Gruskin for helpful comments. This work was not supported by any grant.

References

1. Williams R. *Keywords: A Vocabulary of Culture and Society*. Revised Edn. NY: Oxford University Press, 1983.
2. Krieger N. A glossary for social epidemiology. *J Epidemiol Community Health* 2001;**55**:693–700.
3. Krieger N., Fee E. Man-made medicine and women's health: the biopolitics of sex/gender and race/ethnicity. *Int J Health Serv* 1994;**24**:265–83.
4. Oudshoorn N. *Beyond the Natural Body: An Archeology of Sex Hormones*. London: Routledge, 1994.
5. Hubbard R. Constructing sex differences. In: Hubbard R. *The Politics of Women's Biology*. New Brunswick, NJ: Rutgers University Press, 1990, pp. 136–40.
6. Schiebinger L. *Nature's Body: Gender in the Making of Modern Science*. Boston: Beacon Press, 1993.
7. Doyal L. Sex, gender, and health: the need for a new approach. *BMJ* 2001; **323**:1061–63.
8. Fausto-Sterling A. *Sexing the Body: Gender Politics and the Construction of Sexuality*. New York, NY: Basic Books, 2000.
9. DeBeauvoir S. *The Second Sex*. NY: Vintage Books, 1974 (1952).
10. Institute of Medicine, Committee on Understanding the Biology of Sex and Gender Differences. Wizemann T. M., Pardue M-L. (eds). *Exploring the Biological Contributions to Human Health: Does Sex Matter?* Washington, DC: National Academy Press, 2001.
11. Boling E. P. Gender and osteoporosis: similarities and sex-specific differences. *J Gend Specif Med* 2001;**4**:36–43.

12 Krieger N. Theories for social epidemiology in the 21st century: an ecosocial perspective. *Int J Epidemiol* 2001;**30**:668–77.
13 Ippolito G., Puro V., Heptonstall J., Jagger J., De Carli G., Petrosillo N. Occupational human immunodeficiency virus infection in health care workers: worldwide cases through September 1997. *Clin Infect Dis* 1999;**28**:365–83.
14 Liesegang T. J. Contact lens-related microbial keratitis: Parn I: Epidemiology. *Cornea* 1997;**16**:125–31.
15 Ranke M. G., Saenger P. Turner's syndrome. *Lancet* 2001;**358**:309–14.
16 Aoki Y. Polychlorinated biphenyls, polychlorinated dibenzo-p-dioxins, and polychlorinated dibenzofurans as endocrine disrupters—what we have learned from Yusho disease. *Environ Res* 2001;**86**:2–11.
17 Pickle L. W., Gillum R. F. Geographic variation in cardiovascular disease mortality in US blacks and whites. *J Natl Med Assoc* 1999;**91**:545–56.
18 Van Tongeren M., Nieuwenhuijsen M. J., Gardiner K. *et al.* A job-exposure matrix for potential endocrine-disrupting chemicals developed for a study into the association between maternal occupational exposure and hypospadias. *Ann Occup Hyg* 2002;**46**:465–77.
19 Melvin C. L., Rogers M., Gilbert B. C. *et al.* Pregnancy intention: how PRAMS data can inform programs and policy. *Matern Child Health J* 2000;**4**:197–201.
20 Hader S. L., Smith D. K., Moore J. S., Holmberg S. D. HIV infection in women in the United States: status at the Millennium. *JAMA* 2001;**285**:1186–92.
21 Kravdal O. Is the relationship between childbearing and cancer incidence due to biology or lifestyle? Examples of the importance of using data on men. *Int J Epidemiol* 1995;**4**:477–84.
22 Feldman T., Silver R. Gender differences and the outcome of interventions for acute coronary syndromes. *Cardiol Rev* 2000;**8**:240–47.
23 Wise L. A., Krieger N., Zierler S., Harlow B. L. Lifetime socioeconomic position in relation to onset of perimenopause: a prospective cohort study. *J Epidemiol Community Health* 2002;**56**:851–60.
24 Watts C., Zimmerman C. Violence against women: global scope and magnitude. *Lancet* 2002;**359**:1232–37.
25 Darroch J. Biological synergism and parallelism. *Am J Epidemiol* 1997;**145**:661–68.

3

SHAPING BIOLOGY

Feminism and the idea of 'the biological'

Lynda Birke

Source: S. Williams *et al.* (eds), *Debating Biology*, London: Routledge, 2003, pp. 39–52.

What does the call to 'bring back' the biological mean? Was biology ever in the social sciences in the first place? Being a biologist working on feminist theory has always been a tricky path for me to tread, not least because academic feminism has so long played down the biological. And within feminism, there has been another slippery path: for while the biological processes of the body are largely absent from theory, they are always there – if problematically – in much feminist activism, particularly around women's health.[1] So, if I speak as a biologist or as an activist, I tend to use the language of empirical science, with its reliance on facts and probabilities; but if I move to theory, I must be familiar with the fashionable rhetoric of 'discourses' and 'representation' of the body. Bringing them together, bringing the biological and bodily health, into how we theorize the body, is not an easy task.

Moreover, if we are to debate how (or if) we want to 'bring biology back', then we need to know what it is that we do *not* want (crude genetic determinism, for example). And, importantly, we need to identify *what kind* of biology we want to readmit. 'Biology' is both a subject of study, and a term used to describe set(s) of processes by which organisms work (as in 'human biology'). Some areas of biology-as-practice get a great deal of attention (such as biotechnology and modern genetics), both in scientific literature and in social criticism. Feminist critics of science have focused, for example, on claims made about the power of particular genes to affect human characteristics (and particularly behaviour), as well as the potential harms that might result from genetic manipulation. Another area receiving critical focus is evolution, especially in the form of evolutionary psychology, with its implications that many aspects of our behaviour are hard-wired into us through natural selection.

Yet the study of biology is much more than that. In this chapter, I want to use two areas of inquiry as starting points in order to frame my question about what kind of biology we want to allow back in. One of these is feminist work on the body, and, to a lesser extent, I draw also on ideas about how we think about nonhuman animals. Our ideas about what biology is relies heavily on particular ideas about animals; moreover, how we think about bodies and their processes derives much from experimental procedures involving the bodies of animals. For these reasons we need to bring animals into sociology as much as 'the biological'.

Both of these sources call into question the divisions between biology and the social. Clearly, if feminists are to explore 'the biological', then we do not want that to mean new ways of speaking about biological underpinnings of gender: it is precisely such determinism that we have fought strenuously for so many years. But that struggle cannot deny the biological body altogether – the domain of so much excellent feminist activism throughout the world in women's health (see for example, Shodhini 1997). Nor should it deny the ways in which our knowledge of bodies is derived. So, exploring 'the biological' must also question how and why nonhuman animals always fall into that category, while human behaviour does not – a division which itself reinforces biological determinism (Birke 1994). So, my main focus here is to indicate, first, the meaning(s) of biology that we might want to reject, then, second, to indicate some kinds of biology that might be more acceptable.

Separating ourselves from biology: better things to do with our lives?

Western feminism, like several other of the new social movements, has had an ambivalent relationship with biology.[2] Feminism shares with the social sciences in general a history of rejecting (or at least ignoring) the biological: yet this rejection has added poignancy, for women are so often culturally associated with the messy, abject, body and its biological functions. In that sense, biology poses *particular* problems to feminism over and above the problems it poses to sociology. As Elizabeth Spelman has noted, attending to bodily needs has fallen on women throughout Western history: 'Superior groups, we have been told from Plato on down', she notes, 'have better things to do with their lives' (1988: 127). 'Inferior' groups have tended to become associated with bodily functions, with nature, with animality: small wonder that feminists have sought to avoid the biological – if by 'biological' we imply something fixed, essential and bestial.

In part, this rejection of the biological stems from a politically necessary opposition to crude biological determinism. Women, we have had to assert, are not simply born into the role of housewife. But that rejection assumes a model of the body as somehow fixed and presocial. This assumption in turn is fuelled by the growing power of genetic narratives which, in their most extreme forms, posit bodies as epiphenomena, mere carriers of the genes.

It is hardly surprising, then, that Western feminists of the 1970s and 1980s critiqued crude biological determinism – which is so contrary to the possibilities of social change – and advocated that gender and sexuality were socially constructed. Strategically necessary though that move was, it relied on rather simplistic (and dualistic) notions of gender, separated out from 'sex' as a kind of biological substrate. Later, with the increasing prevalence of postmodernism, a new wave of feminist theory emerged in the 1990s which questioned ideas of sex as substrate, and which prioritized flux and the discursive construction of our ideas about gender/sexuality.

Yet the problems of biological/social dualism remain. The biological body is still treated differently from human behaviour. Feminists tend to object strongly (and with good reason) to claims that, say, women's hormones predispose them to like ironing (see Birke 1999). Yet few of us, I assume, would want to contest that oestrogens affect the uterus, or that evolutionary processes have helped to shape our opposable thumbs. So, the objections to determinism applied only to human behaviour and not to the biological body – a tricky distinction.

Nor did the objections apply to animals. Rather, animals become categorized as belonging to 'biology' in ways that we do not; their behaviour is thus, by default, biologically determined, hard-wired, instinctive, while ours is adaptable and the proper focus of sociological inquiry. But if all animals' behaviour is thus determined, then – unless humans are made of completely different stuff and were dumped on earth by aliens rather than evolving here – it would follow that some of our behaviour must be similarly hard-wired. So, if we want to challenge that claim for humans it means that we have to look again at the claim regarding nonhumans. The two feed off each other. I have argued elsewhere that, if feminists want to challenge biological determinism on all fronts, then one route must be to take on board the growing calls to recognize at least some kinds of nonhuman animals as, clever, adaptable, aware, and cultural – just like us (Bekoff 2002). If we do accept that, then it makes it much more difficult to make claims about simple hard-wiring in our own species.

Another reason why dualism persists is that emerging theory about embodiment – important though that has been – tends to treat the body as an inscribable surface, on which culture acts. For some phenomena – such as body piercing, that may be a valid approach. But it leaves the biological body and its inner processes apart, left in the rag-bag category of 'the biological'. Even if some recent theory seems to dissolve boundaries between bodies and their representations, the *biological* body does not enter social theory. As such, that inner body remains presocial, foundational, while its surface becomes endlessly malleable (Shilling and Mellor 1996). As several critics have noted, however, this focus is problematic, for it marginalizes experience, particularly how the body is *lived* – and particularly in illness. Furthermore, leaving the inner body out leaves little room for understanding the complex ways in which illness is generated across and between social divisions such as class. Can pain, emotion, sexual excitement, ill-health or disability, or the relationships between cardiovascular disease and social histories be understood only in terms of cultural inscription?

Yet messy biological processes do not go away. Just because of hyperbole from some advocates of genetics, can we really deny that genes affect our bodily functions, and hence our health and how we are in the world? Or that we are, indeed, animals, belonging to the primate order? Or – relatedly – that we are products of processes of evolution? In common with many others, I have problems with the rejection of 'biology' that seems to underlie so much feminist theory, for not only does it deny my own bodily experiences (pain and bleeding for instance), but it also puts me in a tricky position with respect to the science that I spent years learning. Like Meera Nanda (1996), I have not found science always abhorrent (critical of it though I may be): it can also be useful, even liberating. And it is in the context of women's health where it can, in principle, become so, when women find ways to challenge medical assumptions and power.[3]

Women and health: 'deviations from the norm'

Even if feminist theory has tended to play down any discussion of the biological, the processes of biology matter to many activists. What kind of biology enters into these debates? For those working on environmental politics, or on health activism, knowing what biology has to say about ecosystems or reproductive health, say, is a crucial part of the political action – even if that knowledge is simultaneously being challenged for its sexism. A substantial part of feminist engagement with issues of health, for example, has addressed the ways in which biomedicine – both as practice and discourse – excludes or marginalizes women. In study after study, women's health needs have been largely defined with respect to male bodies – as well as assumptions made about race and class.[4] As a result, women's bodily processes become the deviations from a norm. The significant exception is reproduction, where it is women's role as reproducers rather than men's that is foregrounded; women thus become defined in terms of reproductive systems.

Although there have been significant changes in the ways that these arguments have run, they remain key concerns. However much we might debate differences among 'women', there is still a substantial literature detailing aspects of *women*'s health (women and smoking, for example).

There is a real dilemma here for feminists, however: on the one hand, we must take issues of women's health seriously. We need to know, for example, if a particular environmental hazard is likely to affect the health of women differentially, or to threaten reproductive capacity. We need to understand how changes in gender and class play out in their impacts on women's health. Yet on the other hand, the 'body' that is at the centre of discussions of health remains quite passive, seeming to be acted upon by these various external agents. So, women's health literature may focus on the impact of (say) environmental toxins *on* fertility. Fertility here (and the organ structures associated with it, such as the uterus) is the substrate, while the biological processes themselves lack agency.

Feminist activism in health starts from women's exclusion from medical knowledge and practice. Activists have pointed to ways in which such exclusion disempowers women, and have therefore sought to promote women's knowledge of how their bodies work as an act of empowerment. Wresting power from the doctors was (and is) central to this kind of politics. In that sense, the self at least has agency in her refusal to accede passively to medical demands.

However, it is not always clear that advocating women's greater knowledge leads to a less passive or negative understanding of the body, not least because the source of much of our understanding about 'how bodies work' comes inevitably from biomedicine itself (Birke 1999), which has been notoriously negative in its descriptions of women's biological processes. Thus one member of the Boston Women's Health Collective lamented that, in writing for *Our Bodies, Ourselves*, she had uncritically repeated the biomedical story of menstruation and menopause as deficiencies – hardly an empowering description, as she later acknowledged (Bell 1994).

So, while feminist theory tends to eschew the biological, biology does enter the debate in some areas of feminist activism, such as environmentalism and health. But that engagement is often ambivalent, moving uneasily between outright rejection and a need to take on board what science says. However much we may, at times, need to accept the science, we can also recognise that the stories science tells are limited, that they recreate the passive body and hard-wired organisms that we want to disavow.

What kind of biology?

The acted-upon body, then, is a product of a biomedicine and related study of biology that has typically seen the individual – human or nonhuman – as separated out from the environment in which s/he lives. That tendency is exacerbated by the way in which physiological data are acquired, often from laboratory studies of highly standardized animals kept under tightly controlled and unvarying conditions. In controlling the laboratory environment, scientific studies thereby separate out the physiology from the more varying environment in which most organisms actually live.

And then, if there are changes in the individual organism and/or its behaviour, biologists routinely seek causes within. Only much later might external causes be added into the picture – if at all. Yet no organism, anywhere on earth, is so isolated: all are deeply embedded in, and part of, multiple environments. Biologists know this in principle, yet all too often treat the organism (or its constituent parts) as existing in a vacuum.

Looking within for causes goes hand in hand with biological determinism. Even if the scientific report tells of genes, hormones, or whatever, influencing some outcome (the development of sexuality, say), it is just a small step to infer that the biological factor(s) cause sexuality to develop in that way. Moreover, many such-studies are done first in nonhuman species: these studies, however, *begin* from the premise that the causes of behaviours lie within. For example, most scientific knowledge about how the sex hormones influence behaviour comes from animal studies, which in turn presume that sex differences in behaviour derive from biological causes. That such differences are also influenced by social factors – even in rats – does not usually enter the equation. Determinism is thus built into the theories in the first place.

Yet what about the kind of biology that we might want to bring into social theory? Clearly we do not want to renew deterministic accounts, however covertly. We need to find ways of acknowledging that internal biology is a factor in our becoming, while at the same time recognizing that there are many other factors too, that influence our becoming who we are, especially in relation to behaviour[5] (see Fausto-Sterling, this volume). Furthermore, we can draw on much wider areas of biological enquiry than the usual Genes 'R' Us story to situate ourselves biologically (ourselves as part of ecosystems for instance). It's not biology that we need to reject wholesale; rather, it is simplistic assumptions that certain biological processes are primary, and that it's the biology of the isolated individual that matters.

An underlying part of the problems facing anyone who wants to conceptualize biology differently is that modern biology seems to be obsessed with genes and molecules. There simply is not a well-developed science of the whole organism (Tauber 1994). So it is frustratingly difficult to find ways of thinking about either biological bodies or animal awareness that do not fall into the abyss of reductionism. But there are ways, and we need to follow them to explore how our biological bodies are both situated in, and part of, a multitude of environments and simultaneously act upon those environments. Only then can we relate our biological bodies to the concerns of feminist politics and sociological theory.

Within recent feminist theory, there have been several recent calls to recognize the materiality of the body – an important step in bringing biology back in. This was, for instance, a feature of Elizabeth Grosz's 1994 book, *Volatile Bodies*. Others have emphasized phenomenological accounts to foreground the lived experience of the body – for example, in relation to pregnancy (see Marshall 1996). Another approach to bodily materiality within recent sociological work draws on Bourdieu's notion of habitus – that is, we learn through social engagement to comport ourselves, to exert control over our bodies (Bourdieu 1984; Lovell 2000). So, social class can influence bodily habitus (through foods eaten, or learning ways of being/moving in the world), and thus the acquisition of cultural capital. Such processes, moreover, could influence our experiencing of our bodies and hence our health.[6]

The idea of habitus is certainly useful, in that such concepts begin to acknowledge bodily materiality. Moreover, culture impacts upon bodily habitus in ways that might in turn affect biological processes. Nonetheless, much of this theory – however sensitive to materiality – seems to me still to ignore the inner workings of the body, which therefore must remain within the purview of biomedicine. So, in order to ponder how habitus might affect what happens inside our bodies, we must necessarily turn to the discourses of natural science: there are few others (although 'alternative' medicine provides less reductionist means of describing the inner body: see Scott, this volume). The concept of habitus does not say much about how habitus is manifest *within* the body: how, for instance, might differences in how we move through the world reflect in differences in bodily functions? In health?[7] And might these differences in being-in-the-world also contribute to different ways of behaving among other species that we like to call hard-wired – to turn the usual logic on its head?

Just as sociologists seeking to theorize the lived body have sought out particular theories that best fit the demand to move beyond the presocial body, so too have some biologists, who have tried to resist, the hegemonic stories of powerful genes.[8] We are not just outcomes of genetic dictates, these authors insist; on the contrary, we are bodily located in particular contexts. They seek to draw on other ways of thinking about biological processes which are less determinist than the story of all-powerful genes and which are potentially more fruitful for thinking about the engagement of sociology and biology.

Thinking about wider contexts is clearly crucial to thinking about the kind of biology on which we want to draw. But a starting point for that development has to be a cross-disciplinary effort to challenge our culture's investment in ideas of discontinuity – that is, the notion that humans are fundamentally and qualitatively different from other species. Both biology and sociology contribute to this belief, despite biology's adherence to evolutionary theory. That is, whenever biologists paint a picture of nonhumans as puppets of their genes or evolutionary heritage, it permits a reading of that picture implying either that humans, too, are puppets of their genes or that humans are different. To bridge the divide, we need to acknowledge and develop further emerging ideas of animal consciousness, emotionality and cultural difference (Bekoff 2002). That is surely a better way of acknowledging evolutionary continuity than the determinist route.

To move towards a more suitable model of biology, we can draw on models of biological systems that emphasise dynamic, rather than static, processes, and that prioritize agency. Steven Rose is one exponent of such a view, insisting that we understand the developmental trajectories of organisms – what he calls their 'lifelines' – as a way of emphasizing the ongoing process of engagement of the organism in its own life history. The organism – any organism, from human to moss to amoeba – thus is not simply *being*, but *becoming* (Rose 1997). It is always in the process of becoming and always making over its environment. So, to understand the sociology of health, we must simultaneously take on board how our bodily health and functions themselves structure the very sociological processes that influence health. What is more, these two-way processes interact throughout our lives, creating different life histories.

This kind of thinking fits with recent feminist scholarship on the body, which has sought to transcend concepts of the bounded body and self by insistence on corporeal fluidity and flow (Grosz 1994). While such approaches seem to play down the biological processes of the body's insides, they share with the biologists' challenges a desire to think about the body as *process(es)* rather than fixed. However, much of this writing emphasizes flows of information (such as genetic or electrical information) in ways that ignore bodily boundaries; like Dawkins's selfish genes, the information is at centre stage and the body becomes epiphenomenal (Birke 1999). Yet we can, as Rose (1997) has argued, think of these processes happening at more than one level simultaneously: genes *and* the body rather than genes instead of the body. Wholeness matters, too.

We can think about 'the body' as existing in, and part of, a nexus of forces, moving through the world and co-creating it. To take that stance de-emphasizes the factors which might 'act upon' the body and prioritizes engagement with the world in which we move. Part of that co-creation is of course how social and cultural forces do indeed write upon the body as surface – but part, too, is how they communicate with the body's inside.

Feminist biologists have been among the voices demanding a more nuanced view of 'the biological' in social theory, seeking to prioritize the engagement of a developing organism with the world in which it lives. We are, these authors insist, not simply emerging out of some blueprint in the DNA; rather a developing embryo is itself part of a process of creation. That co-creation is just as true of an amoeba or a snake or a lion as it is of us. To take the example of how sex differences develop, temperature matters more than genetic dictates for many reptiles.[9] And if you are a newborn rat, how your mother treats you matters as well as hormones in how you exhibit 'gendered' behaviour in later life.

It is that complex engagement throughout life – with biological matter, with the inanimate world, with other social actors – that act together to create (for example) the structures of gender with which we are familiar. To draw on recent feminist insights, we must be aware of the multiple ways in which 'gender' and 'sex' are culturally constructed (including the anthropocentric – or mammalocentric – assumptions that the human way of developing sex is the best one!). Yet we must also be aware of constraints in development, and how those constraints are in turn constructed. Some of these may be the product of social decisions (such as the decision to allocate newborns with phalluses of 'intermediate' length to one or the other sex); others may be products of complex structural processes in embryonic life.[10] But constraints there are.

That call for a new approach to the biological is, however, rather an abstract one and we need to take it further, to avoid ending up with theory that still does not adequately match up the biological and the social. To begin with, sociologists need to engage more overtly with ideas in biology (as this volume attests), and to think through how biological processes might be involved in social ones without assuming that biology equals determinism. So, too, do biologists need to take seriously the complexities of human (and nonhuman) social life without reducing it to simple rules; they need also to recognize the assumptions they make about the causes of behaviour in non-human organisms. But the task is not easy. It is one thing to emphasize what kind of biology we want: it is another to take that further and to figure out how we can develop or use it.

Part of the problem, it seems to me, is that in advocating a more dynamic approach to biology we have not spelled it out enough, so the 'dynamic approach' becomes a kind of magic word. How is that played out in the world of living bodies? What does it mean in relation to the human behaviour that is the foundation of sociological interest? These are important questions which we must address (as other chapters of this book argue).

To spell it out a little more, I will take two concrete examples. These illustrate the complex interactions between social/environmental structures and our biological bodily selves; and they also illustrate, in slightly different ways, how scientific knowledge is generated. The first example is from studies of the immune system. We are now familiar with concepts of 'stress' and how that (whatever it is) can compromise the body's defences. Emily Martin's fascinating study (1994) of concepts of immunity indicates, too, that ideas have changed dramatically over the last thirty years. Where once they relied on analogies of bodies as fortresses, mounting defences, now that has largely given way to discourses of immune systems capable of reacting to their environment – that can be 'tuned up'. These, Martin argues, parallel discursive shifts in the wider culture, particularly in corporate culture.

Now a view of the body's functions that emphasizes its engagement with its environment is (uses by management apart) an improvement. To draw on biology, however, requires making distinctions between conflicting and controversial theories. Weasel (2001), for example, explores major theories of how immune systems work in relation to different feminist epistemologies. In particular, she focuses on the predominant view, which posits a self–other dichotomy and notes how that model, while useful, fails to explain an observation of considerable importance to women, namely, that the foetus ('other' to the mother, biologically) is not normally rejected by maternal physiology. An alternative, and contested, view is the 'danger' theory, whereby the immune system responds to danger signals rather than other-recognition. Weasel considers this theory to be one on which feminist thinking could more usefully draw. Among her reasons for making this claim are that the danger theory better explains the data (including maternal–foetal interactions) and that it is less reductionist in that it acknowledges the situatedness of the immune system.

For some time, it has been widely accepted that the nervous system can influence immunity (the 'stress' argument); more recently, biologists have begun to recognize how the immune system in turn can affect the brain. Thus, Maier and Watkins (1999) for example argue that the immune system can function as a diffuse sense organ, informing the brain about potentially harmful events in the body. But crucially how the organism itself behaves then becomes part of the host's defences (an obvious example is lying down when you have a fever, or changing the diet). So, rather than thinking mainly in terms of how social factors influence long-term health, we could also consider how we as social and biological actors affect the process. Exposure to harm, of any sort, can change the body and so change behaviour. For instance, an infection can trigger release in a vertebrate body of chemicals called cytokines; some of these affect the brain and hence behaviour – the cytokine interleukin-1 for example reduces sexual behaviour in female laboratory rats.

Now I would not wish to imply any simple jump from laboratory findings to the complexities of human behaviour at the social level. I use this rather to underscore (a) how specific examples might illustrate how biology can be 'brought back in', in the sense that biology can pose questions about *how* social engagement impacts upon bodies and health; (b) how some theories might work better for us in connecting to social theory than others; and (c) how tricky it is to talk about biology without falling into the abyss of determinism (just as it's tricky to speak of social processes without falling into the abyss of relativism)! But here, nonetheless, there seems to be fertile ground for exploring ways in which our biological processes are indeed situated within and part of our social world. The functioning of the immune system, particularly, reminds us that we are not, as we sometimes fancy, living in splendid biological isolation – as Basiro Davey aptly reminds us in her chapter.

A second example of the interaction between social engagement and biological processes comes from the recent literature on endocrine disrupters. Until the 1990s, most of the concern about environmental hazards focused on direct risks to health (e.g. from chemicals that might cause cancer). However, it now seems clear that many chemicals to which we are exposed can also adversely affect reproduction without necessarily compromising individual health, even in tiny amounts. They do this by mimicking the effects in the body of the body's own hormones – hence, endocrine disrupters. Media accounts have emphasized how, for example, male Florida alligators have developed tiny penises, and fish in Britain have been reported as changing sex. Chemical spills and sewage effluent were, it seems, the respective culprits in promoting what newspaper reports promptly entitled 'gender bending'; meanwhile, other headlines referred to effects in humans, particularly an alleged decline in male sperm count. Needless to say, these data and their interpretations have also been the subject of much controversy, not only between scientists but also in the public domain (see Birke 2000). Some scientists, for instance, dispute the 'safe' levels of exposure, arguing that we have always been exposed to exogenous hormones (through plant foods for instance).

To other scientists, 'disrupters' is a somewhat misleading term, for it can be read as implying that there was a previous constancy that has been disrupted. This ignores the ways in which every species's physiology (including hormones) has co-evolved with those of other organisms, with the ecosystems of which it is part. There have certainly been hormones around in the water, and in the food we eat, for millennia. To an extent, our endocrine systems have evolved in relation to these – in a fluid and constant interchange, since we excrete steroids into the environment. So, the presence of additional chemicals necessarily shifts that balance, with potential consequences for reproduction.

Indeed, so entwined are these processes, that effects on animal bodies may become cumulative. Arguments about the threshold, or 'safe' level, may he futile for chemicals that mimic molecules occurring normally within bodies; in that case, thresholds are automatically exceeded with exposure (and we are exposed to a multiplicative cocktail of such molecules). Defining 'safe' levels has little meaning in this case. Moreover, effects of disrupters can accumulate over generations, altering hormones in foetuses or eggs, which then grow into adults with altered hormonal sensitivities and reproductive function. Here, again, is an area of biological inquiry with considerable significance for how humans engage with the social world, and for their future health. It is also a salutary lesson in how human activities are changing the world – with consequences for all species, and their futures on this earth.

Now, the examples of such complex interactions I have chosen to discuss are rather arbitrary. My point, however, is to use them to encourage us to think beyond any notions of the biological body as presocial, or primary, and to think about it as engaged, as part of its milieu. These specific details may seem a far cry from rarified social theory about, say, corporeal flows and gender. Yet if we are truly going to bring biology into our thinking about social theory and the body, then I think we are going to have to bother with some of those biological details, to try to understand how those processes operate in (and change) the context of our social engagement. What this means is not only trying to understand how social factors influence bodies (health), but also how bodies and their biology influence social processes. But we must understand these as constantly engaging processes, not as determinants. Endocrine disrupters thus provide an example less of how A affects B (though it is that also) but of how human biology is a dynamic set of processes, nested in among other dynamic sets of processes or systems (and, in this case, the politics of global capitalism and industrial production). To understand health/bodily outcomes of these processes requires a quite different approach to understanding biology than the reductionist one.

Among other things, to emphasize the dynamic agency of biological processes is to acknowledge their own role in their organization. Several theorists now emphasize the significance of self-organization within systems in nature (see discussion in Rose 1997). That is, organization within a system (such as an organism) emerges out of the prior state(s) of that organism. That, it seems to me, offers a compromise between the excesses of genetic determinism and the notion that the body can be understood only discursively or as flows/fluidities. Self-organized systems are fluid and constantly in exchange with their worlds; yet they often appear to be constrained, and highly stable. They are neither fixed nor completely open-ended, they are both/and.

With examples like that of endocrine disrupters, we can begin to see how bodily processes comprise systems fluidly connected to our social and physical environments. More specifically, we can begin to understand better how the impact of social divisions on health can exert effects over generations. As Peter Dickens (2001) notes, there is growing evidence that children from poorer backgrounds are affected biologically before they are even born. These effects (which include those from endocrine disrupting chemicals) in turn influence physiological function, bodily habitus, and future health. Not only does this have nothing to do with genetics (as some determinists would claim), but it is, Dickens argues, an instance of how capitalism may, in the long term, be 'shaping human biology in its own image' (ibid.: 106).

And not only human biology, of course, for other kinds of animals are quite literally and intentionally being reshaped in the service of biotechnology, while others are influenced, just as we are, by the environmental changes to which our bodies are exposed. There are another set of issues here to be concerned about – such as how much the planet's biodiversity is threatened by these processes of reshaping biology, and how much the welfare of individual animals is compromised by new biotechnological creations.

For women, struggles over reproductive rights and issues of control over their own bodies become more acute in a world of growing medical/technological intervention. And reproductive health is further threatened by what some critics see as a barrage of oestrogenic compounds in the environment. In this context, it is crucial that we challenge the biology-as-bedrock arguments, and work towards understanding our biology as part and parcel of our socially engaged selves. We urgently need to 'bring back' *this* kind of biology to the social sciences and to feminism – not only to further our understanding of bodily health but also to counter the seemingly endless claims of biological determinism. This is not only a political or academic challenge, but it is also fundamentally about recognizing the multiple levels of 'our bodies, ourselves'.

Notes

1 This is not to say that such biological processes can necessarily be known without its embeddedness in social and cultural processes. It is just that, while we can acknowledge that intertwining, the literature almost exclusively focuses on those social processes.
2 Yearley (1991) notes how the environmental movement is both hostile to science and technology (which help to create environmental problems) and must call upon scientific knowledge at times to arbitrate environmental disputes. To some extent, this ambivalence applies also to other social movements. Animal rights, tor instance, is hostile to the science that uses laboratory animals, yet must refer to scientific arguments about evolutionary similarities to make their arguments.
3 I don't wish to imply that knowing a bit of science can permit women to take on the medical establishment (would that it were so!). However, women working in women's self-help health groups often do find it emancipatory to take control over access to medical knowledge: my own experience in such groups bears this out.
4 For a general overview, see Whittle and Inhorn 2001. This raises the problem of essentialism, in that all women, irrespective of differences, are subsumed under the term 'women'. There are, however, commonalities, since most women, globally, reproduce. On the impact of difference in relation to women's health research, see Whittle and Inhorn, ibid.
5 Many biologists would accept this, even suggesting that the critics are making mountains out of molehills. However, while biological writing often pays lip service to the interactions between genes and environment, all too often it uses phrases which lend themselves to deterministic interpretations. This is particularly clear when the same research is reported in the media. In the end, the culturally relevant face of biology that emerges from such research is indeed the determinist one. I would also suggest that the enormous interest in genetics and biotechnology among critical scholars working in science studies also helps to fuel the hegemony of genetic discourses. Other areas of biological inquiry are sadly neglected by critics.
6 Social and cultural variation in experience of menarche and menstruation is one example; or the ways in which gender and race can influence how ill health is experienced; see Whittle and Inhorn 2001. Bourdieu did discuss the acquisition of gender in early life, but has been criticized by feminists for binding sex and gender too tightly, of making them over-determined socially (Lovell 2000).
7 And if differences in how we move through the world might become manifest in individual bodies, what does that say about the conclusions drawn from highly standardized studies of very inbred laboratory animals?
8 Among others, these include Rose 1997, Birke 1999 and Fausto-Sterling, this volume.
9 Higher incubation temperatures for many species of turtles and lizards can favour males or females, depending upon the species.
10 In embryonic development, the emergence of structures typically affects – and thereby constrains – the development of further structures. Examples in vertebrates include the pentadactyl limb (with five digits) and the eye.

References

Bekoff, M. (2002) *Minding Animals: Awareness, Emotions and Heart*, Oxford: Oxford University Press.

Bell, S. E. (1994) 'Translating science to the people: Updating *The New Our Bodies, Ourselves*', *Women's Studies International Forum*, 17: 9–18.

Birke, L. (1999) *Feminism and the Biological Body*, Edinburgh: Edinburgh University Press.

Birke, L. (2000) 'Sitting on the fence: biology, feminism, and gender-bending environments', *Women's Studies International Forum*, 23: 587–99.

Bourdieu, P. (1984) *Distinction: A Social Critique of the Judgement of Taste*, London: Routledge.

Dickens, P. (2001) 'Linking the social and the natural sciences: is capital modifying human biology in its own image?' *Sociology*, 35: 93–110.

Grosz, E. (1994) *Volatile Bodies: Toward a Corporeal Feminism*, Bloomington and Indianapolis: Indiana University Press.

Lovell, T. (2000) 'Thinking feminism with and against Bourdieu', *Feminist Theory*, 1: 11–32.

Maier, S. F. and Watkins, L. R. (1999) 'Bidirectional communication between the brain and the immune system: implications for behaviour', *Animal Behaviour*, 57: 741–51.

Marshall, H. (1996) 'Our bodies ourselves: why we should add old fashioned empirical phenomenonology to the new theories of the body', *Women's Studies International Forum*, 19: 253–65.

Martin, E. (1994) *Flexible Bodies: Tracking Immunity in American Culture from the Days of Polio the the Days of AIDS*, Boston: Beacon Press.

Nanda, M. (1996) 'The science quesion in post-colonial feminism', *Economic and Political Weekly*, **April 20–7**, WS2–WS7.

Rose, S. (1997) *Lifelines: Biology, Freedom, Determinism*, Harmondsworth: Penguin.

Shilling, C. and Mellor, P. A. (1996) 'Embodiment, structuration theory and modernity: mind/body dualism and the repression of sensuality', *Body and Society*, 2: 1–15.

Shodhini Collective (1997) *Touch Me, Touch Me Not: Women, Plants and Healing*, New Delhi: Kali for Women.

Spelman, E. (1988) *Inessential Woman: Problems of Exclusion in Feminist Thought*, Boston: Beacon Press.

Tauber, A. I. (1994) *The Immune Self: Theory or Metaphor?*, Cambridge: Cambridge University Press.

Weasel, L. (2001) 'Dismantling the self/other dichotomy in science: towards a feminist model of the immune system', *Hypatia*, 16: 27–44.

Whittle, K. L. and Inhorn, M. C. (2001) 'Rethinking difference: a feminist reframing of gender/race/class for the improvement of women's health research', *International Journal of Health Services*, 31: 147–65.

Yearly, S. (1991) *The Green Case: A Sociology of Environmental Issues, Arguments and Politics*, London: HarperCollins.

4

THE BARE BONES OF SEX
Part 1—sex and gender

Anne Fausto-Sterling

Source: *Signs*, 30:21 (2005), 1491–527.

Here are some curious facts about bones. They can tell us about the kinds of physical labor an individual has performed over a lifetime and about sustained physical trauma. They get thinner or thicker (on average in a population) in different historical periods and in response to different colonial regimes (Molleson 1994; Larsen 1998). They can indicate class, race, and sex (or is it gender—wait and see). We can measure their mineral density and whether on average someone is likely to fracture a limb but not whether a particular individual with a particular density will do so. A bone may break more easily even when its mineral density remains constant (Peacock et al. 2002).[1]

Culture shapes bones. For example, urban ultraorthodox Jewish adolescents have lowered physical activity, less exposure to sunlight, and drink less milk than their more secular counterparts. They also have greatly decreased mineral density in the vertebrae of their lower backs, that is, the lumbar vertebrae (Taha et al. 2001). Chinese women who work daily in the fields have increased bone mineral content and density. The degree of increase correlates with the amount of time spent in physical activity (Hu et al. 1994); weightlessness in space flight leads to bone loss (Skerry 2000); gymnastics training in young women ages seventeen to twenty-seven correlates with increased bone density despite bone resorption caused by total lack of menstruation (Robinson et al. 1995). Consider also some recent demographic trends: in Europe during the past thirty years, the number of vertebral fractures has increased three- to fourfold for women and more than fourfold for men (Mosekilde 2000); in some groups the relative proportions of different parts of the skeleton have changed in recent generations.[2] (See also table 1.)

What are we to make of reports that African Americans have greater peak bone densities than Caucasian Americans (Aloia et al. 1996; Gilsanz et al. 1998),[3] although this difference may not hold when one compares Africans

Table 1 Culture changes bones

Observation	Reference
Vertebral BMD (gm/cm^2) increased in young women during an eight-month program of running or weight-training compared with untrained controls.	Snow-Harter et al. 1992
Two years of aerobics and weight training enhances BMD in young women; gymnastics training improves mechanical competence of skeleton in boys.	Friedlander et al. 1995; Daly et al. 1999
Intensive tennis playing increases bone mineral content, BMAD, and thickness of the humerus of the racket arm; the effect is especially noticeable in players who began at ages 9–10, and the effect is there for both males and females. Later-in-life start-up (29 years) resulted in more marginal effects.	Jones et al. 1977; Haapasalo et al. 1996
Cross-country skiers who train year-round have site-specific increases in BMD (study on females age ~16).	Pettersson et al. 2000
In late-adolescent women, weight-bearing activities are important for determining bone density; high-impact activities modify bone width due to increased muscle strength and lean body mass; lean mass, fat mass, weight, BMI, years of menstruation, and type of physical activity explained 81.6 percent of bone variation.	Soderman et al. 2000
In Japanese women with a genetic variant that impairs vitamin D receptor, exercise, vitamin D, and calcium intake can increase BMD.	Fujita et al. 1999
Long-term exercise improves balance in older osteoarthritic adults (fewer falls).	Messier et al. 2000
In a longitudinal study of youth ages 13–27, maintaining at least an average weight was the best predictor of high BMD in females.	Welton et al. 1994
Premenopausal, but not postmenopausal, women respond to a regime of vertical jumping exercises with increased BMD in their femurs.	Bassey and Ramsdale 1994; Bassey et al. 1998
Physical activity and muscle strength independently predict BMD in total body and in the proximal femur in young men.	Nordstrom, Nordstrom, and Lorentzan 1997
Amateur sports at ages 11–30 improves bone density in a site- or stress-specific fashion (study done on young men).	Nordstrom et al. 1996; Morel et al. 2001
Prepubertal Asian Canadian boys have lowered femoral neck BMC and BMD, ingest 41 percent less calcium, and are 15 percent less active than Caucasian Canadian boys.	McKay et al. 2000
Over three years, men and women over age 65 receiving calcium and vitamin D supplements show less bone loss in the femur and spine and a lower incidence of nonvertebral fractures.	Dawson-Hughes et al. 1997
Ninety percent of adolescent girls and 50 percent of adolescent boys consume less than optimal amounts of dietary calcium.	Bachrach 2001
Fifty percent of 12- to 21-year-olds exercise vigorously and regularly; 25 percent report no vigorous physical activity.	Bachrach 2001
Alcohol consumption correlates with higher BMD, smoking with lower BMD.	Siris et al. 2001
Anorexia nervosa injures bone development and maintenance.	Muñoz and Argente 2002
In the twentieth century, American youth of African, European, and Japanese ancestry increased in height due to changes in sitting height and increase in lower limb length.	Meredith 1978

Note: BMD = bone mineral density, BMAD = bone mineral apparent density (the measure is independent of size), BMI = body mass index, and BMC = bone mineral content.

to British Caucasians (Dibba et al. 1999), or that white women and white men break their hips more often than black women and black men (Kellie and Brody 1990)?[4] How do we interpret reports that Caucasian men have a lifetime fracture risk of 13–25 percent compared with Caucasian women's lifetime risk of 50 percent even though once peak bone mass is attained men and women lose bone at the same rate (Seeman 1997, 1998; NIH Consensus Statement Online 2000)?

Such curious facts raise perplexing questions. Why have bones become more breakable in certain populations? What does it mean to say that a lifestyle behavior such as exercise, diet, drinking, or smoking is a risk factor for osteoporosis? Why do we screen large numbers of women for bone density even though this information does not tell us whether an individual woman will break a bone?[5] Why was a major public policy statement on women's health unable to offer a coherent account of sex (or is it gender?) differences in bone health over the life cycle (Wizemann and Pardue 2001)? Why, if bone fragility is so often considered to be a sex-related trait, do so few studies examine the relationships among childbirth, lactation, and bone development (Sowers 1996; Glock, Shanahan, and McGowan 2000)?

Such curious facts and perplexing questions challenge both feminist and biomedical theory. If "facts" about biology and "facts" about culture are all in a muddle, perhaps the nature/nurture dualism, a mainstay of feminist theory, is not working as it should. Perhaps, too, parsing medical problems into biological (or genetic or hormonal) components in opposition to cultural or lifestyle factors has outlived its usefulness for biomedical theory. I propose that already well-developed dynamic systems theories can provide a better understanding of how social categories act on bone production. Such a framework, especially if it borrows from a second analytic trend called "life course analysis of chronic disease epidemiology" (Kuh and Ben-Shlomo 1997; Ben-Shlomo and Kuh 2002; Kuh and Hardy 2002), can improve our approaches to public health policy, prediction of individual health conditions, and the treatment of individuals with unhealthy bones.[6] To see why we should follow new roads, I consider gender, examining where we—feminist theorists and medical scientists—have recently been. In the second part of this study (Fausto-Sterling in preparation) I will engage with current discussions of biology, race, and medicine to explore claims about racial difference in bone structure and function.

Sex and gender (again)

For centuries, scholars, physicians, and laypeople in the United States and Western Europe used biological models to explain the different social, legal, and political statuses of men and women and people of different hues.[7] When the feminist second wave burst onto the political arena in the early 1970s, we made the theoretical claim that sex differs from gender and that social institutions produce observed social differences between men and women (Rubin 1975). Feminists assigned biological (especially reproductive) differences to the word *sex* and gave to *gender* all other differences.

"Sex," however, has become the Achilles' heel of 1970s feminism. We relegated it to the domain of biology and medicine, and biologists and medical scientists have spent the past thirty years expanding it into arenas we firmly believed to belong to our ally gender. Hormones, we learn (once more), cause naturally more assertive men to reach the top in the workplace (Dabbs and Dabbs 2001). Rape is a behavior that can be changed only with the greatest difficulty because it is wired somehow into men's brains (Thornhill and Palmer 2001). The relative size of eggs and sperm dictate that men are naturally polygamous and women naturally monogamous. And more. (See Zuk 2002; Travis 2003 for a critique of these claims.) Feminist scholars have two choices in response to this spreading oil spill of sex. Either we can contest each claim, one at a time, doing what Susan Oyama calls "hauling the theoretical body back and forth across the sex/gender border" (2000a, 190), or, as I choose to do here, we can reconsider the 1970s theoretical account of sex and gender.

In thinking about both gender and race, feminists must accept the body as simultaneously composed of genes, hormones, cells, and organs—all of which influence health and behavior—and of culture and history (Verbrugge 1997). As a biologist, I focus on what it might mean to claim that our bodies physically imbibe culture. How does experience shape the very bones that support us?[8] Can we find a way to talk about the body without ceding it to those who would fix it as a naturally determined object existing outside of politics, culture, and social change? This is a project already well under way, not only in feminist theoretical circles but in epidemiology, medical sociology, and anthropology as well.

Embodiment merges biology and culture

During the 1990s, feminist reconsideration of the sex/gender problem moved into full swing.[9] Early in the decade Judith Butler argued compellingly for the importance of reclaiming the term *sex* for feminist inquiry but did not delve into the nuts and bolts of how sex and gender materialize in the body. Philosopher Elizabeth Grosz (1994) claimed that sex is neither fixed nor given. In drawing on philosophers such as Maurice Merleau-Ponty (1962) and Alfred North Whitehead ([1929] 1978), Grosz differentiates herself from Butler, holding that materiality is "primordial, not merely the effect of power" (Alcoff 2000, 858). Primordial materiality, however, does not mean that purely biological accounts of human development—no matter how intricate their stories of cellular function—can explain the emergence of lived and differently gendered realities.[10]

Psychologist Elizabeth Wilson offers one of the most interesting and far-reaching critiques of feminist attempts to reclaim the body (Martin 1997; Wilson

1998, 1999). Reaching back to Sigmund Freud's work on hysteria, Wilson emerges with a new purchase on biology itself. Reiterating the varied symptoms produced by psychic trauma (blindness, localized pain, loss of smell, paralysis), she focuses on the "bio-logic" of these physical manifestations (1999). "The neurology, physiology, or biochemistry of hysterical symptomology," she writes, "can be disregarded only in a theoretical milieu that takes certain modes of materiality to be inert" (1999, 10). She suggests that just as "culture," "signification," or "sociality" contribute to the production of complex bodily responses, "biology itself" ought to be investigated as a "site of . . . complex ontological accomplishment" (10). Such investigation, Wilson argues, opens the door for a fundamental reexamination of biomedical analyses of sex differences in physiology and disease patterns. The idea of embodiment as a dynamic system of biocultural formation reaches beyond discussions of gender (e.g., Csordas 1990; Ingold 1998; Williams and Bendelow 1998).[11]

Efforts to reincorporate the body into social theory also come from the field of disability studies. Here too an emphasis on the social construction of disability has been enormously productive. Yet several authors have broached the limitations of an exclusively constructivist approach. At least two different types of critique parallel and foreshadow possible feminist approaches to a reconsideration of the body. The first demands that we recognize the material constraints on the disabled body in its variable forms and that we integrate that recognition into theory (Williams and Busby 2000). The second, more radical move is to suggest that "the disabled body changes the process of representation itself" (Siebers 2001, 738). This latter approach offers a rich resource for feminist theories of representation and another possible entry point into the analysis of materiality in actual, lived-in bodies (see also Schriempf 2001).

Sex and gender in the world of biology and medicine

In contrast to these new feminist explorations of the body, in the field of medicine a more limited view of sex differences prevails. Consider a recent report on sex differences issued by the National Institute of Medicine and, more broadly, the professional movement called "gender-based medicine" promoted by the Society for Women's Health Research (SWHR). The SWHR describes itself as "the nation's only not-for-profit organization whose sole mission is to improve the health of women through research. . . . The Society . . . encourages the study of sex differences that may affect the prevention, diagnosis and treatment of disease and promotes the inclusion of women in medical research studies" (Schachter 2001, 29).[12] The society lobbies Congress, sponsors research conferences, and publishes a peer-reviewed academic journal, the *Journal of Women's Health and Gender-Based Medicine*.

A traditional biomedical model of health and disease provides the intellectual framework for the research conferences (Krieger and Zierler 1995). Although much of the research publicized through such conferences seems strictly to deal with *sex* in the 1970s feminist meaning of the word, sex sometimes strays into arenas that traditional feminists claim for gender. Consider a presentation that was said to provide evidence that prenatal testosterone exposure affects which toys little girls and boys prefer to play with (Berenbaum 2001). Working within a 1970s definition of the sex/gender dualism, the author of this study logically extends the term *sex* into the realm of human behavior.

For those familiar with contemporary feminist theory, it might seem that the large number of biological psychologists who follow similar research programs and the biomedical researchers interested in tracking down all of the medically interesting differences between men and women live in a time warp. But members of the feminist medical establishment, that is, those researchers and physicians for whom the activities and programs of the SWHR make eminent sense, see themselves perched on the forward edge of a nascent movement to bring gender equity to the healthcare system. These feminists work outside of an intellectual milieu that would permit the more revolutionary task proposed by Grosz and Wilson, among others, that of contesting not only "the domination of the body by biological terms but also [contesting] the terms of biology itself" (Grosz 1994, 20).

Within medicine there is a lot of confusion about the terms *sex* and *gender*. Many medical texts use the terms interchangeably, while some scientists apply the term *gender* to the study of nonhuman animals, a problem also debated in the primary biological literature (Pearson 1996; Thomas et al. 2000). Lack of consistent usage promotes confusion among scientists, policy makers, and the general public, in effect foreclosing any space for the analysis of social causes of differences in health outcomes between men and women (Krieger 2003).

Helen Keane and Marsha Rosengarten (2002) have explored the body as a dynamic process out of which gender emerges. In a first example they examine the significance of anabolic steroid use on the alteration of sexed bodies, concluding that "the hormonal body is always in process rather than fixed" (269); they further explore the notion of sex/gender fixity through a discussion of organ transplantation between XX and XY individuals. Finally, they examine "the biological *as* a field of transformations, as active, 'literate matter' as well as an effect *of* mediation and intervention" (275). I have chosen bone development—an area often accepted as an irrefutable site of sex difference—to examine Keane and Rosengarten's formulation. First, to what extent can we understand bone formation as an effect of culture rather than a passive unfolding of biology? Second, can we use dynamic (developmental) systems to ask better research questions and to formulate better public-health responses to bone disease?

Why bones?

Bones are eloquent. Archaeologists read old bone texts to find out how prehistoric peoples lived and worked. A hyperflexed and damaged big toe, a bony growth on the femur, the knee, or the vertebrae, for example, tell bioarchaeologist Theya Molleson that women in a Near Eastern agricultural community routinely ground grain on all fours, grasping a stone grinder with their hands and pushing back and forth on a saddle-shaped stone. The bones of these neolithic people bear evidence of a gendered division of labor, culture, and biology intertwined (Molleson 1994).[13]

Given that modern forensic pathologists also use bones to learn about how people live and die, it seems odd that a report from the National Institute of Medicine, presented as a state-of-the-art account of gender and medicine, deals only superficially with the sexual differentiation of bone disease (Wizeman and Pardue 2001).[14] In a brief three pages on osteoporosis, the monograph cites dramatic statistics on the frequency of osteoporosis in European and Caucasian American women and the dangers of the condition. The report offers a laundry list of factors believed to affect bone health. Jumbled together, with no attempt to understand their interrelationships or their joint, cumulative contributions to bone development and loss, are hormones, diet, exercise, genetic background, vitamin D production, and the bone-destroying effects of drugs such as cortisone, tobacco, and alcohol. In an anemic end-of-chapter recommendation the authors urge researchers to control for all of the above factors as they design their research studies. Indeed, failure to engage the task of formulating new approaches to biology prevented them from making a stronger analysis.

But osteoporosis is a condition that reveals all of the problems of defining sex apart from gender. A close reading of the osteoporosis literature further reveals the difficulties of adding the variable of race to the mix (a point I will develop in a forthcoming paper [Fausto-Sterling in preparation]) while also exemplifying the claim that disease states are socially produced, both by rhetoric and measurement (e.g., Petersen 1998) and by the manner in which cultural practice shapes the very bones in our bodies (Krieger and Zierler 1995).

Of bones and (wo)men

The accuracy of the claim that osteoporosis occurs four times more frequently in women than in men (Glock, Shanahan, and McGowan 2000) depends on how we define osteoporosis, in which human populations (and historical periods) we gather statistics, and what portions of the life cycle we compare. The NIH (2000) defines osteoporosis as a skeletal disorder in which weakened bones increase the risk of fracture. When osteoporosis first wandered onto the medical radar screen, the only signal that a person suffered from it was a bone fracture. Post hoc, a doctor could examine a person with a fracture either using a biopsy to look at the structural competence of the bone or by assessing bone density.

If one looks at lifetime risks for fracture, contemporary Caucasian men range from 13 to 25 percent (Bilezikian, Kurkland, and Rosen 1999) while Caucasian women (who also live longer) have a 50 percent risk. But not all fractures result from osteoporosis. One study looked at fracture incidence in men and women at different ages and found that between the ages of five and forty-five men break more limbs than women.[15] The breaks, however, result from significant work- and sports-related trauma suffered by healthy bones. After the age of fifty, women break their bones more often than men, although after seventy years of age men do their best to catch up (Melton 1988).

The most commonly used medical standard for a diagnosis of osteoporosis no longer depends on broken bones. With the advent of machines called densitometers used to measure bone mineral density (of which more in a moment), the World Health Organization (WHO) developed a new "operational" definition: a woman has osteoporosis if her bone mineral density measures 2.5 times the standard deviation below a peak reference standard for young (white) women. The densitometer manufacturer usually provides the reference data to a screening facility (Seeman 1998), and thus rarely, if ever, do assessments of osteoporosis reflect what Margaret Lock calls "local biologies" (Lock 1998, 39).[16] With the WHO definition, the prevalence of osteoporosis for white women is 18 percent, although there is not necessarily associated pathology, since now, by definition, one can "get" or "have" osteoporosis without ever having a broken bone. The WHO definition is controversial, since bone mineral density (BMD, or grams/cm^2) accounts for approximately 70 percent of bone strength, while the other 30 percent derives from the internal structure of bone and overall bone size. And while women with lower bone density are 2.5 times more likely to experience a hip fracture than women with high bone densities, high risks of hip fracture emerge even in women with high bone densities when five or more other risk factors are present (Cummings et al. 1995).[17] Furthermore, it is hard to know how to apply the criterion, based on a baseline of young white women, to men, children, and members of other ethnic groups. To make matters worse, there is a lack of standardization between instruments and sites at which measurements are taken.[18] Thus it comes as no surprise that "controversy exists among experts regarding the continued use of this [WHO] diagnostic criterion" (NIH Consensus Statement Online 2000, 3).

There is a complicated mixture at play. First, osteoporosis—whether defined as fractures or bone density—is on the rise, even when the increased age of a population is taken into account (Mosekilde 2000). At the same time, it is hard to assess the danger of osteoporosis, in part due to drug company–sponsored "public awareness" campaigns. For example, in preparation for the sales campaign for its new drug, Fosamax, Merck Pharmaceuticals gave a large osteoporosis education grant to the National Osteoporosis Foundation to educate older women about the dangers of osteoporosis (Tanouye 1995).[19] Merck also directly addressed consumers with television ads contrasting frail, pain-wracked older women with lively, attractive seniors, implying the urgent need for older women to use Fosamax (Fugh-Berman, Pearson, Allina, Zones, Worcester, and Whatley 2002).

Mass marketing a new drug, however, requires more than a public awareness campaign. There must also be an easy, relatively inexpensive method of diagnosis. Here the slippage between the new technological measure—bone density—and the old definition of actual fractures and direct assessment of bone structure looms large. Merck promoted affordable bone density testing even before it put Fosamax on the market. The company bought an equipment manufacturing company and ramped up its production of bone density machines while at the same time helping consumers find screening locations by giving a grant to the National Osteoporosis Foundation to push a toll-free number that consumers (presumably alarmed by the Merck TV ads) could call to find a bone density screener in a locale near them (Tanouye 1995; Fugh-Berman, Pearson, Allina, Zones, Worcester, and Whatley 2002).

The availability of a simple technological measure for osteoporosis also made scientific research easier and cheaper. The majority of the thousands upon thousands of research papers on osteoporosis published in the ten years from 1995 to 2005 use BMD as a proxy for osteoporosis. This is true despite a critical scientific literature that insists that the more expensive volumetric measure (grams/cm^3) more accurately measures bone strength and that knowledge of internal bone structure (bone histomorphometry) provides essential information for understanding the actual risk of fracture (Meunier 1988).[20] The explosion of knowledge about osteoporosis codifies a new disorder, still called osteoporosis but sporting a newly simplified account of bone health and disease.[21] Ego Seeman (1997) laments the use of the density measure, which, he argues, "affects the way we conceptualize the skeleton (or fail to), and the way we direct (or misdirect) our research," and "blind[s] us to the biology of bone" (510).

Weaving together these threads—increasing lifetime risk, new disease definitions, and easier measurement—produces an epistemological transformation in our scientific accounts of bones and why they break. The transformation is driven by a combination of cultural forces (why are fracture rates increasing?) and new technologies generated by drug companies interested in creating new markets, disseminated with the help of market forces drummed up by the self-same drug companies, and aided by consumer health movements, including feminist health organizations such as the Society for Women's Research, which argue that gender-based differences in disease have been too long neglected.

Analyzing bone development within the framework of sex versus gender (nature vs. nurture) makes it difficult to understand bone health in men as well as women. Those trying to decide on a proper standard to measure fracture risk in men (should they use a separate male baseline or the only one available, which is for young, white women?) struggle with this problem of gender standardization (Melton et al. 1998). There are differences between men and women, although osteoporosis in men is vastly understudied. In a bibliography of 2,449 citations of papers from 1995 to 1999 (Glock, Shanahan, and McGowan 2000), only 47 (2 percent) addressed osteoporosis in men. But making sense of patterns of bone health for either or both sexes requires a dynamic systems approach. A basic starting place is to ask the development question.

For instance, we find no difference in bone mineral density in (Caucasian) boys and girls under age sixteen but a higher bone mineral density in males than in females thereafter (Zanchetta et al. 1995). This difference (combined with others that develop during middle adulthood) becomes important later in life, since men and women appear to lose bone at the same rate once they have reached a peak bone mass; those starting the loss phase of the life cycle with more bone in place will be less likely to develop highly breakable bones. Researchers offer different explanations for this divergence. Some note that boys continue to grow for an average of two years longer than girls (Seeman 1997). The extra growth period strengthens their bones by adding overall size. Others point additionally to hormones, diet, physical activity, and body weight as contributing to the emerging sex (or is it gender?) difference at puberty (Rizzoli and Bonjour 1999).

So differences in bone mineral density between boys and girls emerge during and after puberty, while for both men and women peak bone mass and strength is reached at twenty-five to thirty years of age (Seeman 1999). Vertebral height is the same in men and women, but vertebral width is greater in men. The volume of the inner latticework does not differ in men and women, but the outer layer of bone (periosteum) is thicker in men. Both width and outer thickness strengthen the bone. In general, sex/gender bone differences at peak are in size rather than density (Bilezikian, Kurkland, and Rosen 1999).

This life-cycle analysis reveals three major differences in the pattern of bone growth and loss in men compared with that in women. First, at peak, men have 20 to 30 percent more bone mass and strength than women. Second, following peak, men but not women compensate for bone loss with new increases in vertebral width that continue to strengthen the vertebrae. Over time both men and women lose 70 to 80 percent of bone strength (Mosekilde 2000), but the pattern of loss differs. In men the decline is gradual, barring secondary causes.[22] In women it is gradual until perimenopause, accelerates for several years during and after the menopause, and then resumes a gradual decline.[23] Lis Moskilde (2000) points out that the rush to link menopause to osteoporosis has led to the neglect of two of the three major differences in the pattern of bone growth between men and women. Yet these two factors are specifically linked to physical activity, and thus amenable to change earlier in life.

Indeed, many studies on children and adolescents address the contribution sociocultural components of bone development make to male-female differences that emerge just after puberty (see table 1). But the overwhelming focus on menopause as the period of the life cycle in which women enter the danger zone steers us away from examining how earlier sociocultural events shape our bones (see Lock 1998). Once menopause enters the picture, the idea that hormones are at the heart of the problem overwhelms other modes of thought.[24] Nor is it clear how hormones affect bone development and loss. In childhood, growth hormone is essential for long bone growth, the gonadal steroids are important for the cessation of bone growth at puberty, and probably both estrogen and testosterone are important for bone health maintenance (Damien, Price, and Lanyon 1998). The details at the cellular level have yet to be understood (Gasperino 1995).

Basic bone biology

In the fetus, cartilage creates the scaffolding onto which bone cells climb before secreting the calcium-containing bone matrix that becomes the hard bone.[25] The cells that secrete the bone matrix are called osteoblasts. As they grow, bones are shaped by the strains and stresses put on them by the activity of their owner. Osteoblasts deposit matrix at some sites, while another cell type, the osteoclast, can chip away at areas of too much growth. Growing bones change shape through this give and take of osteoblast and osteoclast activity in a process called bone remodeling.[26] Long bones increase in length throughout childhood by adding on new material at their growing ends. These growth sites close as a result of hormonal changes during puberty, but bone reshaping continues over the course of a life (Currey 2002).

Bone contains two important types of tissue, which can be seen (fig. 1, *A*) if one cuts it across the middle. The outer dense, hard layer is called compact tissue; the inner layer contains cancellous tissue consisting of a latticework of slender fibers. The fibers of this interior bone lattice fuse into longer structures called trabeculae (Latin for "small beam") that crisscross the interior of the bone. The periosteum (literally, "around the bone"), a layer of tissue through which blood vessels and nerves pass into the interior, covers the bone.

Osteoblasts clinging to the periosteum and around the trabecular struts of the bone's interior can produce new bone in both locations. Osteoblasts can also transform into osteocytes, cells found in large numbers inside the hard bone tissues (Currey 2002). Osteocytes probably play an important role in bone regeneration when they produce chemical signals that tell osteoblasts

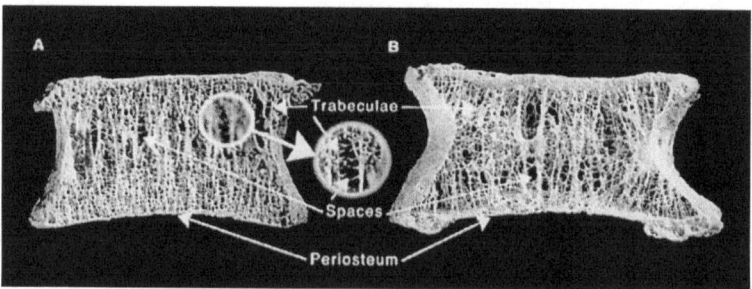

Figure 1 Vertebral structure. Scanning electron micrographs of longitudinal sections of human vertebrae. This image is a modification of one published in Mosekilde 2000. (*A*) Healthy vertebra showing the trabecular structure of the cancellous bone (inset) and the surrounding periosteum. Note the regular vertical arrangement and density of the trabeculae. (*B*) A vertebra exhibiting osteoporosis. Note the increased number and size of spaces where cross struts have broken, as well as the less organized and less dense trabecular structure.

that the bone is under mechanical strain and needs to grow (Mosley 2000). Osteoblasts cannot form new bone unless the surface on which they sit is under a mechanical strain, which explains why exercise remains such an important component of bone health while weightlessness in space or prolonged bed rest result in the loss of bone thickness.[27] Moreover, osteoblasts only add new bone on preexisting surfaces. A person with osteoporosis develops breaks in the tiny cross beams, and these widen into holes that riddle the bone's interior (fig. 1, *B*). A lost strut cannot be replaced because there is no old surface on which to lay down a new mineral layer. A thinning strut, however, can thicken again if the osteoblast produces more new bone than the osteoclast breaks down (Parfitt 1988; Mosekilde 2000).

Bone development, then, is profoundly influenced by what physiologists call functional adaptation. Although a great deal remains to be understood about the biology of use and disuse, some basic principles are already evident. First, both disuse and predictable moderate use result in bone resorption and increased porosity. However, dynamic strain, that is, strain that is unpredictable and of varied impact level, can lead to a linear increase in bone mass (Mosley 2000).[28] Bones may adopt strain thresholds such that only strains above such thresholds induce new bone formation. Strain thresholds may change over the life cycle. Perhaps the decline in estrogen associated with menopause resets the threshold to a higher strain level, thus requiring very high levels of bone stress to stimulate new bone formation. Such dynamic theories allow us to understand how behavior (e.g., changing forms of exercise) and hormonal changes in the body might together produce bone loss or gain (Frost 1986, 1992).

Even such a simplified account of bone development and maintenance shows how hard it can be to understand why people in one group break their bones more often than people in another. Groups may differ in peak bone size even if bone loss later in life is the same. The trabeculae on the bone's inside might be thicker in one group than another, or the outside, compact bone layer might be thicker. There could be less bone loss or a reduction in bone turnover (the balance between osteoclast and osteoblast activity). Trabecular loss could result from thinning rather than perforation, or there could be more new bone formation in the periosteum or less resorption in the bone's interior. What is most striking about the medical literature on osteoporosis is that "whether these differences in bone size, mass, or structure, or bone turnover among ethnic groups or between men and women even partly account for the corresponding group differences in fracture rates is unknown" (Seeman 1997, 517).

Genes, of course, are involved in all of the events described in the previous few paragraphs. Rather than as causes of bone construction and destruction, however, genes are best understood as mediators, suspended in a network of signals (including their own) that induce them to synthesize new molecules.[29] The molecules they make may help to produce more bone or to break down existing bone. Either action may, in turn, be a direct effect (e.g., making a structural element such as collagen) or an indirect effect (e.g., causing the death or sustaining the life of bone-making cells). Researchers have identified over thirty genes that affect bone development either positively or negatively in mice (Peacock et al. 2002), and scientists continue to identify genetic variants affecting bone density in humans (Boyden et al. 2002; Little et al. 2002; Ishida et al. 2003).

Finally, how do hormones fit into all of this? Part of the initial logic of thinking about osteoporosis as a basic biological (sex) difference between men and women derives from the observation that bone thinning increases dramatically around the time of menopause. Most thus assume that declining estrogen causes bone loss. Since estrogen codes in most people's minds as a quintessentially female molecule, it becomes extraordinarily difficult to conceptualize osteoporosis as a disease with many contributors stretching over the entire life cycle. Here, gender constructs (Fausto-Sterling 2000) combined with the profits derived from selling estrogen replacement have contributed mightily to shaping the course of scientific research in this field. Estrogen, though, is only one of a number of hormones linked to bone physiology.

At least three major hormone systems acting both independently of one another and through mutual influence regulate bone formation and loss. Fascinatingly, at least two of these operate at times through the brain and the sympathetic (involuntary) nervous system.[30] The first system includes three major hormones that maintain proper calcium levels throughout the body, dipping into the bone calcium reservoir as needed.[31] The hormones (the active form of vitamin D; parathyroid hormone [PTH], which is made by a small pair of glands called the parathyroid glands; and calcitonin, which is secreted by the thyroid glands) regulate blood calcium levels and bone metabolism.[32] At low concentrations PTH maintains a stable level of mineral turnover in the bone, but at high levels it stimulates osteoclast activity, thus releasing calcium into the bloodstream.[33] Although calcitonin counteracts the effects of PTH on osteoclasts, its functions and mode of action are still poorly understood, but PTH affects bone, kidney, and intestine using vitamin D as an intermediary—a point that returns us to the contributions of sunlight and diet. Our diets and cellular machinery provide inactive forms of vitamin D, but these require the direct energy from sunlight hitting the skin to change into potentially active forms. Final transformations from inactive to active forms of vitamin D occur in the liver and kidney (Bezkorovainy and Rafelson 1996).

Although gonadal hormones—both estrogens and androgens—are clearly important for bone development and maintenance, how they regulate bone metabolism remains uncertain (Kousteni et al. 2001, 2002). Recently, some fascinating studies done on mice have suggested that both androgens and estrogens operate in a fashion unusual for steroid hormones—by preventing the death of bone-forming cells without stimulating new gene activity. Whether these results will hold for humans remains to be seen.[34] Other information from animal models suggests that bone response to mechanical strain requires the presence of an estrogen receptor on the osteoblast cell surface (Lee et al. 2003), but a clear story of the role of estrogens and androgens in bone formation and maintenance throughout the life cycle remains to be told.

Last but certainly not least a hormone called leptin, announced to the world with great fanfare in 1995 as a possible "magic bullet" for weight control (Roush 1995), also affects bone formation. Like the sex steroids, leptin works via a relay system in the hypothalamus, a part of the brain linked to the pituitary gland. Fat tissue produces leptin, which signals specialized nerve cells in the hypothalamus; these activated neurons produce two effects—lowering the appetite and stimulating basal metabolism (via the sympathetic nervous system). In mice, leptin has a second, apparently independent effect, also mediated through the hypothalamus and the sympathetic nervous system. Increased leptin signals nerves in the bone to depress bone formation. This presents an interpretive paradox: obesity provides some protection against osteoporosis. But the more fat cells, the more leptin is made, which in theory ought to depress bone formation. There are several possible explanations for this paradox. In mice it may be that the very overweight body becomes insensitive to its high leptin levels, just as obesity contributes to insulin insensitivity in type 2 diabetes. Or the stimulation of bone formation from the mechanical stress of increased weight might trump the effects of leptin, and/or leptin physiology in mice and humans might differ in important ways.[35]

In the next decade we will surely learn a lot more about the relationships among bone formation, leptin, and the sympathetic nervous system.[36] But we also must learn how to study the balances and interactions among all of the various factors that impinge on bone formation. How do social systems that influence what we eat, how and when we exercise, whether we drink or smoke, what kinds of diseases we get and how they are treated, and how we age, to name some most relevant to bone formation, produce a particular bone structure in a particular individual with a particular life history? To even begin to set up this problem in a manner that can stimulate future work and ultimately bring us better answers, we need to learn how to handle complex, dynamic systems. And so, finally, I turn to a discussion of two overlapping sets of ideas—developmental and dynamic systems theory.

Thinking systematically about bone

There are better ways to think about gender and the bare bones of sex. One cannot easily separate bone biology from the experiences of individuals growing, living, and dying in particular cultures and historical periods and under different regimens of social gender.[37] But how can we integrate the varied information presented in this essay in a manner that helps us ask better research and public policy questions and that, in posing better questions, allows us to find better answers? By *better*, I mean several things: in terms of the science I want to take more of the "curious facts" about bone into account when responding to public health problems. I favor emphasizing lifelong healthful habits that might prevent or lessen the severity of bone problems in late life, but I would also like us to have a better idea of how to help people whose bones are already thin. What dietary changes, what regimens of exercise and sun exposure, what body mass index work best with which medications? How do the medications we choose work? What unintended effects do they have? Finally, *better* includes an ability to predict outcomes for individuals, based on their particular life histories and genetic makeups, rather than merely making probability statements about large and diverse categories of people.

How can we get there from here? Below, I outline in fairly general form the possibilities of dynamic systems and developmental systems approaches. Such formulations allow us to work with the idea that we are always 100 percent nature and 100 percent nurture. I further point to important theoretical and empirical work currently under way by social scientists who study chronic diseases using a life-course approach. Before turning to the specifics of bone development, let me offer a general introduction to these complementary modes of thought.

Figure 2 presents a visual scheme of the larger systems arena. Ludwig von Bertalanffy is usually cited as the originator of "general systems theory," a program for studying complex systems such as organisms as whole entities

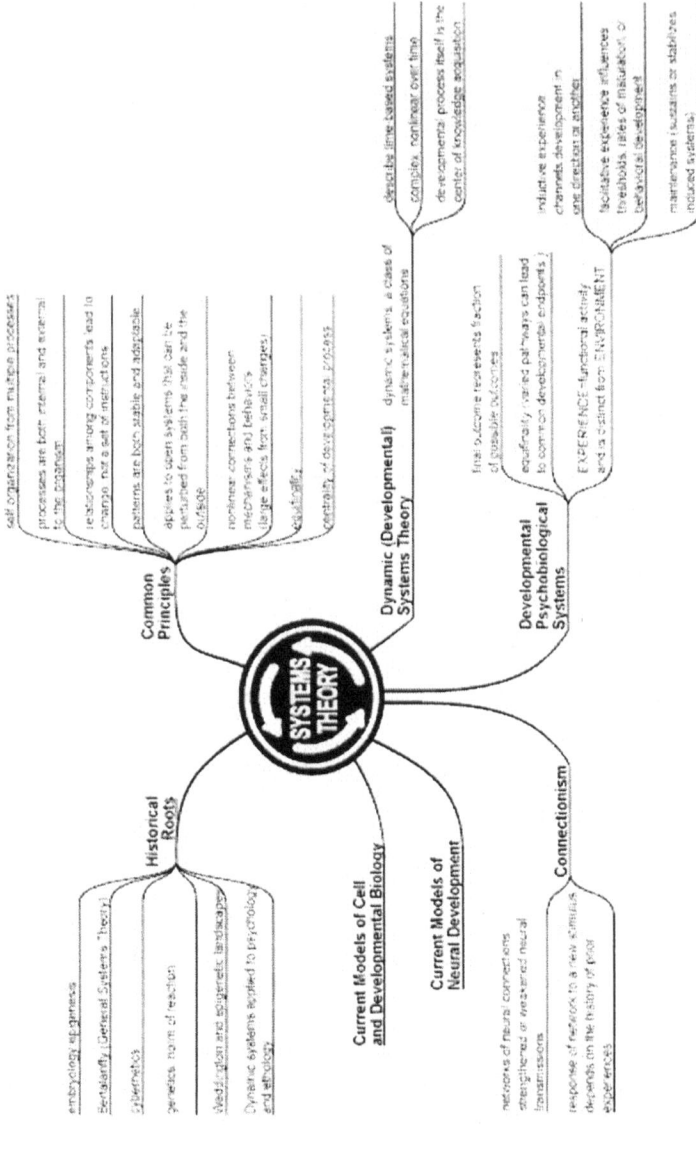

Figure 2 Overview of systems theories.

rather than the traditional approach of reducing the whole to its component parts (Bertalanffy 1969), but the idea of studying developmental outcomes as a result of the combined action of genes and environment began in the early twentieth century before a clear theoretical statement was achieved in the 1940s.[38]

Systems theorists also write about the brain and behavior. D. O. Hebb (1949) linked psychology and physiology by thinking about how functional cellular groups develop in the brain, thus developing a form of systems theory called connectionism. As Esther Thelen and Linda Smith put it, "the connection weights between layers—the response of the network to a particular input—thus depend on the statistical regularities in the network's *history* of experiences" (Thelen and Smith 1998, 580). Thus an organism's current and future behaviors are shaped by past experiences via a direct effect on the strength of connections between cells in the brain.[39]

The varied systems approaches to understanding development share certain features in common. All understand that cells, nervous systems, and whole organisms develop through a process of self-organization rather than according to a preformed set of instructions.[40] The varying relationships among system components lead to change, and new patterns are dynamically stable because the characteristics of the system confer stability. But if the system is sufficiently perturbed, instability ensues and significant fluctuations occur until a new pattern, again dynamically stable, emerges. Bone densities, for example, are often dynamically stable in midlife but destabilize during old age; most medical interventions aim to restabilize the dynamic system that maintains bone density. But we really do not understand how the transition from a stable to an unstable system of bone maintenance occurs.

To address the bare bones of sex, I highlight, in figure 3, seven systems that contribute to bone strength throughout the life cycle.[41] I also describe some of the known interrelationships between them.[42] Each of the seven—physical activity, diet, drugs, bone formation in fetal development, hormones, bone cell metabolism, and biomechanical effects on bone formation—can be analyzed as a complex system in its own right. Bone strength emerges from the interrelated actions of each (and all) of these systems as they act throughout the life cycle. As a first step toward envisioning bone from a systems viewpoint we can construct a theoretical diagram of their interactions. The diagram in systems approaches can be thought of as a theoretical model, to be tested in part or whole and modified as needed.[43] As ways to describe each component system using numerical proxies become available, the pictorial model can provide the framework for a mathematical model. Figure 3 represents one possible diagram of a life-course systems account of bone development.

This feminist systems account embeds the proposed subsystems within the dimensions of gender, socioeconomic position, and culture.[44] Consider the diet system. Generally, of course, diet is shaped by culture and subculture,

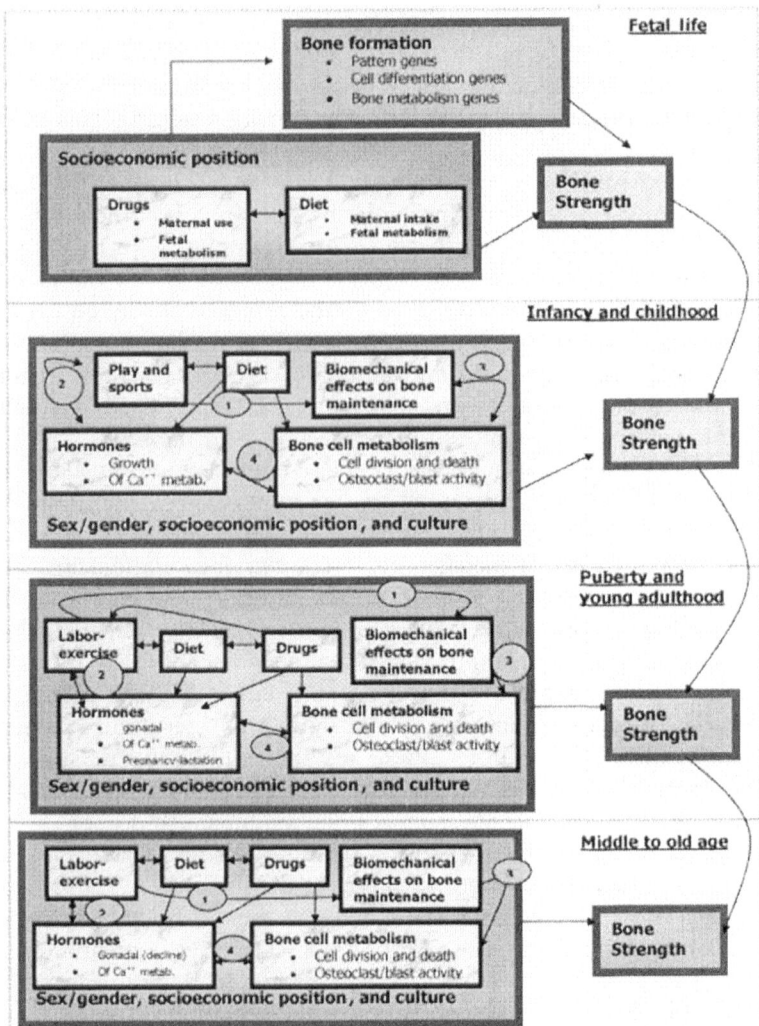

Figure 3 A life history–systems overview of bone development. (1) Physical activity has direct effects on bone cell receptors and indirect effects by building stronger muscles, which exert physical strain on bones, thus stimulating bone synthesis. (2) Physical activity that takes place outdoors involves exposure to sunlight, thus stimulating vitamin D synthesis, part of the hormonal system regulating calcium metabolism. (3) Biomechanical strain affects bone cell metabolism by activating genes concerned with bone cell division and bone (re)modeling. (4) Hormones affect bone cell metabolism by activating genes concerned with bone cell division, cell death, bone (re)modeling, and new hormone synthesis.

including race and ethnicity (Bryant, Cadogan, and Weaver 1999). But gender further influences diet. For example, one study reports that 27 percent of U.S. teenage girls (compared with 10 percent of adolescent boys) who think they weigh the correct amount are nevertheless trying to lose weight (Walsh and Devlin 1998). It may also be true that there are sex/gender differences in basal metabolism rates that influence food intake.

Figure 3 also indicates the cumulative effects of diet on bone formation. Key events may be clustered at certain points in the life cycle.[45] For example, adolescent girls in the United States often diet more and exercise less than during earlier childhood. Diseases such as anorexia nervosa, which have devastating effects on bone development, may also emerge during adolescence. As Yoav Ben-Shlomo and Diana Kuh (2002) point out, such clustering of adverse events is common and may be thought of in terms of "chains of risk" (or benefit). In a life-course approach, prior events set the limits on later ones. If girls and women enter into adulthood with weakened bones, therefore, they can rebuild them, but their peak density may be less than if they had built stronger bones in adolescence.[46] Alternatively, achieving a safe peak bone density might require more sustained and intense work for a person of one history compared with a person of a different history.

Sex/gender, race, class, and culture also differentiate individuals by forms of play in childhood and beyond (Boot et al. 1997), by choices of formal exercise programs, and, in adulthood, by forms of labor, physical and otherwise. In analyzing the system of physical activity one again applies life-course principles by considering that what happens at any one point builds on what has gone before. Important events with regard to bone development may be clustered and interrelated. For both the diet and physical activity systems, it should be possible to design mathematical models based on some measure of bone strength that would incorporate the effects of each of these social systems on bone development throughout the life cycle; once we have plausible models of each system, we can ask questions about their interactions.

The remaining four systems are often considered within the realm of biology, as if biology were separate from culture, although recent work from some medical epidemiologists challenges this distinction (Ellison 1996; Hertzman 1999; Lamont et al. 2000). The system of biomechanical effects on bone synthesis, for example, requires further investigation of all of its inputs (physical strain, activation of genes that stimulate bone cell development or death, etc. [Harada and Rodan 2003]), but these must then be studied in relationship to the gender-differentiated physical activity system. The different body shapes of adult men and women (related to hormones at puberty among other things) may also affect bone biomechanics, and we need, too, to know more about how growth and development affect the number of bone mechanoreceptors—molecules that translate mechanical stress in biochemical activity (Boman et al. 1998; Pavalko et al. 2003).

The impact of hormones on bone development and maintenance requires research attention of a sort currently lacking in the bone literature. We need to know both about the molecular biology of hormones and bone cell hormone receptors and about life-course effects on hormone systems (Ellison 1996; Worthman 2002). Finally, genes involved in bone cell metabolism, pattern formation, hormone metabolism, drug processing, and many other processes contribute importantly to the development of bone strength (Zelzer and Olsen 2003). Understanding how they function within both the local and global (body and sociocultural) networks contributing to bone development requires a systems-level analysis not yet found in the literature.

Conclusion

This article is a call to arms. The sex-gender or nature-nurture accounts of difference fail to appreciate the degree to which culture is a partner in producing body systems commonly referred to as biology—something apart from the social. I introduce an alternative—a life-course systems approach to the analysis of sex/gender. Figure 3 is a research proposal for multiple programs of investigation in several disciplines. We need to ask old questions in new ways so that we can think systematically about the interweaving of bodies and culture. We will not lay bare the bones of sex, but we will come to understand, instead, that our skeletons are part of a life process. If process rather than stasis becomes our intellectual goal, we will improve medical practice and have a more satisfying account of gender and sex as, to paraphrase the phenomenologists, being-in-the-world.

Acknowledgements

Thanks to the members of the Pembroke Seminar on Theories of Embodiment for a wonderful year of thinking about the process of body making and for their thoughtful response to an earlier draft of this essay. Credit for the title goes to Greg Downey. Thanks also to anonymous reviewers from *Signs* for making me sharpen some of the arguments.

Notes

1 Munro Peacock et al. write: "The pathogenesis of a fragility fracture almost always involves trauma and is not necessarily associated with reduced bone mass. Thus, fragility fracture should neither be used synonymously nor interchangeably as a phenotype for osteoporosis" (2002, 303).
2 For example, sitting height reflects trunk length (vertebral height) vs. standing height, which reflects the length of the leg bones. These can change independently of one another. Thus height increases can result from changes in long bone length, vertebral height, or both. See Meredith 1978; Tanner et al. 1982; Malina, Brown, and Zavaleta 1987; Balthazart, Tlemçani, and Ball 1996; Seeman 1997.

3 The use of racial terms such as *Caucasian* and others in this article is fraught. But for the duration of this article I will use the terms as they appear in the sources I cite, leaving an analysis of this problematic terminology to future publications, e.g., Fausto-Sterling 2004.
4 Since a number of studies show no sex difference in hip fracture incidence between African American men and women, the "well-known" gender difference in bone fragility may really only be about white women. As so often happens, the word *gender* excludes women of color (Farmer et al. 1984).
5 Peacock et al. write, "Key bone phenotypes involved in fracture risk relate not only to bone mass but also to bone structure, bone loss, and possibly bone turnover" (2002, 306).
6 I am grateful to Peter Taylor for insisting that I read the work in life-course analysis.
7 Stepan 1982; Russett 1989; Hubbard 1990; Fausto-Sterling 1992.
8 I use the term *experience* rather than the term *environment* here to refer to functional activity. For more detail see Gottlieb, Whalen, and Lickliter 1998.
9 Butler 1990, 1993; Gatens 1996; Kirby 1997; Birke 1999.
10 The "rediscovery" of phenomenology and its application to gendered body image remains a fruitful arena of feminist body theory, e.g., Weiss 1999.
11 Although Thomas J. Csordas (1999) suggests that cultural phenomenological analyses transform understandings of both biology and culture, he is more concerned with how the body changes culture than vice versa. For a different anthropological point of view, see Ingold 1998.
12 Since the society receives both foundation and pharmaceutical company funding, its claim to independence requires scrutiny. The Sex and Gene Expression conferences were funded by Aventis Pharmaceuticals as well as private foundations. Industry and mainstream medical care sponsorship does not unethically direct work, but it limits the permissible ontological and epistemological approaches to the study of women's health and sex differences.
13 Perhaps because the field of archaeology is still struggling to bring gender into the fold, its practitioners often insist on the centrality of the sex/gender distinction. Yet their own conclusions undermine this dualism, precisely because they use a biological product, bone, to draw conclusions about culture and behavior (Ehrenberg 1989; Gero and Conkey 1991; Wright 1996; Armelagos 1998).
14 The validity of using bones to identify race is contested (Goodman 1997).
15 This study (cited in Melton 1988) dates from 1979, and it seems likely that subsequent cultural changes have led to different patterns of breakage; fracture incidence is a moving target.
16 Local biologies reflect local differences in biology. For example, hot flashes are far less frequent in Japan than in the United States, possibly for reasons pertaining to diet. The normalization question here is: Is it best to compare a population to its own group or some group with similar environmental and genetic histories, or to some outgroup standard?
17 These factors include: a mother having broken her hip, especially before age eighty; height at age twenty-five (taller women are more likely to break hips); extreme thinness; sedentary lifestyle; poor vision; high pulse rate; the use of certain drugs; etc.
18 One researcher states: "I think what is also of note, is that the between-center differences are greater than between-sex differences within certain centers" (Lips 1997, 95).
19 Fosamax seems to be able to prevent further bone loss in people who are losing bone and to build back lost bone at least in the hip and spine. In discussing

Merck's campaign, I do not argue that the drug is useless (in fact, I am taking it!), merely (!) that drug companies play an important role in the creation of new "disease" and profit as a result.

20 An association between the change in areal bone density and the change in fracture rates has never been documented" (Seeman 1997, 517). According to the NIH Consensus Statement Online: "Currently there is no accurate measure of overall bone strength" (2000, 5). But BMD is often used as a proxy. The National Women's Health Network cites the pitfalls of using BMD to predict future fractures (Fugh-Berman, Pearson, Allina, Zones, Worcester, Whatley, Massion, et al. 2002), but others cite a strong association between BMD and fracture rate (e.g., Melton et al. 1998; Siris et al. 2001). One overview of studies that attempted to predict osteoporosis-linked fractures with bone mineral density concluded: "Measurements of bone mineral density can predict fracture risk but cannot identify individuals who will have a fracture. We do not recommend a programme of screening menopausal women for osteoporosis by measuring bone density" (Marshall, Johnell, and Wedell 1996, 1254). See also Nelson et al. 2002.

21 For a history of the concept of osteoporosis, see Klinge 1998.

22 A secondary cause might be bone loss due to an eating disorder or a metabolic disease, or the prolonged use of a bone-leaching drug such as cortisone.

23 When I use the words *men* and *women* I refer to particular populations on which these studies were done. These are mostly Caucasian and Northern European or North American. Most of the studies have been done since the 1980s, but bone size, shape, and growth patterns would have differed at the beginning of the twentieth century compared with their appearance at the beginning of the twenty-first. I will not make these points every time I use these words.

24 So powerful is the focus on old age that the long NIH bibliography on menopause completely ignores the possible importance of pregnancy and lactation on bone development. These two processes are profoundly implicated in calcium metabolism, and if there is *no* effect on later bone strength it would be important to find out why. What physiological mechanisms protect the bone of pregnant and lactating women? This is an example of a biological question that lies fallow because of the focus on supposed estrogen deficiency in old age.

25 The bone matrix is made up primarily of a substance called hydroxyapatite that is mostly composed of crystalline forms of the molecules calcium phosphate, calcium carbonate, and small amounts of magnesium, fluoride, and sulfate.

26 One memory device for remembering which cell is which is to think that osteoBlasts Build bone and osteoClasts Chomp on bone.

27 Stress can be from direct impact or from tension placed on the bones by attached muscles. For more details on the importance of mechanical strain on bone development, see Skerry and Lanyon 1995; Mosekilde 2000; Mosley 2000.

28 In animal models it is possible to induce new bone formation (modeling) without first having caused bone resorption (Pead, Skerry, and Lanyon 1988).

29 One review states that mechanical receptors transform signals from deforming bones into changes in the shape of DNA regions that regulate the activities of genes involved in bone formation. The authors write that "bending bone ultimately bends genes" (Pavalko et al. 2003, 104).

30 Physiological functions such as heart and breathing rate and energy metabolism are regulated through involuntary nerves belonging to the sympathetic and parasympathetic nervous systems. These systems balance each other out by stimulating or inhibiting various functions. They are controlled through brain centers without our having to think about them.

31 All cells, but especially nerve and muscle cells, need calcium. So bone is essential not only for structural support but also to maintain healthy calcium levels throughout the body.
32 The active form of vitamin D is 1,25-dihydroxycholecalciferol.
33 Parathyroid hormone also increases Ca^{++} reabsorption in the kidney and absorption in the small intestine.
34 The negative effects of estrogen treatment come from the hormone's more common mode of action—stimulating gene activities after binding to the nucleus. The researchers cited have a compound that has none of the gene-activity-stimulating actions but does behave like androgens and estrogens by preventing the death of osteoblasts. See also Moggs et al. 2003.
35 Ducy et al. 2000; Flier 2002; Takeda et al. 2002; Harada and Rodan 2003.
36 Leptin may also regulate the onset of puberty, thus linking gonadal hormones and the leptin hormone system (Chehab et al. 1997).
37 I found one eloquent but wordless example on the Web in an article on causes of vitamin D deficiency. The short segment titled "Insufficient Exposure to Sunlight" was accompanied by a photograph of two women, standing in the blazing sun, covered from head to toe in burkas, clearly insufficiently exposed to sunlight but not for want of being outdoors in the sun.
38 Brief histories of these ideas as well as accounts of present-day embryology, genetics, and evolution based on systems theory may be found in Waddington 1957; Kauffman 1993; Webster and Goodwin 1996; Schlichting and Pigliucci 1998; van der Weele 1999; Oyama 2000a, 2000b.
39 The implications of these ideas for an integrative theory of the development of gender differences in behavior and psychological skills has not escaped me and is the subject of a work in progress. The explosion of knowledge about the plastic nature of brain development and an increasing understanding of neuroplasticity in adults suggests that far from being destiny, anatomy is dynamic history. A rich literature that joins mathematical models of nonlinear equations (Kelso 1995) has begun to join forces with experimental scientists who study animal behavior (Gottlieb 1997) and those who now use dynamic systems approaches to reconceptualize human behavioral development (Smith and Thelen 1993; Thelen and Smith 1994, 1998; Thelen 1995; Thelen et al. 2001).
40 Among biologists the idea that genes provide such instructions is giving way to a systems account of cell function. The metaphor of the genome (DNA) as a blueprint or set of directions for building cells and organisms is giving way to a new metaphor—genomes as parts list (Vukmirovic and Tilghmann 2000; Tyson, Csikasz-Nagy, and Novak 2002). If the genome lists only the component parts (codes for RNA and protein), the location of the assembly directions becomes uncertain: one needs to specify a cell or organism's past history and current conditions in order to predict a current developmental event accurately. Cell biologists have now turned in earnest to complexity and systems theory to help learn the rules by which organisms are assembled. (See entire December 2002 issue of *Bioessays* devoted to "Modeling Complex Biological Systems.") In another example, authors extend and twist the book metaphor: "Just as words must be assembled into sentences, paragraphs, chapters and books to make sense, vital cellular functions are performed by structured ensembles of proteins ... not by freely diffusing and occasionally colliding proteins" (Sali et al. 2003, 216).
41 I use Peter Taylor's definition of systems as "units that have clearly defined boundaries, coherent internal dynamics, and simply mediated relations with their external context" (personal communication 2003).

42 This choice of systems emerges from the data presented earlier in this article. Since this is a model, others might argue for dividing the pie in a different way. To keep the diagram readable and the discussion manageable, I have not emphasized that the entire grouping of systems is embedded in a larger system I call "general health." There are many disease states that secondarily affect bone (e.g., kidney disease or endocrine disorders) by affecting calcium metabolism or preventing exercise. The relationships among the systems affecting bone strength would be shifted in dramatic ways worthy of study in their own right under such circumstances.

43 Choice of model has profound implications. For a discussion of a lifestyle model of disease that emphasizes individual choice vs. a "social production model," see Krieger and Zierler 1995. For an update on current theories of social epidemiology, see Krieger 2001.

44 To the extent that race is a legitimate category separate from class and culture, I will incorporate it into the bone systems story in pt. 2 of this work. For a model of social pathways in childhood that lead to adult health, see Kuh and Ben-Shlomo 1997.

45 Bonjour et al. 1997; Boot et al. 1997; Perry 1997; Wang et al. 2003.

46 For the effects of dietary calcium later in life, see Heaney 2000.

References

Alcoff, Linda Martín. 2000. "Philosophy Matters: A Review of Recent Work on Feminist Philosophy." *Signs: Journal of Women in Culture and Society* 25(3): 841–82.

Aloia, J. F., A. N. Vaswani, J. K. Yeh, and E. Flaster. 1996. "Risk for Osteoporosis in Black Women." *Calcified Tissue International* 59(6):415–23.

Armelagos, George J. 1998. "Introduction: Sex, Gender and Health Status in Prehistoric and Contemporary Populations." In *Sex and Gender in Paleopathological Perspective*, ed. Anne L. Grauer and Patricia Stuart-Macadam, 1–10. Cambridge: Cambridge University Press.

Bachrach, Laura K. 2001. "Acquisition of Optimal Bone Mass in Childhood and Adolescence." *Trends in Endocrinology and Metabolism* 12(1):22–28.

Balthazart, Jacques, Omar Tlemçani, and Gregory F. Ball. 1996. "Do Sex Differences in the Brain Explain Sex Differences in Hormonal Induction of Reproductive Behavior? What 25 Years of Research on the Japanese Quail Tells Us." *Hormones and Behavior* 30(4):627–61.

Bassey, E. J., and S. J. Ramsdale. 1994. "Increase in Femoral Bone Density in Young Women Following High-Impact Exercise." *Osteoporosis International* 4:72–75.

Bassey, E. J., M. C. Rothwell, J. J. Littlewood, and D. W. Pye. 1998. "Pre- and Post-menopausal Women Have Different Bone Mineral Density Responses to the Same High-Impact Exercise." *Journal of Bone and Mineral Research* 13(12): 1805–13.

Ben-Shlomo, Yoav, and Diana Kuh. 2002. "A Life Course Approach to Chronic Disease Epidemiology: Conceptual Models, Empirical Challenges, and Interdisciplinary Perspectives." *International Journal of Epidemiology* 31(2):285–93.

Berenbaum, Sheri. 2001. "Prenatal Androgen Effects on Cognitive and Social Development." Paper presented at the Second Annual Conference on Sex and Gene Expression, March 8–11, Winston-Salem, North Carolina.

Bertalanffy, Ludwig von. 1969. *General System Theory: Foundations, Development, Applications*. New York: Braziller.
Bezkorovainy, Anatoly, and Max E. Rafelson. 1996. *Concise Biochemistry*. New York: Dekker.
Bilezikian, John P., Etah S. Kurland, and Clifford S. Rosen. 1999. "Male Skeletal Health and Osteoporosis." *Trends in Endocrinology and Metabolism* 10(6):244–50.
Birke, Lynda. 1999. *Feminism and the Biological Body*. Edinburgh: Edinburgh University Press.
Boman, U. Wide, A. Möller, and K. Albertsson-Wikland. 1998. "Psychological Aspects of Turner Syndrome." *Journal of Psychosomatic Obstetrics and Gynaecology* 19(1):1–18.
Bonjour, Jean-Phillippe, Anne-Lise Carrie, Serge Ferrari, Helen Clavien, Daniel Slosman, and Gerald Theintz. 1997. "Calcium-Enriched Foods and Bone Mass Growth in Prepubertal Girls: A Randomized, Double-Blind, Placebo-Controlled Trial." *Journal of Clinical Investigation* 99(6):1287–94.
Boot, Annemieke M., Maria A. J. de Ridder, Huibert A. P. Pols, Eric P. Krenning, and Sabine M. P. F. de Muinck Keizer-Schrama. 1997. "Bone Mineral Density in Children and Adolescents: Relation to Puberty, Calcium Intake, and Physical Activity." *Journal of Clinical Endocrinology and Metabolism* 82(1):57–62.
Boyden, Lynn M., Junhao Mao, Joseph Belsky, Lyle Mitzner, Anita Farhi, Mary A. Mitnick, Dianqing Wu, Karl Insogna, and Richard P. Lifton. 2002. "High Bone Density Due to a Mutation in LDL-Receptor-Related Protein 5." *New England Journal of Medicine* 346(20):1513–21.
Bryant, Rebecca J., Jo Cadogan, and Connie M. Weaver. 1999. "The New Dietary Reference Intakes for Calcium: Implications for Osteoporosis." *Journal of the American College of Nutrition* 18(5):S406–S412.
Butler, Judith. 1990. *Gender Trouble: Feminism and the Subversion of Identity*. New York: Routledge.
———. 1993. *Bodies That Matter: On the Discursive Limits of "Sex."* New York: Routledge.
Chehab, Farid F., Khalid Mounzih, Ronghua Lu, and Mary E. Lim. 1997. "Early Onset of Reproductive Function in Normal Female Mice Treated with Leptin." *Science* 275 (January 3): 88–90.
Csordas, Thomas J. 1990. "Embodiment as a Paradigm for Anthropology." *Ethos* 18(1):5–47.
———. 1999. "Embodiment and Cultural Phenomenology." In *Perspectives on Embodiment: The Intersections of Nature and Culture*, ed. Gail Weiss and Honi Fern Haber, 143–62. New York: Routledge.
Cummings, Steven R., Michael C. Nevitt, Warren S. Browner, Katie Stone, Kathleen M. Fox, Kristine E. Ensrud, Jane Cauley, Dennis Black, and Thomas M. Vogt. 1995. "Risk Factors for Hip Fracture in White Women." *New England Journal of Medicine* 332(12):767–73.
Currey, John D. 2002. *Bones: Structure and Mechanics*. Princeton, N.J.: Princeton University Press.
Dabbs, James McBride, and Mary Godwin Dabbs. 2001. *Heroes, Rogues, and Lovers: Testosterone and Behavior*. New York: McGraw-Hill.
Daly, Robin M., Peter A. Rich, Rudi Klein, and Shona Bass. 1999. "Effects of High-Impact Exercise on Ultrasonic and Biochemical Indices of Skeletal Status:

A Prospective Study in Young Male Gymnasts." *Journal of Bone and Mineral Research* 14(7):1222–30.

Damien, E., J. S. Price, and L. E. Lanyon. 1998. "The Estrogen Receptor's Involvement in Osteoblasts' Adaptive Response to Mechanical Strain." *Journal of Bone and Mineral Research* 13(8):1275–82.

Dawson-Hughes, Bess, Susan S. Harris, Elizabeth A. Krall, and Gerard E. Dallal. 1997. "Effect of Calcium and Vitamin D Supplementation on Bone Density in Men and Women 65 Years of Age or Older." *New England Journal of Medicine* 337 (September 4): 670–76.

Dibba, Bakary, Ann Prentice, Ann Laskey, Dot Stirling, and Tim Cole. 1999. "An Investigation of Ethnic Differences in Bone Mineral, Hip Axis Length, Calcium Metabolism and Bone Turnover between West African and Caucasian Adults Living in the United Kingdom." *Annals of Human Biology* 26(3): 229–42.

Ducy, Patricia, Michael Amling, Shu Takeda, Matthias Priemel, Arndt F. Schilling, Frank T. Beil, Jianhe Shen, Charles Vinson, Johannes M. Rueger, and Gerard Karsenty. 2000. "Leptin Inhibits Bone Formation through a Hypothalamic Relay: A Central Control of Bone Mass." *Cell* 100(2):197–207.

Ehrenberg, Margaret. 1989. *Women in Prehistory*. London: British Museum Press.

Ellison, Peter T. 1996. "Developmental Influences on Adult Ovarian Hormonal Function." *American Journal of Human Biology* 8(6):725–34.

Farmer, Mary E., Lon R. White, Jacob A. Brody, and Kent R. Bailey. 1984. "Race and Sex Differences in Hip Fracture Incidence." *American Journal of Public Health* 74(12):1374–80.

Fausto-Sterling, Anne. 1992. *Myths of Gender: Biological Theories about Women and Men*. 2d ed. New York: Basic Books.

———. 2000. *Sexing the Body: Gender Politics and the Construction of Sexuality*. New York: Basic Books.

———. 2004. "Refashioning Race: DNA and the Politics of Health Care." *differences: A Journal of Feminist Cultural Studies*. In press.

———. In preparation. "The Bare Bones of Sex: Part II—Race."

Flier, Jeffrey S. 2002. "Physiology: Is Brain Sympathetic to Bone?" *Nature* 420(6916):619, 620–22.

Friedlander, Anne L., Harry K. Genant, Steven Sadowsky, Nancy Byl, and Claus-C. Gluer. 1995. "A Two-Year Program of Aerobics and Weight Training Enhances Bone Mineral Density of Young Women." *Journal of Bone and Mineral Research* 10(4):574–85.

Frost, Harold M. 1986. *Intermediary Organization of the Skeleton*. Vols. 1 and 2. Boca Raton, Fla.: CRC Press.

———. 1992. "The Role of Changes in Mechanical Usage Set Points in the Pathogenesis of Osteoporosis." *Journal of Bone and Mineral Research* 7(3):253–61.

Fugh-Berman, Adriane, C. K. Pearson, Amy Allina, Jane Zones, Nancy Worcester, and Mariamne Whatley. 2002. "Manufacturing Need, Manufacturing 'Knowledge.'" *Network News* (May/June):1, 4.

Fugh-Berman, Adriane, C. K. Pearson, Amy Allina, Jane Zones, Nancy Worcester, Mariamne Whatley, Charlea Massion, and Ellen Michaud. 2002. "Hormone Therapy and Osteoporosis: To Prevent Fractures and Falls, There Are Better Options than Hormones." *Network News* (July/August): 4–5.

Fujita, Y., K. Katsumata, A. Unno, T. Tawa, and A. Tokita. 1999. "Factors Affecting Peak Bone Density in Japanese Women." *Calcified Tissue International* 64(2):107–11.

Gasperino, James. 1995. "Androgenic Regulation of Bone Mass in Women." *Clinical Orthopaedics and Related Research* 311:278–86.

Gatens, Moira. 1996. *Imaginary Bodies: Ethics, Power, and Corporeality*. London: Routledge.

Gero, Joan M., and Margaret W. Conkey, eds. 1991. *Engendering Archeology: Women in Prehistory*. Oxford: Blackwell.

Gilsanz, Vicente, David L. Skaggs, Arzu Kovanlikaya, James Sayre, M. Luiza Loro, Francine Kaufman, and Stanley G. Korenman. 1998. "Differential Effect of Race on the Axial and Appendicular Skeletons of Children." *Journal of Clinical Endocrinology and Metabolism* 83(5):1420–27.

Glock, Martha, Kathleen A. Shanahan, Joan A. McGowan, and compilers, eds. 2000. "Osteoporosis [Bibliography Online]: 2,449 Citations from January 1995 through December 1999." Available online at http://www.nlm.nih.gov/pubs/cbm/osteoporosis.html. Last accessed May 5, 2004.

Goodman, Alan H. 1997. "Bred in the Bone?" *Sciences* 37(2):20–25.

Gottlieb, Gilbert. 1997. *Synthesizing Nature-Nurture: Prenatal Roots of Instinctive Behavior*. Mahwah, N.J.: Erlbaum.

Gottlieb, Gilbert, Richard E. Whalen, and Robert Lickliter. 1998. "The Significance of Biology for Human Development: A Developmental Psychobiological Systems View." In *Handbook of Child Psychology*, ed. Richard M. Lerner, 233–73. New York: Wiley.

Grosz, Elizabeth. 1994. *Volatile Bodies: Toward a Corporeal Feminism*. Bloomington: Indiana University Press.

Haapasalo, Heidi, Hard Sievanen, Pekka Kannus, Ari Heinonen, Pekka Oja, and Ilkka Vuori. 1996. "Dimensions and Estimated Mechanical Characteristics of the Humerus after Long-Term Tennis Loading." *Journal of Bone and Mineral Research* 11(6):864–72.

Harada, Shun-ichi, and Gideon A. Rodan. 2003. "Control of Osteoblast Function and Regulation of Bone Mass." *Nature* 423 (May 15): 349–55.

Heaney, Robert P. 2000. "Calcium, Dairy Products, and Osteoporosis." *Journal of the American College of Nutrition* 19(2):S83–S99.

Hebb, D. O. 1949. *The Organization of Behavior: A Neuropsychological Theory*. New York: Wiley.

Hertzman, Clyde. 1999. "The Biological Embedding of Early Experience and Its Effects on Health in Adulthood." *Annals of the New York Academy of Science* 896:85–95.

Hu, J. F., X. H. Zhao, J. S. Chen, J. Fitzpatrick, B. Parpia, and T. C. Campbell. 1994. "Bone Density and Lifestyle Characteristics in Premenopausal and Postmenopausal Chinese Women." *Osteoporosis International* 4:288–97.

Hubbard, Ruth. 1990. *The Politics of Women's Biology*. New York: Routledge.

Ingold, Tim. 1998. "From Complementarity to Obviation: On Dissolving the Boundaries between Social and Biological Anthropology, Archeology and Psychology." *Zeitschrift für Ethnologie* 123(1):21–52.

Ishida, Ryota, Mitsuru Emi, Yoichi Ezura, Hironori Iwasaki, Hideyo Yoshida, Takao Suzuki, Takayuki Hosoi et al. 2003. "Association of a Haplotype (196phe/532ser) in the Interleukin-1-Receptor Associated Kinase (Iraki) Gene with Low Radial Bone Mineral Density in Two Independent Populations." *Journal of Bone and Mineral Research* 18(3):419–32.

Jones, Henry H., James D. Priest, Wilson C. Hayes, Carol Chin Tichenor, and Donald A. Nagel. 1977. "Humeral Hypertrophy in Response to Exercise." *Journal of Bone and Joint Surgery* 59-A(2):204–8.

Kauffman, Stuart. 1993. *The Origins of Order: Self-Organization and Selection in Evolution.* New York: Oxford University Press.

Keane, Helen, and Marsha Rosengarten. 2002. "On the Biology of Sexed Subjects." *Australian Feminist Studies* 17(39):261–79.

Kellie, Shirley E., and Jacob A. Brody. 1990. "Sex-Specific and Race-Specific Hip Fracture Rates." *American Journal of Public Health* 80(3):326–28.

Kelso, J. A. Scott. 1995. *Dynamic Patterns: The Self-Organization of Brain and Behavior.* Cambridge, Mass.: MIT Press.

Kirby, Vicki. 1997. *Telling Flesh: The Substance of the Corporeal.* New York: Routledge.

Klinge, Ineke. 1998. "Gender and Bones: The Production of Osteoporosis, 1941–1996." Ph.D. dissertation, University of Utrecht.

Kousteni, S., T. Bellido, L. Plotkin, C. A. O'Brien, D. L. Bodenner, L. Han, G. B. DiGregorio et al. 2001. "Nongenotropic, Sex-Nonspecific Signaling through the Estrogen or Androgen Receptors: Dissociation from Transcriptional Activity." *Cell* 104(5):719–30.

Kousteni, S., J.-R. Chen, T. Bellido, L. Han, A. A. Ali, C. A. O'Brien, L. Plotkin et al. 2002. "Reversal of Bone Loss in Mice by Nongenotropic Signaling of Sex Steroids." *Science* 298(5594):843–46.

Krieger, Nancy. 2001. "Theories for Social Epidemiology in the Twenty-First Century: An Ecosocial Perspective." *International Journal of Epidemiology* 30(4): 668–77.

———. 2003. "Genders, Sexes, and Health: What Are the Connections—Why Does It Matter?" *International Journal of Epidemiology* 32(4):652–57.

Krieger, Nancy, and Sally Zierler. 1995. "Accounting for Health of Women." *Current Issues in Public Health* 1:251–56.

Kuh, Diana, and Yoav Ben-Shlomo, eds. 1997. *A Life Course Approach to Chronic Disease Epidemiology.* Oxford: Oxford University Press.

Kuh, Diana, and Rebecca Hardy, eds. 2002. *A Life Course Approach to Women's Health.* Oxford: Oxford University Press.

Lamont, Douglas, Louise Parker, Martin White, Nigel Unwin, Stuart M. A. Bennett, Melanie Cohen, David Richardson, Heather O. Dickinson, K. G. M. M. Alberti, and Alan W. Kraft. 2000. "Risk of Cardiovascular Disease Measured by Carotid Intima-Media Thickness at Age 49–51: A Lifecourse Study." *British Medical Journal* 320 (January 29): 273–78.

Larsen, Clark Spencer. 1998. "Gender, Health, and Activity in Foragers and Farmers in the American Southeast: Implications for Social Organization in the Georgia Bight." In *Sex and Gender in Paleopathological Perspective,* ed. Anne L. Grauer and Patricia Stuart-Macadam, 165–87. Cambridge: Cambridge University Press.

Lee, Karla, Helen Jessop, Rosemary Suswillo, Gul Zaman, and Lance E. Lanyon. 2003. "Bone Adaptation Requires Oestrogen Receptor-Alpha." *Nature* 424 (6947):389.

Lips, Paul. 1997. "Epidemiology and Predictors of Fractures Associated with Osteoporosis." *American Journal of Medicine* 103(2A):S3–S11.

Little, Randall D., John P. Carulli, Richard G. Del Mastro, Josée Dupuis, Mark Osborne, Colleen Folz, Susan P. Manning et al. 2002. "A Mutation in the LDL Receptor-Related Protein 5 Gene Results in the Autosomal Dominant High-Bone-Mass Trait." *American Journal of Human Genetics* 70(1):11–19.

Lock, Margaret. 1998. "Anomalous Ageing: Managing the Postmenopausal Body." *Body and Society* 4(1):35–61.

Malina, Robert M., Kathryn H. Brown, and Antonio N. Zavaleta. 1987. "Relative Lower Extremity Length in Mexican American and in American Black and White Youth." *American Journal of Physical Anthropology* 72:89–94.

Marshall, Deborah, Olof Johnell, and Hans Wedel. 1996. "Meta-analysis of How Well Measures of Bone Mineral Density Predict Occurrence of Osteoporotic Fractures." *British Medical Journal* 312(7041):1254–59.

Martin, Biddy. 1997. "Success and Its Failures." *differences: A Journal of Feminist Cultural Studies* 9(3):102–31.

McKay, H. A., M. A. Petit, K. M. Khan, and R. W. Schutz. 2000. "Lifestyle Determinants of Bone Mineral: A Comparison between Prepubertal Asian- and Caucasian-Canadian Boys and Girls." *Calcified Tissue International* 66(5): 320–24.

Melton, L. Joseph, III. 1988. "Epidemiology of Fractures." In *Osteoporosis: Etiology, Diagnosis, and Management*, ed. B. Lawrence Riggs and L. Joseph Melton, III, 133–54. New York: Raven.

Melton, L. Joseph, III, Elizabeth J. Atkinson, Michael K. O'Connor, W. Michael O'Fallon, and B. Lawrence Riggs. 1998. "Bone Density and Fracture Risk in Men." *Journal of Bone and Mineral Research* 13(12):1915–23.

Meredith, Howard V. 1978. "Secular Change in Sitting Height and Lower Limb Height of Children, Youths, and Young Adults of Afro-Black, European, and Japanese Ancestry." *Growth* 42(1):37–41.

Merleau-Ponty, Maurice. 1962. *Phenomenology of Perception*. Trans. Colin Smith. New York: Humanities Press.

Messier, Stephen P., Todd D. Royer, Timothy E. Craven, Mary L. O'Toole, Robert Burns, and Walter H. Ettinger. 2000. "Long-Term Exercise and Its Effects on Balance in Older, Osteoarthritic Adults: Results from Fitness, Arthritis, and Seniors Trial (Fast)." *Journal of the American Geriatrics Society* 48(2):131–38.

Meunier, Pierre J. 1988. "Assessment of Bone Turnover by Histormorphometry." In *Osteoporosis: Etiology, Diagnosis, and Management*, ed. B. Lawrence Riggs and L. Joseph Melton III, 317–32. New York: Raven.

Moggs, Jonathan G., Damian G. Deavall, and George Orphanides. 2003. "Sex Steroids, Angels, and Osteoporosis." *BioEssays* 25(3):195–99.

Molleson, Theya. 1994. "The Eloquent Bones of Abu Hureyra." *Scientific American* 2:70–75.

Morel, J., B. Combe, J. Fracisco, and J. Bernard. 2001. "Bone Mineral Density of 704 Amateur Sportsmen Involved in Different Physical Activities." *Osteoporosis International* 12(2):152–57.

Mosekilde, Lis. 2000. "Age-Related Changes in Bone Mass, Structure, and Strength—Effects of Loading." *Zeitschrift für Rheumatologie* 59 (Supplement 1): I/1–I/9.

Mosley, John R. 2000. "Osteoporosis and Bone Functional Adaptation: Mechano-biological Regulation of Bone Architecture in Growing and Adult Bone." *Journal of Rehabilitation Research and Development* 37(2):189–200.

Muñoz, M. T., and J. Argente. 2002. "Anorexia Nervosa in Female Adolescents: Endocrine and Bone Mineral Density Disturbances." *European Journal of Endocrinology* 147(3):275–86.

Nelson, Heidi D., Mark Helfand, Steven H. Woolf, and Janet D. Allan. 2002. "Screening for Postmenopausal Osteoporosis: A Review of the Evidence for the U.S. Preventive Services Task Force." *Annals of Internal Medicine* 137(6):529–41.

NIH Consensus Statement Online. 2000. 17(1):1–36.

Nordstrom, P., K. Thorsen, E. Bergstrom, and R. Lorentzon. 1996. "High Bone Mass and Altered Relationships between Bone Mass, Muscle Strength, and Body Constitution in Adolescent Boys on a High Level of Physical Activity." *Bone* 19(2):189–95.

Nordstrom, P., G. Nordstrom, and R. Lorentzon. 1997. "Correlation of Bone Density to Strength and Physical Activity in Young Men with a Low or Moderate Level of Physical Activity." *Calcified Tissue International* 60(4):332–37.

Oyama, Susan. 2000a. *Evolution's Eye: A System's View of the Biology-Culture Divide.* Durham, N.C.: Duke University Press.

———. 2000b. *The Ontogeny of Information: Developmental Systems and Evolution.* Durham, N.C.: Duke University Press.

Parfitt, A. M. 1988. "Bone Remodeling: Relationship to the Amount and Structure of Bone, and the Pathogenesis and Prevention of Fractures." In *Osteoporosis: Etiology, Diagnosis, and Management*, ed. B. Lawrence Riggs and L. Joseph Melton, III, 45–93. New York: Raven.

Pavalko, Fred M., Suzanne M. Norvell, David B. Burr, Charles H. Turner, Randall L. Duncan, and Joseph P. Bidwell. 2003. "A Model for Mechanotransduction in Bone Cells: The Load-Bearing Mechanosomes." *Journal of Cellular Biochemistry* 88(1):104–12.

Peacock, Munro, Charles H. Turner, Michael J. Econs, and Tatiana Foroud. 2002. "Genetics of Osteoporosis." *Endocrine Reviews* 23(3):303–26.

Pead, Matthew J., Timothy M. Skerry, and Lance E. Lanyon. 1988. "Direct Transformation from Quiesence to Bone Formation in the Adult Periosteum Following a Single Brief Period of Bone Loading." *Journal of Bone and Mineral Research* 3(6):647–56.

Pearson, G. A. 1996. "Of Sex and Gender." *Science* 274(5286):324–29.

Perry, Ivan J. 1997. "Fetal Growth and Development: The Role of Nutrition and Other Factors." In Kuh and Ben-Shlomo 1997, 145–68.

Petersen, Alan. 1998. "Sexing the Body: Representations of Sex Differences in *Gray's Anatomy*, 1858 to the Present." *Body and Society* 4(1):1–15.

Pettersson, U., H. Alfredson, P. Nordstrom, K. Henriksson-Larsen, and R. Lorentzon. 2000. "Bone Mass in Female Cross-Country Skiers: Relationship between Muscle Strength and Different BMD Sites." *Calcified Tissue International* 67(3):199–206.

Rizzoli, R., and J.-P. Bonjour. 1999. "Determinants of Peak Bone Mass and Mechanisms of Bone Loss." *Osteoporosis International 9* (Supplement 2): S17–S23.

Robinson, T. L., C. Snow-Harter, D. R. Taaffe, D. Gillis, J. Shaw, and R. Marcus. 1995. "Gymnasts Exhibit Higher Bone Mass than Runners despite Similar Prevalence of Amenorrhea and Oligomenorrhea." *Journal of Bone and Mineral Research* 10(1):26–35.

Roush, Wade. 1995. "'Fat Hormone' Poses Hefty Problem for Journal Embargo." *Science* 269 (August 4): 672.

Rubin, Gayle. 1975. "The Traffic in Women: Notes on the 'Political Economy' of Sex." In *Toward an Anthropology of Women*, ed. Rayna R. Reiter, 157–210. New York: Monthly Review Press.

Russett, Cynthia Eagle. 1989. *Sexual Science: The Victorian Construction of Womanhood*. Cambridge, Mass.: Harvard University Press.

Sali, Andrej, Robert Glaeser, Thomas Earnest, and Wolfgang Baumeister. 2003. "From Words to Literature in Structural Proteins." *Nature* 422(6928):216–55.

Schacter, Beth. 2001 "About the Society for Women's Health Research." Proceedings from the Second Annual Conference on Sex and Gene Expression, March 8–11. Winston-Salem, North Carolina.

Schlichting, Carl D., and Massimo Pigliucci. 1998. *Phenotypic Evolution: A Reaction Norm Perspective*. Sunderland, Mass.: Sinauer Associates.

Schriempf, Alexa. 2001. "(Re)fusing the Amputated Body: An Interactionist Bridge for Feminism and Disability." *Hypatia* 16(4):53–79.

Seeman, E. 1997. "Perspective: From Density to Structure: Growing Up and Growing Old on the Surfaces of Bone." *Journal of Bone and Mineral Research* 12(4):509–21.

———. 1998. "Editorial: Growth in Bone Mass and Size—Are Racial and Gender Differences in Bone Mineral Density More Apparent than Real?" *Journal of Clinical Endocrinology and Metabolism* 83(5):1414–19.

———. 1999. "The Structural Basis of Bone Fragility in Men." *Bone* 25(1):143–17.

Siebers, Tobin. 2001. "Disability in Theory: From Social Constructionism to the New Realism of the Body." *American Literary History* 13(4):737–54.

Siris, Ethel S., Paul D. Miller, Elizabeth Barrett-Connor, Kenneth G. Faulkner, Lois E. Wehren, Thomas A. Abbott, Marc L. Berger, Arthur C. Santora, and Louis M. Sherwood. 2001. "Identification and Fracture Outcomes of Undiagnosed Low Bone Mineral Density in Postmenopausal Women: Results from the National Osteoporosis Risk Assessment." *Journal of the American Medical Association* 286(22):2815–22.

Skerry, Tim. 2000. "Biomechanical Influences on Skeletal Growth and Development." In *Development, Growth, and Evolution: Implications for the Study of the Hominid Skeleton*, ed. Paul O'Higgins and Martin J. Cohn, 29–39. London: Academic Press.

Skerry, Tim, and Lance E. Lanyon. 1995. "Interruption of Disuse by Short Duration Walking Exercise Does Not Prevent Bone Loss in the Sheep Calcaneus." *Bone* 16(2):269–74.

Smith, Linda B., and Esther Thelen, eds. 1993. *A Dynamic Systems Approach to Development: Applications*. Cambridge, Mass.: MIT Press.

Snow-Harter, Christine, Mary L. Bouxsein, Barbara Lewis, Dennis Carter, and Robert Marcus. 1992. "Effects of Resistance and Endurance Exercise on Bone Mineral Status of Young Women: A Randomized Exercise Intervention Trial." *Journal of Bone and Mineral Research* 7(7):761–69.

Soderman, K., E. Bergstrom, R. Lorentzon, and H. Alfredson. 2000. "Bone Mass and Muscle Strength in Young Female Soccer Players." *Calcified Tissue International* 67(4):297–303.

Sowers, Maryfran. 1996. "Pregnancy and Lactation as Risk Factors for Subsequent Bone Loss and Osteoporosis." *Journal of Bone and Mineral Research* 11(8):1052–60.

Stepan, Nancy. 1982. *The Idea of Race in Science: Great Britain, 1800–1960*. London: Macmillan.
Taha, Wael, Daisy Chin, Arnold Silverberg, Larisa Lashiker, Naila Khateeb, and Henry Anhalt. 2001. "Reduced Spinal Bone Mineral Density in Adolescents of an Ultra-Orthodox Jewish Community in Brooklyn." *Pediatrics* 107(5):e79–e85.
Takeda, Shu, Florent Elefteriou, Regis Levasseur, Xiuyun Liu, Liping Zhao, Keith L. Parker, Dawna Armstrong, Patricia Ducy, and Gerard Karsenty. 2002. "Leptin Regulates Bone Formation via the Sympathetic Nervous System." *Cell* 111(3): 305–17.
Tanner, J. M., T. Hayashi, M. A. Preece, and N. Cameron. 1982. "Increase in Length of Leg Relative to Trunk in Japanese Children and Adults from 1957 to 1977: Comparison with British and Japanese Children." *Annals of Human Biology* 9(5):411–23.
Tanouye, Elyse. 1995. "Merck's Osteoporosis Warnings Pave the Way for Its New Drug." *Wall Street Journal*, June 28, B1, B4.
Thelen, Esther. 1995. "Motor Development: A New Synthesis." *American Psychologist* 50(2):79–95.
Thelen, Esther, Gregor Schöner, Christian Scheier, and Linda B. Smith. 2001. "The Dynamics of Embodiment: A Field Theory of Infant Perseverative Reaching." *Behavioral and Brain Sciences* 24(1):1–86.
Thelen, Esther, and Linda B. Smith. 1994. *A Dynamic Systems Approach to the Development of Cognition and Action*. Cambridge, Mass.: MIT Press.
———. 1998. "Dynamic Systems Theories." In *Handbook of Child Psychology: Theoretical Models of Human Development*, ed. Richard M. Lerner, 563–634. New York: Wiley.
Thomas, Mark G., Tudor Parfitt, Deborah A. Weiss, Karl Skorecki, James F. Wilson, Magdel le Roux, Neil Bradman, and David B. Goldstein. 2000. "Y Chromosomes Traveling South: The Cohen Modal Haplotype and the Origins of the Lemba—the 'Black Jews of Southern Africa.'" *American Journal of Human Genetics* 66(2):674–86.
Thornhill, Randy, and Craig T. Palmer. 2001. *A Natural History of Rape*. Cambridge, Mass.: MIT Press.
Travis, Cheryl Brown, ed. 2003. *Evolution, Gender, and Rape*. Cambridge, Mass.: MIT Press.
Tyson, John J., Attila Csikasz-Nagy, and Bela Novak. 2002. "The Dynamics of Cell Cycle Regulation." *BioEssays* 24:(12):1095–1109.
Van der Weele, Cor. 1999. *Images of Development: Environmental Causes of Ontogeny*. Albany: State University of New York Press.
Verbrugge, Martha H. 1997. "Recreating the Body: Women's Physical Education and the Science of Sex Differences in America, 1900–1940." *Bulletin of the History of Medicine* 71(2):273–304.
Vukmirovic, Ognenka Gog, and Shirley M. Tilghmann. 2000. "Exploring Genome Space." *Nature* 405(6793):820–22.
Waddington, C. H. 1957. *The Strategy of the Genes: A Discussion of Some Aspects of Theoretical Biology*. London: Allen & Unwin.
Walsh, Timothy B., and Michael J. Devlin. 1998. "Eating Disorders: Progress and Problems." *Science* 280(5638):1387–90.

Wang, May-Choo, Patricia B. Crawford, Mark Hudes, Marta Van Loan, Kirstin Siemering, and Laura K. Bachrach. 2003. "Diet in Midpuberty and Sedentary Activity in Prepuberty Predict Peak Bone Mass." *American Journal of Clinical Nutrition* 77(2):495–503.

Webster, Gerry, and Brian Goodwin. 1996. *Form and Transformation: Generative and Relational Principles in Biology*. Cambridge: Cambridge University Press.

Weiss, Gail. 1999. *Body Images: Embodiment as Intercorporeality*. New York: Routledge.

Welton, D. C., H. C. G. Kemper, G. B. Post, W. Van Mechelen, J. Twisk, P. Lips, and G. J. Teule. 1994. "Weight-Bearing Activity during Youth Is a More Important Factor for Peak Bone Mass than Calcium Intake." *Journal of Bone and Mineral Research* 9(7):1089–96.

Whitehead, Alfred North. (1929) 1978. *Process and Reality: An Essay in Cosmology*. New York: Macmillan.

Williams, Gareth, and Helen Busby. 2000. "The Politics of 'Disabled' Bodies." In *Health, Medicine and Society: Key Theories, Future Agendas*, ed. Simon J. Williams, Jonathan Gabe, and Michael Calnan, 169–85. London: Routledge.

Williams, Simon J., and Gilliam Bendelow. 1998. *The Lived Body: Sociological Themes, Embodied Issues*. London: Routledge.

Wilson, Elizabeth, 1998. *Neural Geographies: Feminism and the Microstructure of Cognition*. New York: Routledge.

———. 1999. "Introduction: Somatic Compliance—Feminism, Biology, and Science." *Australian Feminist Studies* 14(29):7–18.

Wizemann, Theresa M., and Mary-Lou Pardue, eds. 2001. *Exploring the Biological Contributions to Human Health: Does Sex Matter?* Washington, D.C.: National Academy Press.

Worthman, Carol M. 2002. "Endocrine Pathways in Differential Well-Being across the Life Course." In Kuh and Hardy 2002, 197–216.

Wright, Rita P., ed. 1996. *Gender and Archeology*. Philadelphia: University of Pennsylvania Press.

Zanchetta, J. R., H. Plotkin, and M. L. Alvarez Filgueira. 1995. "Bone Mass in Children: Normative Values for the 2–20-Year-Old Population." *Bone* 16 (Supplement 4): S393–S399.

Zelzer, Elazar, and Bjorn R. Olsen. 2003. "The Genetic Basis for Skeletal Diseases." *Nature* 423(6937):343–48.

Zuk, Marlene. 2002. *Sexual Selections: What We Can and Can't Learn about Sex from Animals*. Berkeley: University of California Press.

5

BODIES, HEALTH, GENDER— BRIDGING FEMINIST THEORIES AND WOMEN'S HEALTH

Ellen Kuhlmann and Birgit Babitsch

Source: *Women's Studies International Forum*, 25:4 (2002), 433–42.

Synopsis

In this article, we discuss body concepts in recent feminist theories and women's health research. We argue that a dissociation process has occurred between women's and gender studies, on the one hand, and research and activism on women's health issues, on the other. These findings are chosen as a starting point for considering the material body. In a comparative approach we sketch statements on the body in the works of Judith Butler, Donna Haraway, and Elisabeth Grosz followed by summaries of developments within key areas of women's health research. The article argues that no single perspective offers completely satisfying answers to the issues of the materiality of the sexed body and the processes of health and illness. We propose the bridging of divergent perspectives to bring the material body back into feminist theory and to further new concepts that take the living and changing body into account.
© 2002 Elsevier Science Ltd. All rights reserved.

Introduction

Postmodern theories raise new questions about the body. Traditional certainties about the relationship between nature and culture and their contingent variations are being supplanted by far-reaching uncertainties about the nature of the body. These uncertainties touch on a sore point within feminist theorizing. The body and embodiment were once seen as stable points of reference within feminism and as promising counter-concepts to a Cartesian mind–body model. Now, the search for common points of reference in recent feminist theorizing has proven to be much more complex. The body has become a zone of uncertainty and thus, the category of *sex/gender* must also be re-negotiated. Furthermore, the fact that the reference system body/gender has been called into question has furthered the drifting apart of women's and gender studies, on the one hand, and research and activism on women's health issues, on the other. The women's health movement of the 1970s and early 1980s is generally considered to have had significant influence on the direction taken by feminist theorizing (see Dresser, 1996; Gordon & Thorne, 1996, p. 323; for a retrospective critique, see Bell, 1994; Marshall, 1996). Such an influence can no longer be readily demonstrated for recent women's health research and policy-making. To date, this development has not been discussed from either perspective. Instead, representatives of each field have tended to ignore the concepts and empirical results of the other (see the contributions in Price & Shildrick, 1999).

This dissociation process has also been due to the differentiation of feminist theory and the establishment of women's health research as an academic field with several locations in the academy—especially within public health research, medical sociology and applied social science. This gap has also been widened by difficulties in transferring research results to praxis and the general lack of links between the levels of policy-making and service delivery and women's health research, due very often to time constraints and deficits in practical knowledge on the part of academic women.

In our opinion, however, this dissociation also points to fundamental problems with the materialization of the (sexual) body. In recent years, this topic has been the focus of an elaborate discourse on the issue of the sex/gender difference. In particular, the now extensive debates about the work of Judith Butler (1990, 1993) have sharpened the controversy. Until now, however, all attempts to reduce the anatomically differentiated body to a cultural construction have produced unsatisfying results. Although the "ontological leftovers" of body and gender elicit feelings of unease, it would be impossible to begin to think about the questions raised by health and illness, reproduction, bodily perceptions, and knowledge of bodies without these "leftovers." Women's health research has not entered these debates to date but has instead, in a sense, undermined these controversies by concentrating on the empirical connections between health, gender, and socio-cultural influences. This strategy, however, bears a significant risk of promoting latent biologism which can enter the research process unrecognized. Linda Birke shows that "the ghost of biology still haunts us" (Birke, 1999a, p. 42). But, she argues, "ignoring or omitting the biological body does not help; indeed, it merely serves indirectly to reinforce biological determinism" (Birke, 1999b, p. 175).

In this article, our starting point will be the divergent developments in dealing with the body within recent feminist theories, on the one hand, and women's health research, on the other. We will attempt to elucidate the theoretical implications which are implicit in these two perspectives. What are the implications of recent feminist body discourse for women's health research, a field with a twofold obligation to the categories of body and gender? Do health-related concepts and empirical studies of women's health research harbor an explanatory potential which might be of value for furthering feminist theorizing about the body?

In attempting to crystallize two divergent developmental directions from the plethora of recent, western-located feminist theories (e.g., Benhabib, Butler, Cornel, & Fraser, 1995; Haraway, 1997) and the broad spectrum of women's health research (e.g., Doyal, 2000; Mahowald, 2000; Pollard & Hyatt, 1999), we are, of course, aware of how problematic such a reduction is. But we view such a comparative approach to questions of the body's materiality as a useful attempt to focus on the blind spots, the potential, and the limits of each perspective on the body and gender. We aim to sound out the possible amplifying effects of the various feminist perspectives without allowing one explanatory model to "swallow up" the other and without advocating an arbitrary link. We cannot and do not intend to present the entire spectrum of research but have instead chosen certain works with the aim of marking diverse approaches. We would like to introduce new aspects into a sometimes static debate, in which there is a seemingly uncompromising and irreconcilable confrontation between those who enthusiastically welcome the dismantling of boundaries between nature and culture, between the artificial and the organic, and those who worry about the "disembodiment" of women.

We will begin by briefly sketching the main statements on the body in the works of Judith Butler (1990, 1993), Donna Haraway (1991, 1997), and Elisabeth Grosz (1994). We have chosen these three authors because they place the body at the center of their analysis and because they have initiated influential debates in western-related feminist theory. Furthermore and this point is decisive—although their theoretical proposals differ, their work shares the common goal of attempting to overcome essentialist concepts of the body, dualism and binaries. It is this common aim which leads us to believe that the work of these three scholars will prove more fruitful for women's health research than that of other authors, who base their thinking on a fixed and ahistorical concept of sex difference, however they may define it (e.g., Greer, 1999). In our opinion, the question of how corporeality can be brought back into the debate without biological reductionism is decisive for women's health research. Nonetheless, our choice of authors and discussion of these issues should be understood as an example and not as an exhaustive treatment of the possible links between feminist theories and women's health issues.

These sections will be followed by brief summaries of developments within two areas of women's health research: health behavior and links between health and social situation. These areas were the focus of research in the early days of women's health research (e.g., Ehrenreich & English, 1974; Lewin & Oleson, 1985; Schneider, 1981; Waldron, 1980) and have undergone interesting developments in the meantime. We deal with these issues from our situated perspective as German feminist health researchers (e.g., Babitsch, 1997, 2000; Kuhlmann, 1997, in press) and take several examples from this field. Finally, we will discuss questions for further study and possible explanatory models which come into play when each area of work is open to reflecting on the others' work.

The body as text—performative acts

Judith Butler has most radically questioned the boundaries drawn between biological sex and gender as socially constructed sex. Working within an analytical framework based on Foucault and discourse theory, Butler rejects the search for the origins of gender identity. She views "the boundary and surface of bodies as politically constructed" in order "to denaturalize and resignify bodily categories" (Butler, 1990, p. X). She sees performances and subversive actions as strategies for deconstructing the categories of body and gender which produce multiplicity beyond the binary framework. "Gender ought not to be conceived as the cultural inscription of meaning on a given sex (a juridical conception); gender must also designate the very apparatus of production whereby the sexes themselves are established. (. . .) gender is also the discursive/cultural means by which 'sexed nature' or a 'natural sex' is produced and established as 'prediscursive,' prior to culture, a politically neutral surface *on which* culture acts" (Butler, 1990, p. 7, italics in the original). The body, according to Butler, is always interpreted through cultural meanings and, therefore, anatomy is also defined as gender identity. In Butler's view, "'the body' is itself a construction, as are the myriad 'bodies' that constitute the domain of gendered subjects. Bodies cannot be said to have a signifiable existence prior to the mark of their gender; the question then emerges: To what extent does the body *come into being* in and through the mark(s) of gender?" (Butler, 1990, p. 8, italics in the original). Butler sees "the construal of 'sex' no longer as a bodily given on which the construct of gender is artificially imposed, but as a cultural norm which governs the materialization of bodies" (Butler, 1993, pp. 2–3).

Her call for "denaturalizing critique, critique that reveals the contingent, performatively constructed character of what passes for necessary and unalterable" (Fraser, 1995, p. 161) inspires others to take a critical look at supposed certainties about the body and the sexes. But in the final analysis, Butler reduces bodies to language and discourse. Here, the work of authors who have emphasized the complexity, ambivalence, and transience of concepts of nature, culture, and gender (e.g., MacCormack & Strathern, 1980) offer new insights. Ludmilla Jordanova, for example, has used historical material to show that "since the eighteenth century the polarities seem to have hardened, yet the lived experience to which they supposedly relate was extremely complex" (Jordanova, 1999, p. 157). According to her work "different parts of the body were emphasized at different periods, and from different points of view," and "the association of women with nature had a positive and a negative side" (Jordanova, 1999, pp. 162–163). Emily Martin's empirical studies (1987, 1994) have revealed the complexity of the links between the lived body, social position, and cultural inscriptions. Martin describes the multitude of possible ways in which women can respond in their daily lives to the scientific metaphors of medicine about their bodies and how these responses are related to the specific life situation of each woman shaped by class, ethnic background and other factors (Martin, 1987). In her study of the immune system, Martin shows how medicine's interpretive patterns change and how these interpretations are integrated into individual perceptions in daily life. They serve to structure bodies, organizations, and society in similar ways and in doing so again have an influence on bodies (Martin, 1994).

Seen from the perspective of this work, the critique of "disembodiment"— or formulated more moderately: the denial of the reality of bodies—as characteristic of recent feminist theories is fed by Butler's theories, but this critique falls short. In fact, Butler pursues a dualistic ontology in which—and this is perhaps the new element in her argument—the "mind" no longer dominates the body, but instead the body is reduced to cultural practices. In other words, Butler radicalizes the supremacy of the mind which is found throughout Western tradition. Touching, feeling, perceiving and having specific bodily knowledge have no autonomous place in her theoretical schemes.

Hybrid bodies—cyborg visions

Donna Haraway (1991) presents an epistemological concept of "situated knowledge," which adheres to the embodiment and partiality of all knowledge. Her model is characterized by the linkage of materialistic theorems with the perspectives of discourse theory and cultural theory. Haraway assumes that the body, gender, and nature have a non-discursive basis. She views the body as "made," but also as an active epistemological object. The body is "anything but a blank page for social inscriptions, including those of biological discourse. (. . .) The *body*, the object of biological discourse, itself becomes a most engaging being" (Haraway, 1991, pp. 197–199, italics in the original). It is an agent and not a resource; bodies as objects of knowledge are "material–semiotic generative nodes. Their *boundaries* materialize in social interaction. Boundaries are drawn by mapping practices; 'objects' do not preexist as such. Objects are boundary projects" (Haraway, 1991, p. 200f, italics in the original).

The aim is to break open an ongoing naturalizing discourse which "continues to justify 'social' orders in terms of 'natural' legitimations" (Haraway, 1997, p. 108). The metaphor of vision is present as an alternative to a polarizing understanding of nature/culture, mind/body, sex/gender, etc. The latter attempts to conceal its own position, its own claims to power, behind universalism and relativism and thus attempts to deny responsibility. Haraway would like to "insist on the embodied nature of all vision, and so reclaim the sensory system that has been used to signify a leap out of the marked body into a conquering gaze from nowhere. (. . .) This gaze signifies the unmarked positions of Man and White" (Haraway, 1991, p. 188).

Haraway contrasts these unmarked positions by positing a feminist objectivity which is not based on transcendence and the subject/object divide. She questions both the human/animal delimitation and the distinction between machine and organism. To date, she is the most radical proponent of the dissolution of the boundaries between nature and technology, based on the figure of the cyborg, a creature with a hybrid body which cannot be described with the usual polarized categories (Haraway, 1997). Haraway welcomes this dissolution of borders as an opportunity to pull the legitimatory rug out from under naturalizing discourses. If one follows her argument, then making boundaries disappear can lead to a deconstruction of gender dualism and help overcome hierarchies. But her call for dissolving the borders between humans/animals/machine also conjures up significant ethical risks. Haraway is unable to define criteria for ethically responsible action or provide normative points of reference. She is also unable to determine the social position of the body within power relations. Her suggestions open up "if brought to their radical conclusion, the gates for the total manipulation of human and non-human nature" (Kollek, 1996, p. 150; see also Birke, 1999b). Thus, we must face the question of what price we are willing to pay in exchange for the delimitation of naturalized categories.

Volatile bodies—the call for an "embodied" feminism

Elisabeth Grosz (1994) sets the materiality of bodies at center stage, but soundly rejects essentialist interpretations. She criticizes the fact that feminist theories distance themselves from the body and aims, in contrast, to describe the body "so that it can now be understood as the very 'stuff of subjectivity'" (Grosz, 1994, p. ix). According to Grosz, focusing on the body is advantageous for feminist concerns, since it unavoidably leads to the question of sexual difference. The body must be seen as capable of doing much more than culture allows. "Being a body is something that we must come to accommodate psychically, something that we must live" (Grosz, 1994, p. xiii). The human body is able "to transform or rewrite its environment, to continually augment its powers and capacities through the incorporation into the body's own spaces and modalities of objects that, while external, are internalized, added to, supplemented by the 'organic body'" (Grosz, 1994, p. 188). In her model, the levels of the psyche/the social, body/mind, subject/object enter into multi-layered links, they neither oppose one another nor do they form hierarchies. "It is not enough to reformulate the body in non-dualist and non-essentialist terms. It must also be reconceived in specifically *sexed* terms" (Grosz, 1995, p. 84, italics in the original).

Grosz counters the visions of liberation from materiality and the limitations of bodies with a body concept which can be thought as material, but nonetheless flowing: "the metaphoric of flow is simply one among a number of ways in which sexual difference may be thought" (Grosz, 1994, p. xiii). For Grosz, sexual difference is to be understood as the horizon that "is implied in the very possibility of an entity, an identity, a subject, an other and their relations" (Grosz, 1994, p. 209). She emphasizes conceiving of the body in "terms that may grant women the capacity for independence and autonomy, which thus far have been attributed only to men" (Grosz, 1994, p. xiii).

Grosz offers positive points of reference for female sexual difference which are located directly within bodies. In her opinion, this opens up an opportunity for confronting hegemonical male interpretations with an autonomous, independent female bodily existence. But as Marie-Louise Angerer (1999, p. 67) has pointed out, Grosz, like Butler, bases her concept on the assumption that the categorization of bodies according to gender is not unequivocal and requires permanent confirmation and repetition. Grosz' proposals leave a number of questions unanswered: although she avoids essentialist arguments, she does not offer a satisfying differentiation of universal categories. By focusing on *the* bodies, she distracts from the differences which characterize these bodies and the historical conditions of their process of "becoming"—for black, white, old, young, healthy, ill bodies, and their various intermediates. Perhaps due to the lack of a perspective which adequately reflects processes in society, the author utilizes an undifferentiated concept of autonomy, one which does not encompass historical and situative elements.

Performance, cyborgs and flow—what do they offer to women's health research?

The work briefly summarized here radically questions the stability of bodies and sex and sketches new models for the links between nature and culture as the central metaphors of dichotomy and binary thinking. Butler views "the body" as a construction and "sex" as a cultural norm; both can be changed by performance and subversive actions. In Haraway's view, in contrast, the body is "made" *and* active, an agent and not a resource. Haraway rejects any kind of drawing of borders based on supposedly "natural" traits and instead presents the figure of the cyborg, as a hybrid entity. Grosz emphasizes sexual difference and the body as the "stuff' of subjectivity. Working from a psychoanalytical perspective, she challenges static and hierarchical concepts with the metaphoric of flow and multilayered connections between subject and object, which are never fixed or solid. Taken together, these proposals offer important insights for women's health research; they are especially useful for critically analyzing scientific "facts" about bodies, health, and gender and enable us "to re-think the traditional claims of medical practice to cure and care" (Shildrick & Price, 1999, p. 8). Various feminist scholars have analyzed the social processes through which medical knowledge is constructed and have shown how this knowledge dominates the practice of health care and leads to the devaluation of women and the neglect of their health care needs (e.g., Birke, 1999b: Hubbard & Wald, 1993; Spanier, 1995).

But beyond this, the usefulness of feminist theoretical debates for women's health has been limited. Feminist theorists relate their work to the issues and results of women's health research either marginally or not at all. Butler shows no interest in questions of health; Haraway and Grosz do take up health and medical issues but do not relate them to women's health research. In some work on women's health issues, the theoretical concepts of these two authors are discussed (e.g., Bell, 1994; Birke, 2000). Conceptualizing the body as transformable and transforming offers new opportunities for understanding the links between factors "outside" and "inside" the body.

Thus, the dissociation process which we described above has not proceeded symmetrically. Scholars in the area of women's health research have been more active in searching for common ground than feminist theorists. However, most authors remain skeptical about suggestions of hybridization (e.g., Birke, 1999b; Davis-Floyd, 1998; Kollek, 2000). A central "fault line" seems to be the issue of whether the body is recognized as possessing its own materiality, beyond cultural inscriptions and social process of production. This issue ties into the question of whether or not and how processes occurring within the body can be measured and analyzed. A further fundamental problem is the fact that neither Haraway nor Grosz have developed a conceptual approach to the realm of subjective experience. In a study on cosmetic surgery, Kathy Davis (1997) has presented an impressive portrayal of the ambivalence and tensions between subjective perception and women's needs and social judgement. In general, however, it is still impossible to predict what the consequences of transformation and hybridization between and within bodies will be for the health of different women with different social and cultural backgrounds. We can only expect reliable answers to such questions from empirical studies.

In summary, our answer to the question of what feminist theories have to offer for women's health research is as follows: for some questions, feminist theories can produce important new insights, but they fall short of telling the bigger story which must be grasped in order to gain a deeper understanding of women's health issues.

The sexual body in health research

Women's health research confronts the interpretative power of biomedical discourse and biomedical structures with a complex understanding of health and experienced-based competence in dealing with health and illness. Researchers in this field (e.g., Doyal, 2000; Macintyre, Hunt, & Sweeting, 1996) emphasize the significance of the conditions of social life and clearly reject biomedicine's fixation on individual risks and behavior as the main factors influencing health and illness. This perspective is based on an empirical, praxis-oriented concept which questions the naturalization of health and illness and instead highlights social and cultural factors. A large number of very different studies have demonstrated the usefulness of these approaches, as will be shown below.

Within this spectrum, an important area of work focuses on individual health-related behavior. Health behavior is conceptualized as social behavior expressed through the body, which plays out or questions the social order of the sexes and interpretations of "femininity" and "masculinity" (see Saltonstall, 1993; Stein-Hilbers, 1995). Robin Saltonstall (1993) writes of "doing health" as a form of "doing gender." In research carried out in Germany, the concept of "somatic culture" has been formulated. Cornelia Helfferich (1994), for example, views the body as "a vehicle for cultural forms of expression" (Helfferich, 1994, p. 9) and somatic culture as "one aspect of the culture of sexual dualism" (Helfferich, 1994, p. 58). Petra Kolip (1999) also discusses the forms in which somatic culture and its individual components manifest themselves as a specific way of dealing with the body which reflects the confrontation with a variety of gender-specific stress factors. In this context, health risk behavior is "the individual and collective attempt to produce femininity and masculinity in dealings with the body" (Kolip, 1999. p. 301). In this perspective, empirically substantiated differences between men and women with respect to health and illness represent above all an expression of the social norms for "femininity" and "masculinity" and of living conditions which vary according to gender (see Kuhlmann, 1997).

The concepts of "doing gender" (West & Fenstermaker, 1995; West & Zimmerman, 1991) and "somatic culture" point to the links between the two spheres, but ultimately, culture dominates "body." By focusing on interaction, the significance of the body is reduced to a specific, pre-existing framework (e.g., Saltonstall, 1993). The body becomes a passive background, an object which carries out actions and generates classifications.

A further important direction taken in research on women's health highlights structural issues. Studies in this area have taken up work done in epidemiology and the sociology of inequality (e.g., Doyal, 2000; Macintyre et al., 1996) and asked "how the living conditions of women in our society and the burdens, discrimination, and contradictions they entail influence the health and wellbeing of women and their health behavior" (Maschewsky-Schneider,

1994, p. 30). By analyzing the variation in people's social situation with greater precision, researchers are now able to determine specific profiles of health-related lifestyles and health status. However, these interactions are extremely complex and cannot be described as binary or linear relationships (Babitsch, 1997, 2000). Macintyre et al. (1996) ask whether gender differences in health are really as simple as they seem; and indeed, the data raise more questions than they can answer. Some studies (e.g., Doyal, 2000; Matthews, Manor, & Power, 1999) have described health-relevant differences between men and women which are closely linked to social conditions and lifestyles; others (e.g., Arber, 1990; Macran, Clarke, & Joshi, 1996) report on differences and similarities within the individual groups of women studied. These results and the research perspectives which have evolved from them offer opportunities for developing differentiated understandings of the categories "woman," "gender," "health," and their multi-faceted interactions (see Hunt & Annandale, 1999; Macintyre et al., 1996; Matthews et al., 1999; McDonough & Walters, 2001). Such research on social conditions incorporates concepts from social theory which focus on the interactions between health and gender. However, these concepts generally remain on the macro-sociological level and are not always formulated explicitly. As we have shown above, work by Davis (1997); Martin (1994), and others has resulted in a better understanding of the interactions between social conditions and individual perceptions.

Women's health research has formulated convincing critiques of the biomedical model and has successfully influenced structures within the sphere of health care, in particular in the areas of gynecology and obstetrics and preventive health care (e.g., Bell, 1994; The Boston Women's Health Collective, 1973). But these achievements have been secured at the cost of limiting the analysis of interactions between health and social context to what happens beyond the skin, outside of the body. This critique is strongly emphasized by the work of Linda Birke (1999b; see also Fausto-Sterling, 2000; Hubbard, 1994; Martin, 1994). Thus, central fields of research into women's health concerns utilize precisely those theoretical approaches which do *not* include a specific conceptualization of the body.

Body, gender, health—shifting categories

Feminist theories and women's health research share the common intention of reflecting critically on biology as a stable and fixed framework for the categories "body" and "gender." Both areas of research have undergone a process of radicalization—each in its own way—and each is in itself very heterogeneous. The main differences between the two fields are twofold: (1) the extent to which they fundamentally question a given material framework of reference and (2) the levels on which the body and health are conceptualized and reformulated. The theoretical models and empirical results sketched here point to an apparent paradox: research on women's health, as the discipline which is unavoidably concerned with the body, avoids for the most part theoretical debates about the materiality of the body and instead focuses its analyses on social position and/or symbolic practices. While this may appear to be an understandable pragmatic reaction to discourses which leave no room for health and illness, from a theoretical standpoint it means that opportunities for new insights lie fallow. There are, however, some authors who have undertaken more in-depth analyses of the links between what is "outside" and "inside" the body; such work especially has focused on breast cancer (e.g., Hubbard & Wald, 1993; Stacey, 1997), reproductive health (e.g., Birke, 2000; Rapp, 1999) and osteoporosis (e.g., Klinge, 1997).

A mere transfer of feminist concepts to women's health research, such as was attempted with the concept of patriarchy in the early days of the field, can hardly be the goal of future work. As Anne Balsamo (1996) points out, it is significant "that feminist approaches to 'the body' resist the easy dissolution or dematerialization of the body offered by postmodernist theorists." She asserts that "it is time for feminism to crash the postmodern party" (Balsamo, 1996, pp. 31, 40). This is especially true of Butler's proposals, which, seen on the backdrop of debates about "virtual reality" (see Braidotti, 1998), strengthen unmistakable tendencies to disqualify the body's sensory perceptions and experiences. Viewed with the tunnel vision of (de-)constructionist debates about the body, health becomes a "black box," bodies become objects to be designed and modeled. Thus, it would seem that women's health research would be well advised to keep a critical distance from certain elements of discourse-oriented and poststructuralist theory, without, however, rejecting them outright. We have to bear in mind that "our beliefs about gender affect what kinds of knowledge scientists produce about sex in the first place" (Fausto-Sterling, 2000, p. 3).

Grosz and Haraway, among others, have shown that constructivist and materialized perspectives on the body must not necessarily be in opposition to each other. In spite of the essential differences between these two approaches, both authors conceptualize the body as flexible, volatile, transformable, but nonetheless as something material. Radical attempts to re-conceive the relationship between nature and culture and the many variegated metaphorical representations of this relationship harbor opportunities for a dynamic materialization of the body. The promise of new insights resulting from this process have been recognized by a number of authors in other fields of research.

Linda Birke (1999a), for example, conceives of the body as "changing and changeable, as transformable (. . .) Living the body means experiencing it as transformable, not only as cultural meanings/readings, but also within itself" (Birke, 1999a, p. 45). Her work on the interaction between chemicals thought to damage reproduction and hormones clearly demonstrates the deeper insights into bodily processes to be gained by this approach (Birke,

2000; see also Oudshoorn, 1996). These opportunities for changing the body "within itself have been neglected or dealt with inadequately within women's health research. On the other hand, empirically established links between health, social situation, and sex and, in particular, the differences within groups with similar life conditions, must be seen as indications of the fact that the body is more than a mere surface for the inscription of discourses and that the body does not merely react to social contexts but instead also itself acts as an "agent" (Haraway). The problem is that, to date, we know little about how this action unfolds.

Despite their differences, the approaches developed by Grosz and Haraway are characterized by a similar problem: neither of them offers a clearly formulated positioning of the body within social theory. In Grosz' work, this results in an inadequate differentiation within the category "women" as a whole. Furthermore, she fails to explicate the epistemological grounds for her assumption that sexual relations which guarantee women's autonomy can be realized on the basis of non-hierarchical constructions of gender which recognize sexual difference. In contrast to Grosz, Haraway questions all naturalizing differentiations and emphasizes their potential for creating hierarchy. By doing so, however, she loses sight of the social and ethical consequences of dissolving or shifting borders, as well as of the ambivalence of such borders. In the face of biomedicine's—and in particular genetics'—increasing appropriation of the body, this issue has become especially crucial. It is presumably no coincidence that the risks of overstepping borders have been emphasized by German authors, who approach these issues with the heightened awareness resulting from German history (see Braun, 1998; Gransee, 1999; Kollek, 2000). An adequate answer to the attempts of human genetics to define bodies according to their genetic makeup and to shape, manipulate, and re-design them on this basis should, however, utilize the explanatory potential of constructivist theories, since they offer "instruments for visualizing the cultural and social interweavings of supposedly natural categories as fetus, gene, or DNA" (Hofmann, 1999, p. 272; see Hubbard, 1994; Nelkin & Lindee, 1995; Spanier, 1995). But such an answer must also include critical reflection on the risks involved.

Dissolving traditional boundaries does not guarantee that new boundaries will be negotiated and established or where these new boundaries will be drawn, nor allow us to predict what consequences this will have for gender relations. This raises a problem common to all kinds of (de-)constructivist approaches: the failure to make the necessary distinctions between difference and hierarchy (see Kuhlmann, 1999), a shortcoming which can lead to untenable epistemological links between gender constructions and gender relations within society. The creation and the dissolution of borders depends not only on technological opportunities. These processes are equally dependent on power constellations within society, or, in other words, on which social actors with what specific interests successfully acquire powers of definition in negotiating new/old/transcendent boundaries. If we follow Balsamo's argument, then "the question is how to empower technological agents so that they work on behalf of the right kind of social change" (Balsamo, 1996, p. 156).

The selection of a variety of theoretical and empirical approaches sketched in this article demonstrates that no single perspective offers completely satisfying answers to these problems; each has its specific risks and blind spots. For this reason, we propose that researchers interested in these issues cooperate in intensifying the search for new answers and join in integrating concepts of health and illness into the debates on the body. Furthermore, we consider it essential that feminist theorists take empirical data gathered by women's health research and the multi-faceted individual dimensions of bodily perceptions into account when formulating their concepts. The value of such a development would be twofold: theorists would (again) take on responsibility for women's health concerns and empirically oriented researchers and those involved in policy-making would discover new links between their problems and the debates within feminist theory.

We hope that our examples have revealed relevant "fault lines" between theoretical debates and women's health research and thus contributed to the search for common issues and interests on both sides. However, we agree with Birke's (2000) assessment, that this is a project which will be difficult to realize in full and that it means that theorists, as well as empirical researchers and activists will have to get used to "sitting on the fence" (Birke, 2000, p. 587). Nonetheless, in our opinion, such an uncomfortable position would seem to be the most promising standpoint from which we might begin comprehending such divergent dimensions as cultural inscriptions, medical discourse, living conditions, and individual feelings and perceptions as well as biological processes inside the body, as factors which all contribute to the very different ways we are embodied.

Acknowledgement

We wish to thank the editor and the anonymous referees for their inspiring comments.

References

Angerer, Marie-Luise (1999). The body of gender: Or the body of what? Zur Leere des Geschlechts und seiner Fassade (The body of gender: Or the body of what? The emptiness of sex and its facade). In Genus, Münsteraner Arbeitskreis für gender studies (Eds.), *Kultur, Geschlecht, Körper* (Culture, gender, bodies) (pp. 64–76). Münster: Agenda Verlag.

Arber, Sarah (1990). Revealing women's health. Re-analysing the General Household Survey. In Helen Roberts (Ed.), *Women's health counts* (pp. 63–92). London: Routledge.

Babitsch, Birgit (1997). Soziale Ungleichheit und Gesundheit bei Frauen in Westdeutschland (Social inequality and health status of women in Western Germany). In Wolfgang Ahrens, Bärbel-Maria Bellach, & Karl-Heinz Jöckel (Eds.), *Messung soziodemographischer Merkmale in der Epidemiologie* (Measuring socio-demographic traits in epidemiology) (pp. 95–112). München: MMV Medizin Verlag.

Babitsch, Birgit (2000). Soziale Lage, Frauen und Gesundheit (Social situation, women, and health). In Uwe Helmert, Karin Bammann, Walter Voges, & Rainer Müller (Eds.), *Müssen Arme früher sterben? Soziale Ungleichheit und Gesundheit in Deutschland* (Must the poor die earlier? Social inequality and health in Germany) (pp. 63–73). Weinheim: Juventa.

Balsamo, Anne (1996). *Technologies of the gendered body. Reading cyborg women.* Durham: Duke University Press.

Bell, Susan E. (1994). Translating science to the people. Updating the new our bodies, ourselves. *Women's Studies International Forum 17*(1), 9–18.

Benhabib, Seyla, Butler, Judith, Cornel, Drucilla, & Fraser, Nancy (Eds.) (1995). *Feminist contentions: A philosophical exchange.* New York: Routledge.

Birke, Linda (1999a). Bodies and biology. In Janet Price & Margrit Shildrick (Eds.), *Feminist theory and the body* (pp. 42–49). New York: Routledge.

Birke, Linda (1999b). *Feminism and the biological body.* Edinburgh: Edinburgh University Press.

Birke, Linda (2000). Sitting on the fence: Biology, feminism and gender-bending environments. *Women's Studies International Forum 23*(5), 587–599.

Braidotti, Rosi (1998). *Cyberfeminism with a difference.* (www.let.ruu.nl/womens_studies/rosi/cyberfem.htm).

Braun, Katrin (1998). Mensch, Tier, Schimäre: Grenzauflösungen durch Technologie (Human, animal, chimera: Dissolving borders with technology). In Gudrun-Axeli Knapp (Ed.), *Kurskorrekturen* (Correcting the course). (pp. 153–177). Frankfurt: Campus.

Butler, Judith (1990). *Gender trouble.* New York: Routledge.

Butler, Judith (1993). *Bodies that matter: On the discursive limits of "sex".* London: Routledge.

Davis, Kathy (1997). My body is my art: Cosmetic surgery as feminist utopia? In Kathy Davis (Ed.), *Embodied practices. Feminist perspectives on the body* (pp. 168–181). London: Sage.

Davis-Floyd, Robbie (1998). From technobirth to cyborg babies. In Robbie Davis-Floyd & Joseph Dumit (Eds.), *Cyborg babies. From techno-sex to techno-tots* (pp. 255–282). New York: Routledge.

Doyal, Lesley (2000). Gender equity in health: Debates and dilemmas. *Social Science & Medicine 51*(6), 931–939.

Dresser, Rebecca (1996). What bioethics can learn from the women's health movement. In Susan M. Wolf (Ed.), *Feminism and bioethics. Beyond reproduction* (pp. 143–159). New York: Oxford University Press.

Ehrenreich, Barbara, & English, Deidre (1974). *Complaints and disorders: The sexual politics of sickness.* London: Compendium.

Fausto-Sterling, Anne (2000). *Sexing the body.* New York: Basic Books.

Fraser, Nancy (1995). Pragmatism, feminism and the linguistic turn. In Seyla Benhabib, Judith Butler, Drucilla Fraser, & Nancy Fraser (Eds.), *Feminist contentions: A philosophical exchange* (pp. 157–171). New York: Routledge.

Gordon, Linda, & Thorne, Barry (1996). Women's bodies and feminist subversions. *Contemporary Sociology* 25(3), 322–325.

Gransee, Carmen (1999). *Grenz-Bestimmungen. Zum Problem identitätslogischer Konstruktionen von "Natur" und "Geschlecht"* (Defining boundaries. The problem of identitarian constructions of "nature" and "gender"). Tübingen: Edition Diskord.

Greer, Germaine (1999). *The whole woman*. London: Doubleday.

Grosz, Elisabeth (1994). *Volatile bodies. Towards a corporeal feminism*. Australia: Allen & Unwin.

Grosz, Elisabeth (1995). *Space, time, and perversion. Essays on the politics of bodies*. New York: Routledge.

Haraway, Donna J. (1991). *Simians, cyborgs, and women: The reinvention of nature*. New York and London: Routledge.

Haraway, Donna J. (1997). *Modest_Witness@Second_Millenium.FemaleMan©_Meets_Oncomouse*™. New York and London: Routledge.

Helfferich, Cornelia (1994). *Jugend, Körper und Geschlecht* (Adolescence, body and gender). Opladen: Leske+Budrich.

Hofmann, Heidi (1999). *Die feministischen Diskurse über Reproduktionstechnologien* (Feminist discourse of reproductive technologies). Frankfurt: Campus.

Hubbard, Ruth (1994). Constructs of genetic difference: Race and sex. In Robert F. Weir, Susan C. Lawrence, & Evan Fales (Eds.), *Genes and human self-knowledge* (pp. 195–206). Iowa: University of Iowa Press.

Hubbard, Ruth, & Wald, Elijah (1993). *Exploding the gene myth*. Boston: Beacon Press.

Hunt, Kate, & Annandale, Ellen (1999). Relocating gender and morbidity: Examining men's and women's health in contemporary Western societies. *Social Science & Medicine* 48(1), 1–5.

Jordanova, Ludmilla (1999). 'Natural facts': A historical perspective on science and sexuality. In Janet Price & Margrit Shildrick (Eds.), *Feminist theory and the body* (pp. 157–168). New York: Routledge.

Klinge, Ineke (1997). Female bodies and brittle bones: Medical interventions in osteoporosis. In Kathy Davis (Ed.), *Embodied practices. Feminist perspectives on the body* (pp. 59–72). London: Sage.

Kolip, Petra (1999). Riskierte Körper: Geschlechtsspezifische somatische Kulturen im Jugendalter (Risking the body. Gendered body culture in adolescence). In Bettina Dausien, Mechtild Oechsle, Christiane Schmerl, & Marlene Stein-Hilbers (Eds.), *Erkenntnisprojekt Geschlecht* (The epistemological project of sex/gender) (pp. 291–303). Opladen: Leske+Budrich.

Kollek, Regine (1996). Metaphern, Strukturbilder, Mythen—Zur symbolischen Bedeutung des menschlichen Genoms (Metaphors, structural images, myths—On the symbolic meaning of the human genome). In Lisbeth N. Trallori (Ed.), *Die Eroberung des Lebens* (The conquest of life) (pp. 137–153). Wien: Verlag für Gesellschaftskritik.

Kollek, Regine (2000). Technicalisation of human procreation and social living conditions. In Hille Haker & Deryck Beyleveld (Eds.), *The ethics of genetics in human procreation* (pp. 139–179). Aldershot: Ashgate.

Kuhlmann, Ellen (1997). Geschlecht—ein Gesundheitsrisiko? Eine Anwendung des gendering—Konzepts in der Gesundheitsforschung (The concept of "doing gender" in health research). *Feministische Studien* 15(1), 138–147.

Kuhlmann, Ellen (1999). Differenz und Hierarchie—(k)ein symbiotisches Verhältnis (Difference and hierarchy—(in)dependent categories?). In Ayla Neusel & Angelika Wetterer (Eds.), *Vielfältige Verschiedenheiten. Geschlechterverhältnisse in Hochschule, Studium und Beruf* (Multi-facetted differences. Gender relations in the academy, education and workplace). (pp. 285–304). Frankfurt: Campus.

Kuhlmann, Ellen (in press). Humangenetik und Geschlecht. Formationen zwischen Hegemonie und Autonomiekonstrukten (Human genetics and gender. Formations between hegemony and constructions of autonomy). In Ellen Kuhlmann & Regine Kollek (Eds.), *Konfiguration des Menschen. Biowissenschaften als Arena der Geschlechterpolitik* (Configuration of the human. Gender politics in biosciences). Opladen: Leske+Budrich.

Lewin, Ellen, & Oleson, Virginia (Eds.) (1985). *Women, health and healing.* New York: Travistock.

MacCormack, Carol, & Strathern, Marilyn (Eds.) (1980). *Nature, culture and gender.* Cambridge: Cambridge University Press.

Macintyre, Sally, Hunt, Kate, & Sweeting, Helen (1996). Gender differences in health. Are things really as simple as they seem? *Social Science & Medicine 42*(4), 617–624.

Macran, Susan, Clarke, Lynda, & Joshi, Heather (1996). Women's health. Dimensions and differentials. *Social Science & Medicine 42*(9), 1203–1216.

Mahowald, Mary B. (2000). *Genes, women, equality.* New York: Oxford University Press.

Marshall, Helen (1996). Our bodies, our selves: Why we should add old fashioned empirical phenomenology to the new theories of the body. *Women's Studies International Forum 19*(3), 253–265.

Martin, Emily (1987). *The woman in the body.* Milton Keynes: Open University Press.

Martin, Emily (1994). *Flexible bodies.* Boston: Beacon Press.

Maschewsky-Schneider, Ulrike (1994). Frauen leben länger als Männer. Sind sie auch gesünder? (Women live longer than men. Are they also more healthy?). *Zeitschrift für Frauenforschung 12*(4), 28–38.

Matthews, Sharon, Manor, Orly, & Power, Chris (1999). Social inequalities. Are there gender differences? *Social Science & Medicine 48*(1), 49–60.

McDonough, Peggy, & Walters, Vivienne (2001). Gender and health: Reassessing patterns and explanations. *Social Science & Medicine 52*(4), 547–559.

Nelkin, Dorothy, & Lindee, Susan M. (1995). *The DNA mystique. The genes as cultural icon.* New York: Freeman.

Oudshoorn, Nelly (1996). The decline of the one-size-fits-all paradigm, or, how reproductive scientists try to cope with postmodernity. In Nina Lykke & Rosi Braidotti (Eds.), *Between monsters, goddesses and cyborgs* (pp. 153–172). London: Zed Books.

Pollard, Tessa M., & Hyatt, Susan Brin (Eds.) (1999). *Sex, gender and health.* Cambridge: Cambridge University Press.

Price, Janet, & Shildrick, Margrit (Eds.) (1999). *Feminist theory and the body.* New York: Routledge.

Rapp, Rayna (1999). *Testing women, testing the fetus. The social impact of amniocentesis in America.* New York: Routledge.

Saltonstall, Robin (1993). Healthy bodies, social bodies: Men's and women's concepts and practices of health in everyday life. *Social Science & Medicine 36*(1), 7–14.

Schneider, Ulrike (Ed.) (1981). *Was macht Frauen krank? Ansätze zu einer frauenspezifischen Gesundheitsforschung* (What makes women sick? Approaches to women's health research). Frankfurt: Campus.

Shildrick, Margrit, & Price, Jannet (1999). Openings on the body. In Jannet Price & Margrit Shildrick (Eds.), *Feminist theory and the body* (pp. 1–14). New York: Routledge.

Spanier, Bonnie B. (1995). *Im/partial science. Gender ideology in molecular biology*. Bloomington: Indiana University Press.

Stacey, Jackie (1997). *Teratologies. A cultural study of cancer*. London: Routledge.

Stein-Hilbers, Marlene (1995). Geschlechterverhältnisse und somatische Kulturen (Gender relations and body culture). *Jahrbuch für kritische Medizin 15*(24), 62–81.

The Boston Women's Health Book Collective (1973). *Our bodies, our selves*. New York: Simon & Schuster.

Waldron, Ingrid (1980). Employment and women's health. An analysis of causal relationship. *International Journal of Health Services 10*(3), 435–454.

West, Candace, & Fenstermaker, Sarah (1995). Doing difference. *Gender and Society 9*(1), 8–37.

West, Candace, & Zimmerman, Don (1991). Doing gender. In Judith Lorber & Susan A. Farrell (Eds.), *The social construction of gender* (pp. 13–37). Newbury Park: Sage.

6
THE EGG AND THE SPERM
How science has constructed a romance based on stereotypical male-female roles

Emily Martin

Source: *Signs*, 16:3 (1991), 485–501.

> The theory of the human body is always a part of a world-picture.... The theory of the human body is always a part of a *fantasy*.
> [JAMES HILLMAN, *The Myth of Analysis*][1]

As an anthropologist, I am intrigued by the possibility that culture shapes how biological scientists describe what they discover about the natural world. If this were so, we would be learning about more than the natural world in high school biology class; we would be learning about cultural beliefs and practices as if they were part of nature. In the course of my research I realized that the picture of egg and sperm drawn in popular as well as scientific accounts of reproductive biology relies on stereotypes central to our cultural definitions of male and female. The stereotypes imply not only that female biological processes are less worthy than their male counterparts but also that women are less worthy than men. Part of my goal in writing this article is to shine a bright light on the gender stereotypes hidden within the scientific language of biology. Exposed in such a light, I hope they will lose much of their power to harm us.

Egg and sperm: a scientific fairy tale

At a fundamental level, all major scientific textbooks depict male and female reproductive organs as systems for the production of valuable substances, such as eggs and sperm.[2] In the case of women, the monthly cycle is described as being designed to produce eggs and prepare a suitable place for them to be fertilized and grown—all to the end of making babies. But the enthusiasm ends there. By extolling the female cycle as a productive enterprise, menstruation must necessarily be viewed as a failure. Medical texts describe menstruation as the "debris" of the uterine lining, the result of necrosis, or death of tissue. The descriptions imply that a system has gone awry, making products of no use, not to specification, unsaleable, wasted, scrap. An illustration in a widely used medical text shows menstruation as a chaotic disintegration of form, complementing the many texts that describe it as "ceasing," "dying," "losing," "denuding," "expelling."[3]

Male reproductive physiology is evaluated quite differently. One of the texts that sees menstruation as failed production employs a sort of breathless prose when it describes the maturation of sperm: "The mechanisms which guide the remarkable cellular transformation from spermatid to mature sperm remain uncertain.... Perhaps the most amazing characteristic of spermatogenesis is its sheer magnitude: the normal human male may manufacture several hundred million sperm per day."[4] In the classic text *Medical Physiology*, edited by Vernon Mountcastle, the male/female, productive/destructive comparison is more explicit: "Whereas the female *sheds* only a single gamete each month, the seminiferous tubules *produce* hundreds of millions of sperm each day" (emphasis mine).[5] The female author of another text marvels at the length of the microscopic seminiferous tubules, which, if uncoiled and placed end to end, "would span almost one-third of a mile!" She writes, "In an adult male these structures produce millions of sperm cells each day." Later she asks, "How is this feat accomplished?"[6] None of these texts expresses such intense enthusiasm for any female processes. It is surely no accident that the "remarkable" process of making sperm involves precisely what, in the medical view, menstruation does not: production of something deemed valuable.[7]

One could argue that menstruation and spermatogenesis are not analogous processes and, therefore, should not be expected to elicit the same kind of response. The proper female analogy to spermatogenesis, biologically, is ovulation. Yet ovulation does not merit enthusiasm in these texts either. Textbook descriptions stress that all of the ovarian follicles containing ova are already present at birth. Far from being *produced*, as sperm are, they merely sit on the shelf, slowly degenerating and aging like overstocked inventory: "At birth, normal human ovaries contain an estimated one million follicles [each], and no new ones appear after birth. Thus, in marked contrast to the male, the newborn female already has all the germ cells she will ever have. Only a few, perhaps 400, are destined to reach full maturity during her active productive life. All the others degenerate at some point in their development so that few, if any, remain by the time she reaches menopause at approximately 50 years of age."[8] Note the "marked contrast" that this description sets up between male and female: the male, who continuously produces fresh germ cells, and the female, who has stockpiled germ cells by birth and is faced with their degeneration.

Nor are the female organs spared such vivid descriptions. One scientist writes in a newspaper article that a woman's ovaries become old and worn out from ripening eggs every month, even though the woman herself is still relatively young: "When you look through a laparoscope . . . at an ovary that has been through hundreds of cycles, even in a superbly healthy American female, you see a scarred, battered organ."[9]

To avoid the negative connotations that some people associate with the female reproductive system, scientists could begin to describe male and female processes as homologous. They might credit females with "producing" mature ova one at a time, as they're needed each month, and describe males as having to face problems of degenerating germ cells. This degeneration would occur throughout life among spermatogonia, the undifferentiated germ cells in the testes that are the long-lived, dormant precursors of sperm.

But the texts have an almost dogged insistence on casting female processes in a negative light. The texts celebrate sperm production because it is continuous from puberty to senescence, while they portray egg production as inferior because it is finished at birth. This makes the female seem unproductive, but some texts will also insist that it is she who is wasteful.[10] In a section heading for *Molecular Biology of the Cell*, a best-selling text, we are told that "Oogenesis is wasteful." The text goes on to emphasize that of the seven million oogonia, or egg germ cells, in the female embryo, most degenerate in the ovary. Of those that do go on to become oocytes, or eggs, many also degenerate, so that at birth only two million eggs remain in the ovaries. Degeneration continues throughout a woman's life: by puberty 300,000 eggs remain, and only a few are present by menopause. "During the 40 or so years of a woman's reproductive life, only 400 to 500 eggs will have been released," the authors write. "All the rest will have degenerated. It is still a mystery why so many eggs are formed only to die in the ovaries."[11]

The real mystery is why the male's vast production of sperm is not seen as wasteful.[12] Assuming that a man "produces" 100 million (10^8) sperm per day (a conservative estimate) during an average reproductive life of sixty years, he would produce well over two trillion sperm in his lifetime. Assuming that a woman "ripens" one egg per lunar month, or thirteen per year, over the course of her forty-year reproductive life, she would total five hundred eggs in her lifetime. But the word "waste" implies an excess, too much produced. Assuming two or three offspring, for every baby a woman produces, she wastes only around two hundred eggs. For every baby a man produces, he wastes more than one trillion (10^{12}) sperm.

How is it that positive images are denied to the bodies of women? A look at language—in this case, scientific language—provides the first clue. Take the egg and the sperm.[13] It is remarkable how "femininely" the egg behaves and how "masculinely" the sperm.[14] The egg is seen as large and passive.[15] It does not *move* or *journey*, but passively "is transported," "is swept,"[16] or even "drifts"[17] along the fallopian tube. In utter contrast, sperm are small, "streamlined,"[18] and invariably active. They "deliver" their genes to the egg, "activate the developmental program of the egg,"[19] and have a "velocity" that is often remarked upon.[20] Their tails are "strong" and efficiently powered.[21] Together with the forces of ejaculation, they can "propel the semen into the deepest recesses of the vagina."[22] For this they need "energy," "fuel,"[23] so that with a "whiplashlike motion and strong lurches"[24] they can "burrow through the egg coat"[25] and "penetrate" it.[26]

At its extreme, the age-old relationship of the egg and the sperm takes on a royal or religious patina. The egg coat, its protective barrier, is sometimes called its "vestments," a term usually reserved for sacred, religious dress. The egg is said to have a "corona,"[27] a crown, and to be accompanied by "attendant cells."[28] It is holy, set apart and above, the queen to the sperm's king. The egg is also passive, which means it must depend on sperm for rescue. Gerald Schatten and Helen Schatten liken the egg's role to that of Sleeping Beauty: "a dormant bride awaiting her mate's magic kiss, which instills the spirit that brings her to life."[29] Sperm, by contrast, have a "mission,"[30] which is to "move through the female genital tract in quest of the ovum."[31] One popular account has it that the sperm carry out a "perilous journey" into the "warm darkness," where some fall away "exhausted." "Survivors" "assault" the egg, the successful candidates "surrounding the prize."[32] Part of the urgency of this journey, in more scientific terms, is that "once released from the supportive environment of the ovary, an egg will die within hours unless rescued by a sperm."[33] The wording stresses the fragility and dependency of the egg, even though the same text acknowledges elsewhere that sperm also live for only a few hours.[34]

In 1948, in a book remarkable for its early insights into these matters, Ruth Herschberger argued that female reproductive organs are seen as biologically interdependent, while male organs are viewed as autonomous, operating independently and in isolation:

> At present the functional is stressed only in connection with women: it is in them that ovaries, tubes, uterus, and vagina have endless interdependence. In the male, reproduction would seem to involve "organs" only.
>
> Yet the sperm, just as much as the egg, is dependent on a great many related processes. There are secretions which mitigate the urine in the urethra before ejaculation, to protect the sperm. There is the reflex shutting off of the bladder connection, the provision of prostatic secretions, and various types of muscular propulsion. The sperm is no more independent of its milieu than the egg, and yet from a wish that it were, biologists have lent their support to the notion that the human female, beginning with the egg, is congenitally more dependent than the male.[35]

Bringing out another aspect of the sperm's autonomy, an article in the journal *Cell* has the sperm making an "existential decision" to penetrate the egg: "Sperm are cells with a limited behavioral repertoire, one that is directed toward fertilizing eggs. To execute the decision to abandon the haploid state, sperm swim to an egg and there acquire the ability to effect membrane fusion."[36] Is this a corporate manager's version of the sperm's activities—"executing decisions" while fraught with dismay over difficult options that bring with them very high risk?

There is another way that sperm, despite their small size, can be made to loom in importance over the egg. In a collection of scientific papers, an electron micrograph of an enormous egg and tiny sperm is titled "A Portrait of the Sperm."[37] This is a little like showing a photo of a dog and calling it a picture of the fleas. Granted, microscopic sperm are harder to photograph than eggs, which are just large enough to see with the naked eye. But surely the use of the term "portrait," a word associated with the powerful and wealthy, is significant. Eggs have only micrographs or pictures, not portraits.

One depiction of sperm as weak and timid, instead of strong and powerful —the only such representation in western civilization, so far as I know— occurs in Woody Allen's movie *Everything You Always Wanted To Know About Sex* *But Were Afraid to Ask*. Allen, playing the part of an apprehensive sperm inside a man's testicles, is scared of the man's approaching orgasm. He is reluctant to launch himself into the darkness, afraid of contraceptive devices, afraid of winding up on the ceiling if the man masturbates.

The more common picture—egg as damsel in distress, shielded only by her sacred garments; sperm as heroic warrior to the rescue—cannot be proved to be dictated by the biology of these events. While the "facts" of biology may not *always* be constructed in cultural terms, I would argue that in this case they are. The degree of metaphorical content in these descriptions, the extent to which differences between egg and sperm are emphasized, and the parallels between cultural stereotypes of male and female behavior and the character of egg and sperm all point to this conclusion.

New research, old imagery

As new understandings of egg and sperm emerge, textbook gender imagery is being revised. But the new research, far from escaping the stereotypical representations of egg and sperm, simply replicates elements of textbook gender imagery in a different form. The persistence of this imagery calls to mind what Ludwik Fleck termed "the self-contained" nature of scientific thought. As he described it, "the interaction between what is already known, what remains to be learned, and those who are to apprehend it, go to ensure harmony within the system. But at the same time they also preserve the harmony of illusions, which is quite secure within the confines of a given thought style."[38] We need to understand the way in which the cultural content in scientific descriptions changes as biological discoveries unfold, and whether that cultural content is solidly entrenched or easily changed.

In all of the texts quoted above, sperm are described as penetrating the egg, and specific substances on a sperm's head are described as binding to the egg. Recently, this description of events was rewritten in a biophysics lab at Johns Hopkins University—transforming the egg from the passive to the active party.[39]

Prior to this research, it was thought that the zona, the inner vestments of the egg, formed an impenetrable barrier. Sperm overcame the barrier by mechanically burrowing through, thrashing their tails and slowly working their way along. Later research showed that the sperm released digestive enzymes that chemically broke down the zona; thus, scientists presumed that the sperm used mechanical *and* chemical means to get through to the egg.

In this recent investigation, the researchers began to ask questions about the mechanical force of the sperm's tail. (The lab's goal was to develop a contraceptive that worked topically on sperm.) They discovered, to their great surprise, that the forward thrust of sperm is extremely weak, which contradicts the assumption that sperm are forceful penetrators.[40] Rather than thrusting forward, the sperm's head was now seen to move mostly back and forth. The sideways motion of the sperm's tail makes the head move sideways with a force that is ten times stronger than its forward movement. So even if the overall force of the sperm were strong enough to mechanically break the zona, most of its force would be directed sideways rather than forward. In fact, its strongest tendency, by tenfold, is to escape by attempting to pry itself off the egg. Sperm, then, must be exceptionally efficient at *escaping* from any cell surface they contact. And the surface of the egg must be designed to trap the sperm and prevent their escape. Otherwise, few if any sperm would reach the egg.

The researchers at Johns Hopkins concluded that the sperm and egg stick together because of adhesive molecules on the surfaces of each. The egg traps the sperm and adheres to it so tightly that the sperm's head is forced to lie flat against the surface of the zona, a little bit, they told me, "like Br'er Rabbit getting more and more stuck to tar baby the more he wriggles." The trapped sperm continues to wiggle ineffectually side to side. The mechanical force of its tail is so weak that a sperm cannot break even one chemical bond. This is where the digestive enzymes released by the sperm come in. If they start to soften the zona just at the tip of the sperm and the sides remain stuck, then the weak, flailing sperm can get oriented in the right direction and make it through the zona—provided that its bonds to the zona dissolve as it moves in.

Although this new version of the saga of the egg and the sperm broke through cultural expectations, the researchers who made the discovery continued to write papers and abstracts as if the sperm were the active party who attacks, binds, penetrates, and enters the egg. The only difference was that sperm were now seen as performing these actions weakly.[41] Not until August 1987, more than three years after the findings described above, did these researchers reconceptualize the process to give the egg a more active role. They began to describe the zona as an aggressive sperm catcher, covered with adhesive molecules that can capture a sperm with a single bond and clasp it to the zona's surface.[42] In the words of their published account: "The innermost vestment, the *zona pellucida*, is a glyco-protein shell, which captures and tethers the sperm before they penetrate it. . . . The sperm is captured at the initial contact between the sperm tip and the *zona*. . . . Since the thrust [of the sperm] is much smaller than the force needed to break a single affinity bond, the first bond made upon the tip-first meeting of the sperm and *zona* can result in the capture of the sperm."[43]

Experiments in another lab reveal similar patterns of data interpretation. Gerald Schatten and Helen Schatten set out to show that, contrary to conventional wisdom, the "egg is not merely a large, yolk-filled sphere into which the sperm burrows to endow new life. Rather, recent research suggests the almost heretical view that sperm and egg are mutually active partners."[44] This sounds like a departure from the stereotypical textbook view, but further reading reveals Schatten and Schatten's conformity to the aggressive-sperm metaphor. They describe how "the sperm and egg first touch when, from the tip of the sperm's triangular head, a long, thin filament shoots out and harpoons the egg." Then we learn that "remarkably, the harpoon is not so much fired as assembled at great speed, molecule by molecule, from a pool of protein stored in a specialized region called the acrosome. The filament may grow as much as twenty times longer than the sperm head itself before its tip reaches the egg and sticks."[45] Why not call this "making a bridge" or "throwing out a line" rather than firing a harpoon? Harpoons pierce prey and injure or kill them, while this filament only sticks. And why not focus, as the Hopkins lab did, on the stickiness of the egg, rather than the stickiness of the sperm?[46] Later in the article, the Schattens replicate the common view of the sperm's perilous journey into the warm darkness of the vagina, this time for the purpose of explaining its journey into the egg itself: "[The sperm] still has an arduous journey ahead. It must penetrate farther into the egg's huge sphere of cytoplasm and somehow locate the nucleus, so that the two cells' chromosomes can fuse. The sperm dives down into the cytoplasm, its tail beating. But it is soon interrupted by the sudden and swift migration of the egg nucleus, which rushes toward the sperm with a velocity triple that of the movement of chromosomes during cell division, crossing the entire egg in about a minute."[47]

Like Schatten and Schatten and the biophysicists at Johns Hopkins, another researcher has recently made discoveries that seem to point to a more interactive view of the relationship of egg and sperm. This work, which Paul Wassarman conducted on the sperm and eggs of mice, focuses on identifying the specific molecules in the egg coat (the zona pellucida) that are involved in egg-sperm interaction. At first glance, his descriptions seem to fit the model of an egalitarian relationship. Male and female gametes "recognize one another," and "interactions . . . take place between sperm and egg."[48] But the article in *Scientific American* in which those descriptions appear begins with a vignette that presages the dominant motif of their presentation: "It has been more than a century since Hermann Fol, a Swiss zoologist, peered into his microscope and became the first person to see a sperm penetrate an egg, fertilize it and form the first cell of a new embryo."[49] This portrayal of the sperm as the active party—the one that *penetrates* and *fertilizes* the egg and *produces* the embryo—is not cited as an example of an earlier, now outmoded view. In fact, the author reiterates the point later in the article: "Many sperm can bind to and penetrate the zona pellucida, or outer coat, of an unfertilized mouse egg, but only one sperm will eventually fuse with the thin plasma membrane surrounding the egg proper (*inner sphere*), fertilizing the egg and giving rise to a new embryo."[50]

The imagery of sperm as aggressor is particularly startling in this case: the main discovery being reported is isolation of a particular molecule *on the egg coat* that plays an important role in fertilization! Wassarman's choice of language sustains the picture. He calls the molecule that has been isolated, ZP3, a "sperm receptor." By allocating the passive, waiting role to the egg, Wassarman can continue to describe the sperm as the actor, the one that makes it all happen: "The basic process begins when many sperm first attach loosely and then bind tenaciously to receptors on the surface of the egg's thick outer coat, the zona pellucida. Each sperm, which has a large number of egg-binding proteins on its surface, binds to many sperm receptors on the egg. More specifically, a site on each of the egg-binding proteins fits a complementary site on a sperm receptor, much as a key fits a lock."[51] With the sperm designated as the "key" and the egg the "lock," it is obvious which one acts and which one is acted upon. Could this imagery not be reversed, letting the sperm (the lock) wait until the egg produces the key? Or could we speak of two halves of a locket matching, and regard the matching itself as the action that initiates the fertilization?

It is as if Wassarman were determined to make the egg the receiving partner. Usually in biological research, the *protein* member of the pair of binding molecules is called the receptor, and physically it has a pocket in it rather like a lock. As the diagrams that illustrate Wassarman's article show, the molecules on the sperm are proteins and have "pockets." The small, mobile molecules that fit into these pockets are called ligands. As shown in the diagrams, ZP3 on the egg is a polymer of "keys"; many small knobs stick out. Typically, molecules on the sperm would be called receptors and molecules on the egg would be called ligands. But Wassarman chose to name ZP3 on the egg the receptor and to create a new term, "the egg-binding protein," for the molecule on the sperm that otherwise would have been called the receptor.[52]

Wassarman does credit the egg coat with having more functions than those of a sperm receptor. While he notes that "the zona pellucida has at times been viewed by investigators as a nuisance, a barrier to sperm and hence an impediment to fertilization," his new research reveals that the egg coat "serves as a sophisticated biological security system that screens incoming sperm, selects only those compatible with fertilization and development, prepares sperm for fusion with the egg and later protects the resulting embryo from polyspermy [a lethal condition caused by fusion of more than one sperm with a single egg]."[53] Although this description gives the egg an active role, that role is drawn in stereotypically feminine terms. The egg *selects* an appropriate mate, *prepares* him for fusion, and then *protects* the resulting offspring from harm. This is courtship and mating behavior as seen through the eyes of a sociobiologist: woman as the hard-to-get prize, who, following union with the chosen one, becomes woman as servant and mother.

And Wassarman does not quit there. In a review article for *Science*, he outlines the "chronology of fertilization."[54] Near the end of the article are two subject headings. One is "Sperm Penetration," in which Wassarman describes how the chemical dissolving of the zona pellucida combines with the "substantial propulsive force generated by sperm." The next heading is "Sperm-Egg Fusion." This section details what happens inside the zona after a sperm "penetrates" it. Sperm "can make contact with, adhere to, and fuse with (that is, fertilize) an egg."[55] Wassarman's word choice, again, is astonishingly skewed in favor of the sperm's activity, for in the next breath he says that sperm *lose* all motility upon fusion with the egg's surface. In mouse and sea urchin eggs, the sperm enters at the *egg*'s volition, according to Wassarman's description: "Once fused with egg plasma membrane [the surface of the egg], how does a sperm enter the egg? The surface of both mouse and sea urchin eggs is covered with thousands of plasma membrane-bound projections, called microvilli [tiny "hairs"]. Evidence in sea urchins suggests that, after membrane fusion, a group of elongated microvilli cluster tightly around and interdigitate over the sperm head. As these microvilli are resorbed, the sperm is drawn into the egg. Therefore, sperm motility, which ceases at the time of fusion in both sea urchins and mice, is not required for sperm entry."[56] The section called "Sperm Penetration" more logically would be followed by a section called "The Egg Envelops," rather than "Sperm-Egg Fusion." This would give a parallel—and more accurate—sense that both the egg and the sperm initiate action.

Another way that Wassarman makes less of the egg's activity is by describing components of the egg but referring to the sperm as a whole entity. Deborah Gordon has described such an approach as "atomism" ("the part is independent of and primordial to the whole") and identified it as one of the "tenacious assumptions" of Western science and medicine.[57] Wassarman employs atomism to his advantage. When he refers to processes going on within sperm, he consistently returns to descriptions that remind us from whence these activities came: they are part of sperm that penetrate an egg or generate propulsive force. When he refers to processes going on within eggs, he stops there. As a result, any active role he grants them appears to be assigned to the parts of the egg, and not to the egg itself. In the quote above, it is the microvilli that actively cluster around the sperm. In another example, "the driving force for engulfment of a fused sperm comes from a region of cytoplasm just beneath an egg's plasma membrane."[58]

Social implications: thinking beyond

All three of these revisionist accounts of egg and sperm cannot seem to escape the hierarchical imagery of older accounts. Even though each new account gives the egg a larger and more active role, taken together they bring into play another cultural stereotype: woman as a dangerous and aggressive threat. In the Johns Hopkins lab's revised model, the egg ends up as the female aggressor who "captures and tethers" the sperm with her sticky zona, rather like a spider lying in wait in her web.[59] The Schatten lab has the egg's nucleus "interrupt" the sperm's dive with a "sudden and swift" rush by which she "clasps the sperm and guides its nucleus to the center."[60] Wassarman's description of the surface of the egg "covered with thousands of plasma membrane-bound projections, called microvilli" that reach out and clasp the sperm adds to the spiderlike imagery.[61]

These images grant the egg an active role but at the cost of appearing disturbingly aggressive. Images of woman as dangerous and aggressive, the femme fatale who victimizes men, are widespread in Western literature and culture.[62] More specific is the connection of spider imagery with the idea of an engulfing, devouring mother.[63] New data did not lead scientists to eliminate gender stereotypes in their descriptions of egg and sperm. Instead, scientists simply began to describe egg and sperm in different, but no less damaging, terms.

Can we envision a less stereotypical view? Biology itself provides another model that could be applied to the egg and the sperm. The cybernetic model—with its feedback loops, flexible adaptation to change, coordination of the parts within a whole, evolution over time, and changing response to the environment—is common in genetics, endocrinology, and ecology and has a growing influence in medicine in general.[64] This model has the potential to shift our imagery from the negative, in which the female reproductive system is castigated both for not producing eggs after birth and for producing (and thus wasting) too many eggs overall, to something more positive. The female reproductive system could be seen as responding to the environment (pregnancy or menopause), adjusting to monthly changes (menstruation), and flexibly changing from reproductivity after puberty to nonreproductivity later in life. The sperm and egg's interaction could also be described in cybernetic terms. J. F. Hartman's research in reproductive biology demonstrated fifteen years ago that if an egg is killed by being pricked with a needle, live sperm cannot get through the zona.[65] Clearly, this evidence shows that the egg and sperm *do* interact on more mutual terms, making biology's refusal to portray them that way all the more disturbing.

We would do well to be aware, however, that cybernetic imagery is hardly neutral. In the past, cybernetic models have played an important part in the imposition of social control. These models inherently provide a way of thinking about a "field" of interacting components. Once the field can be seen, it can become the object of new forms of knowledge, which in turn can allow new forms of social control to be exerted over the components of the field. During the 1950s, for example, medicine began to recognize the psychosocial *environment* of the patient: the patient's family and its psychodynamics. Professions such as social work began to focus on this new environment, and the resulting knowledge became one way to further control the patient. Patients began to be seen not as isolated, individual bodies, but as psychosocial entities located in an "ecological" system: management of "the patient's psychology was a new entree to patient control."[66]

The models that biologists use to describe their data can have important social effects. During the nineteenth century, the social and natural sciences strongly influenced each other: the social ideas of Malthus about how to avoid the natural increase of the poor inspired Darwin's *Origin of Species*.[67] Once the *Origin* stood as a description of the natural world, complete with competition and market struggles, it could be reimported into social science as social Darwinism, in order to justify the social order of the time. What we are seeing now is similar: the importation of cultural ideas about passive females and heroic males into the "personalities" of gametes. This amounts to the "implanting of social imagery on representations of nature so as to lay a firm basis for reimporting exactly that same imagery as natural explanations of social phenomena."[68]

Further research would show us exactly what social effects are being wrought from the biological imagery of egg and sperm. At the very least, the imagery keeps alive some of the hoariest old stereotypes about weak damsels in distress and their strong male rescuers. That these stereotypes are now being written in at the level of the *cell* constitutes a powerful move to make them seem so natural as to be beyond alteration.

The stereotypical imagery might also encourage people to imagine that what results from the interaction of egg and sperm—a fertilized egg—is the result of deliberate "human" action at the cellular level. Whatever the intentions of the human couple, in this microscopic "culture" a cellular "bride" (or femme fatale) and a cellular "groom" (her victim) make a cellular baby. Rosalind Petchesky points out that through visual representations such as sonograms, we are given "*images* of younger and younger, and tinier and tinier, fetuses being 'saved.'" This leads to "the point of visibility being 'pushed back' *indefinitely*."[69] Endowing egg and sperm with intentional action, a key aspect of personhood in our culture, lays the foundation for the point of viability being pushed back to the moment of fertilization. This will likely lead to greater acceptance of technological developments and new forms of scrutiny and manipulation, for the benefit of these inner "persons"; court-ordered restrictions on a pregnant woman's activities in order to protect her fetus, fetal surgery, amniocentesis, and rescinding of abortion rights, to name but a few examples.[70]

Even if we succeed in substituting more egalitarian, interactive metaphors to describe the activities of egg and sperm, and manage to avoid the pitfalls of cybernetic models, we would still be guilty of endowing cellular entities with personhood. More crucial, then, than what *kinds* of personalities we bestow on cells is the very fact that we are doing it at all. This process could ultimately have the most disturbing social consequences.

One clear feminist challenge is to wake up sleeping metaphors in science, particularly those involved in descriptions of the egg and the sperm. Although the literary convention is to call such metaphors "dead," they are not so much dead as sleeping, hidden within the scientific content of texts—and all the more powerful for it.[71] Waking up such metaphors, by becoming aware of when we are projecting cultural imagery onto what we study, will improve our ability to investigate and understand nature. Waking up such metaphors, by becoming aware of their implications, will rob them of their power to naturalize our social conventions about gender.

Acknowledgements

Portions of this article were presented as the 1987 Becker Lecture, Cornell University, I am grateful for the many suggestions and ideas I received on this occasion. For especially pertinent help with my arguments and data I thank Richard Cone, Kevin Whaley, Sharon Stephens, Barbara Duden, Susanne Kuechler, Lorna Rhodes, and Scott Gilbert. The article was strengthened and clarified by the comments of the anonymous *Signs* reviewers as well as the superb editorial skills of Amy Gage.

Notes

1 James Hillman, *The Myth of Analysis* (Evanston, Ill.: Northwestern University Press, 1972), 220.
2 The textbooks I consulted are the main ones used in classes for undergraduate premedical students or medical students (or those held on reserve in the library for these classes) during the past few years at Johns Hopkins University. These texts are widely used at other universities in the country as well.

3 Arthur C. Guyton, *Physiology of the Human Body*, 6th ed. (Philadelphia: Saunders College Publishing, 1984), 624.
4 Arthur J. Vander, James H. Sherman, and Dorothy S. Luciano, *Human Physiology: The Mechanisms of Body Function*, 3d ed. (New York: McGraw Hill, 1980), 483–84.
5 Vernon B. Mountcastle, *Medical Physiology*, 14th ed. (London: Mosby, 1980), 2:1624.
6 Eldra Pearl Solomon, *Human Anatomy and Physiology* (New York: CBS College Publishing, 1983), 678.
7 For elaboration, see Emily Martin, *The Woman in the Body: A Cultural Analysis of Reproduction* (Boston: Beacon, 1987), 27–53.
8 Vander, Sherman, and Luciano, 568.
9 Melvin Konner, "Childbearing and Age," *New York Times Magazine* (December 27, 1987), 22–23, esp. 22.
10 I have found but one exception to the opinion that the female is wasteful: "Smallpox being the nasty disease it is, one might expect nature to have designed antibody molecules with combining sites that specifically recognize the epitopes on smallpox virus. Nature differs from technology, however: it thinks nothing of wastefulness. (For example, rather than improving the chance that a spermatozoon will meet an egg cell, nature finds it easier to produce millions of spermatozoa.)" (Niels Kaj Jerne, "The Immune System," *Scientific American* 229, no, 1 [July 1973]: 53). Thanks to a *Signs* reviewer for bringing this reference to my attention.
11 Bruce Alberts et al., *Molecular Biology of the Cell* (New York: Garland, 1983), 795.
12 In her essay "Have Only Men Evolved?" (in *Discovering Reality: Feminist Perspectives on Epistemology, Metaphysics, Methodology, and Philosophy of Science*, ed. Sandra Harding and Merrill B. Hintikka [Dordrecht: Reidel, 1983], 45–69, esp. 60–61), Ruth Hubbard points out that sociobiologists have said the female invests more energy than the male in the production of her large gametes, claiming that this explains why the female provides parental care. Hubbard questions whether it "really takes more 'energy' to generate the one or relatively few eggs than the large excess of sperms required to achieve fertilization." For further critique of how the greater size of eggs is interpreted in sociobiology, see Donna Haraway, "Investment Strategies for the Evolving Portfolio of Primate Females," in *Body/Politics*, ed. Mary Jacobus, Evelyn Fox Keller, and Sally Shuttleworth (New York: Routledge, 1990), 155–56.
13 The sources I used for this article provide compelling information on interactions among sperm. Lack of space prevents me from taking up this theme here, but the elements include competition, hierarchy, and sacrifice. For a newspaper report, see Malcolm W. Browne, "Some Thoughts on Self Sacrifice," *New York Times* (July 5, 1988), C6. For a literary rendition, see John Barth, "Night-Sea Journey," in his *Lost in the Funhouse* (Garden City, N.Y.: Doubleday, 1968), 3–13.
14 See Carol Delaney, "The Meaning of Paternity and the Virgin Birth Debate," *Man* 21, no. 3 (September 1986): 494–513. She discusses the difference between this scientific view that women contribute genetic material to the fetus and the claim of long-standing Western folk theories that the origin and identity of the fetus comes from the male, as in the metaphor of planting a seed in soil.
15 For a suggested direct link between human behavior and purportedly passive eggs and active sperm, see Erik H. Erikson, "Inner and Outer Space: Reflections on Womanhood," *Daedalus* 93, no. 2 (Spring 1964): 582–606, esp. 591.

16 Guyton (n. 3 above), 619; and Mountcastle (n. 5 above), 1609.
17 Jonathan Miller and David Pelham, *The Facts of Life* (New York: Viking Penguin, 1984), 5.
18 Alberts et al., 796.
19 Ibid., 786.
20 See, e.g., William F. Ganong, *Review of Medical Physiology*, 7th ed. (Los Altos, Calif.: Lange Medical Publications, 1975), 322.
21 Alberts et al. (n. 11 above), 796.
22 Guyton, 615.
23 Solomon (n. 6 above), 683.
24 Vander, Sherman, and Luciano (n. 4 above), 4th ed. (1985), 580.
25 Alberts et al., 796.
26 All biology texts quoted above use the word "penetrate."
27 Solomon, 700.
28 A. Beldecos et al., "The Importance of Feminist Critique for Contemporary Cell Biology," *Hypation* 3, no. 1 (Spring 1988): 61–76.
29 Gerald Sehatten and Helen Schatten, "The Energetic Egg," *Medical World News* 23 (January 23, 1984): 51–53, esp. 51.
30 Alberts et al., 796.
31 Guyton (n. 3 above), 613.
32 Miller and Pelham (n. 17 above), 7.
33 Alberts et al. (n. 11 above), 804.
34 Ibid., 801.
35 Ruth Herschberger, *Adam's Rib* (New York: Pelligrini & Cudaby, 1948), esp. 84. I am indebted to Ruth Hubbard for telling me about Herschberger's work, although at a point when this paper was already in draft form.
36 Bennett M. Shapiro, "The Existential Decision of a Sperm," *Celt* 49, no. 3 (May 1987): 293–94, esp. 293.
37 Lennart Nilsson, "A Portrait of the Sperm," in *The Functional Anatomy of the Spermatozoan*, ed. Bjorn A. Afzelius (New York: Pergamon, 1975), 79–82.
38 Ludwik Fleck, *Genesis and Development of a Scientific Fact*, ed. Thaddeus J. Trenn and Robert K. Merton (Chicago: University of Chicago Press, 1979), 38.
39 Jay M. Baltz carried out the research I describe when he was a graduate student in the Thomas C. Jenkins Department of Biophysics at Johns Hopkins University.
40 Far less is known about the physiology of sperm than comparable female substances, which some feminists claim is no accident. Greater scientific scrutiny of female reproduction has long enabled the burden of birth control to be placed on women. In this case, the researchers' discovery did not depend on development of any new technology. The experiments made use of glass pipettes, a manometer, and a simple microscope, all of which have been available for more than one hundred years.
41 Jay Baltz and Richard A. Cone, "What force Is Needed to Tether a Sperm?" (abstract for Society for the Study of Reproduction, 1985), and "Flagellar Torque on the Head Determines the Force Needed to Tether a Sperm" (abstract for Biophysical Society, 1986).
42 Jay M. Baltz, David F. Katz, and Richard A. Cone, "The Mechanics of the Sperm-Egg Interaction at the Zona Pellucida," *Biophysical Journal* 54, no. 4 (October 1988): 643–54. Lab members were somewhat familiar with work on metaphors in the biology of female reproduction. Richard Cone, who runs the lab, is my husband, and he talked with them about my earlier research on the subject

from time to time. Even though my current research focuses on biological imagery and I heard about the lab's work from my husband every day, I myself did not recognize the role of imagery in the sperm research until many weeks after the period of research and writing I describe. Therefore, I assume that any awareness the lab members may have had about how underlying metaphor might be guiding this particular research was fairly inchoate.

43 Ibid., 643, 650.
44 Schatten and Schatten (n. 29 above), 51.
45 Ibid., 52.
46 Surprisingly, in an article intended for a general audience, the authors do not point out that these are sea urchin sperm and note that human sperm do not shoot out filaments at all.
47 Schatten and Schatten, 53.
48 Paul M. Wassarman, "Fertilization in Mammals," *Scientific American* 259, no. 6 (December 1988): 78–84, esp. 78, 84.
49 Ibid., 78.
50 Ibid., 79.
51 Ibid., 78.
52 Since receptor molecules are relatively *immotile* and the ligands that bind to them relatively *motile*, one might imagine the egg being called the receptor and the sperm the ligand. But the molecules in question on egg and sperm are immotile molecules. It is the sperm as a *cell* that has motility, and the egg as a cell that has relative immotility.
53 Wassarman, 78–79.
54 Paul M. Wassarman, "The Biology and Chemistry of Fertilization," *Science* 235, no. 4788 (January 30, 1987): 553–60, esp. 554.
55 Ibid., 557.
56 Ibid., 557–58. This finding throws into question Schatten and Schatten's description (n. 29 above) of the sperm, its tail beating, diving down into the egg.
57 Deborah R. Gordon, "Tenacious Assumptions in Western Medicine," in *Biomedicine Examined*, ed. Margaret Lock and Deborah Gordon (Dordrecht: Kluwer, 1988), 19–56, esp. 26.
58 Wassarman, "The Biology and Chemistry of Fertilization," 558.
59 Baltz, Katz, and Cone (n. 42 above), 643, 650.
60 Schatten and Schatten, 53.
61 Wassarman, "The Biology and Chemistry of Fertilization," 557.
62 Mary Ellman, *Thinking about Women* (New York: Harcourt Brace Jovanovich, 1968), 140; Nina Auerbach, *Woman and the Demon* (Cambridge, Mass.: Harvard University Press, 1982), esp. 186.
63 Kenneth Alan Adams, "Arachnophobia: Love American Style," *Journal of Psychoanalytic Anthropology* 4, no. 2 (1981): 157–97.
64 William Ray Arney and Bernard Bergen, *Medicine and the Management of Living* (Chicago: University of Chicago Press, 1984).
65 J. F. Hartman, R. B. Gwatkin, and C. F. Hutchison, "Early Contact Interactions between Mammalian Gametes *In Vitro*," *Proceedings of the National Academy of Sciences (U.S.)* 69, no. 10 (1972): 2767–69.
66 Arney and Bergen, 68.
67 Ruth Hubbard, "Have Only Men Evolved?" (n. 12 above), 51–52.
68 David Harvey, personal communication, November 1989.
69 Rosalind Petchesky, "Fetal Images: The Power of Visual Culture in the Politics of Reproduction," *Feminist Studies* 13, no. 2 (Summer 1987): 263–92, esp. 272.

70 Rita Arditti, Renate Klein, and Shelley Minden, *Test-Tube Women* (London: Pandora, 1984); Ellen Goodman, "Whose Right to Life?" *Baltimore Sun* (November 17, 1987); Tamar Lewin, "Courts Acting to Force Care of the Unborn," *New York Times* (November 23, 1987), A1 and B10; Susan Irwin and Brigitte Jordan, "Knowledge, Practice, and Power: Court Ordered Cesarean Sections," *Medical Anthropology Quarterly* 1, no. 3 (September 1987): 319–34.

71 Thanks to Elizabeth Fee and David Spain, who in February 1989 and April 1989, respectively, made points related to this.

Part 2

FROM WOMEN'S HEALTH TO GENDER AND HEALTH: QUESTIONING BINARY THINKING

7

SEXISM, FEMINISM AND MEDICALISM

A decade review of literature on gender and illness

Juanne N. Clarke

Source: *Sociology of Health and Illness*, 5:1 (1983), 62–82.

Abstract

Do we really have a dependent variable in our study of the sex differences in illness and sex differences in the explanations for illness? The purpose of this paper, which reviews the literature in this area over the past decade, is to argue that because of both conceptual and methodological difficulties in the definition of health/illness, there are serious problems in the available analyses to date. Confusions between medical and lay definitions, mental and physical illness, illness *per se* and illness behaviour are among the issues raised with respect to the first issue: conceptual and definitional incommensurability. Proxy respondents, distinctions between males and females in illness experience, and improper rate calculation are among the issues discussed in the section concerning methodology.

Introduction

In a seminal article Constance Nathanson (1975) reviewed the literature published to that date, which explored the causes of sex differences in morbidity and mortality. That women have been regarded as more likely to be ill while men have been found to be more likely to have high rates of mortality is and was one of the most consistent findings in the literature dealing with sex, morbidity and mortality. Women's surplus in illness rates appeared in Nathanson's review to exist with regards to rates of mental illness, physical illness and use of health services. Much-repeated and yet infrequently tested explanatory models for this finding were thought to be the following:

(1) women report more illness than men because it is culturally more acceptable for them to be ill; (2) the sick role is more compatible with women's other role responsibilities; and (3) women have more illness than men because their assigned social roles are more stressful.

(Nathanson, 1975:57)

Nathanson's study is based on a large and growing literature concerned with the relationships between sex and morbidity and sex and mortality.[1]

Despite the plethora of studies on sex and illness, one would have an exceedingly difficult task should one want to describe the differences in the morbidity experience of men and women. When explanations as to the supposed difference are offered, the confusion mounts. The difficulty in describing the health situations of men and women arises from the lack of conceptual and methodological clarity in the very definition and measurement of morbidity and gender. A variety of theoretical and methodological limitations is responsible for the fact that the numerous empirical studies have not led to an increase in understanding the significant aspects of the distinct morbidity/mortality situations of men and women. Thus this paper will not present a summary of the findings from the last decade but rather will attempt to review first the conceptual and then the methodological issues which describe this literature.

The conceptualization of illness and gender

One major difficulty in the conceptualizations of illness and gender[2] is that social scientists have often accepted the categorizations of illness given them by the medical profession and the prevalent sociological versions of gender given them by this male-dominated discipline. This is a problem for two reasons. First, because sociologists have been willing to adopt the models of health and illness prescribed by the powerful medical profession and thus have ignored the unique contribution which the sociological imagination provides. Second, because one group of males (physicians) has dictated to another group of males (sociologists) interpretations of the experiences of women. One example of the implications of the first problem is in the distinction in the sociological literature between mental and physical illness. This distinction is a direct derivative of the specialities evolved by the medical profession. That this is not a necessary differentiation can be illustrated in two different ways. First, it is common for persons to talk about, to explain health, in a holistic manner. People often speak of the way in which particular stress has caused a headache, nervous stomach, sweating palms and so on. Second, there is a growing body of literature demonstrating the irreducible unity of the mind and body (see Herbert Benson, 1979, for example).

The problems which result from the fact that male doctors or male sociologists define women's experience has been amply demonstrated by a number of feminist scholars. Classic examples of this literature are provided in the work of Ehrenreich and English (1973, 1978). Ehrenreich and English argue, in this series of works which are based on historical research, that medicine has made a prime contribution to a sexist description of women as sick, particularly with respect to their reproductive functions and their emotions, and as sickening to men. They demonstrate the ways in which attributing illness to women has served the interests of male doctors. As the authors put it, 'The myth of female frailty, and the very real cult of female hypochondria that seemed to support the myth, played directly to the financial interests of the medical profession'. In the late nineteenth and early twentieth centuries, the regular AMA doctors (members of the American Medical Association – the intellectual ancestors of today's doctors) still had no legal monopoly over medical practice and no legal control over the number of people who called themselves 'doctors'. Competition from lay healers of both sexes, and from what the AMA saw as an excess of naturopaths, osteopaths and other non-allopathic physicians, had doctors running scared. A good part of the competition was female; women lay healers and midwives dominated the urban ghettos and the countryside and in many areas suffragists were beating on the doors of medical school.

For the doctors, the myth of female frailty served two purposes. It helped disqualify women as healers but made women highly qualified as patients (Ehrenreich and English, 1973:23). Contemporary medical practice is based on these historical facts: women's illnesses now tend to be thought (by male doctors) psychogenic in origin, related to women's neurosis and to women's hazardous menstrual and reproductive cycles. Psychotropic drug use which predominates amongst women provides some evidence of the tendency of male doctors to see women's complaints as 'unreal'. Cooperstock and Leonard's (1979) study of the social meaning of the tranquillizer use has shown us how women (and men with somewhat different problems) use mood-altering drugs to help them cope with their unsatisfactory lives and relationships, roles and relationships which are structurally determined.

Women's reproduction and its prevention are major causes of the attendance of women at the offices of physicians. The medicalization of childbirth has generated a great deal of doctoring of women who in contemporary obstetrical practice are obliged by their doctors to have monthly, bimonthly and weekly check-ups during pregnancy and who are increasingly likely to be subjected to Caesarian sections, forceps deliveries and scheduled births.

> The modern ob-gyn emphasizes surgery rather than primary care, a policy that promotes the financial and professional interests of physicians. The belief that female reproductive organs are expendable equipment, dangerous and dysfunctional outside of childbearing,

continues to provide justification for aggressive surgical practices. ... This is organizational deviance and it is institutionalized amongst ob-gyn doctors.

(Scully, 1980: 233–4)

It must be noted here that the evidence is that the involvement of the male doctor in what was once the work of the female midwife has not served the health of the mother or of the baby. Maternal and infant mortality figures which compare historical and societal rates of these variables note the prophylactic value of the midwife.

(Haire, 1972; Arms, 1975)

Recent research sponsored by the AMA has shown that the hysterectomy has become the most frequent operation in the United States and now outranks the tonsillectomy and the appendectomy, the former top surgical contenders (Scully, 1980:17). Equally disturbing is the 1977 editorial cited by Scully in the prestigious *New England Journal of Medicine*, which states that some physicians are recommending prophylactic mastectomies for women with precancerous breast disease even though the definition of 'precancerous' is indeterminate.

Currently, an increasing number of women are entering medical school. We might suppose that when more women become doctors medical care will change. Unfortunately, the effect of this change will be slow to come, because of the present overwhelming dominance of men, and masculine ideologies in the care and cure involved in medicine. That the dominant sex is embedded in the dominant institutional position with respect to health care (Navarro, 1975) has had significant implications for women's notions of their health, bodies and childbirth. Women from the same elite background as our contemporary cadres of male physicians would, in this view, be expected to adopt the values and social conduct of their class equals. Change, in this view, in the medical profession would require an increase in the number of persons of working-class background in medical school.

Indeed, women's illnesses and bodies are regarded as so unusual that a speciality has evolved designed specifically to deal with them (Ob.-Gyn.). Scully and Bart (1981) examined gynaecology texts published from 1943 to 1973 in the United States and noted persistent paternalistic and often condescending attitudes of doctors of this speciality towards female patients. One illustration of this is the following comment regarding women who work in the paid labour force,

> The very recent widening of the sphere of feminine activities, with the assumption of the male function of protection and maintenance, has led to a further weakening of the reproductive urge, resulting in the modern 'smart' type – sexless, frigid, self-sufficient.

The acceptance of the notion that gender is coincidental with sex and that both are bipolar variables is another source of harrowing complications in understanding of the ways in which sex/gender leads to different sorts and levels of illness. The assumption has been that biological sex and sociological gender are each unitary concepts (Tresemer, 1975). A biological male has been thought to be a social male and a biological female a social female. There are several problems here.

> First, biological differentiation is not conclusive proof of gender identity. Boys without penises may become normal males; girls with penises but without uteruses may come to see themselves as female. Socialization, can, at times, reverse the disturbing effects of mixed physical characteristics.
>
> (Eshleman and Clarke, 1978:35)

(See Eshleman and Clarke, 1978 for a more complete discussion of this.) Gender and sex, as many have agreed (see Clarke, 1978 and Eshleman and Clarke, 1978 for a further discussion), are not coincidental. Nor is it correct to think of either sex or gender as unitary concepts. According to John Money there are six crucial determinants in the distinction between male and female: (1) the chromosomes, (2) the hormone balance, (3) the internal genitalia, (4) the external genitalia, (5) the gonads, and (6) the sex of assignment and socialization. Congruity amongst all six elements generally leads to the development of a successful unitary gender identity in a person. Incongruity can lead to a sense of discomfort with the assigned gender, hermaphroditism, or a mixture of 'typically' male and female behaviours in one individual. The maleness and femaleness of these six qualities are not necessarily distinct; one's sex identity is determined by a combination (Eshleman and Clarke, 1978:32). That gender role is not coincidental with sex has been demonstrated in numerous ways, in for instance studies of androgyny, role-reversal, cross-sexuals, and transsexuality. Both gender and sex, as historically defined by male sociologists in male-dominated societies, are conceptually problematic.

Mental illness and gender

Let us turn now to the complexities involved in the meaning of illness and briefly discuss mental illness. Gove and Tudor (1974), define mental illness in an idiosyncratic way to exclude some of the kinds of problems which bring people into psychiatric treatment. They refine and exclude categories until the definition of mental illness refers to a single range of problems only – feelings, emotions or mental states.

> A disorder which involves personal discomfort (as indicated by distress, anxiety, etc.) and/or mental disorganization (as indicated by

confusion, thought blockage, motor retardation, and, in the more extreme cases, by hallucinations and delusions) that is *not* caused by an *organic* or *toxic* condition.

(1974:69, my emphasis)

This definition is useful to their particular hypothesis testing; it allows them to support it. But it does not apply to the way that mental illness is defined by the lay population, by the mental health professionals, those who take censuses of mental illness data, nor to other sociological researchers (e.g. Smith, 1975; Dohrenwend and Dohrenwend, 1976). In addition, physicians have acknowledged women's feelings, moods and so on more than those of men. Women's illnesses are not taken seriously, and are not as likely to be seen as having a biological cause (see Diana Scully for instance, for a discussion of the ways that contemporary Ob.-Gyn. doctors see women's problems, 1980:94–100). Scully observed residents, interns and doctors who were specializing in Ob.-Gyn. for three years and was led to conclude, 'Residents were encouraged to suspect that many "female complaints", including menstrual pain, were psychosomatic' (p. 95).

As Dohrenwend and Dohrenwend declare (1976:1339), Gove and Tudor's (1974) definition 'excludes types of disorders that most experienced psychiatrists and clinical psychologists would include, while including symptomatic distress that experienced clinicians would exclude and combining disparate types of disorders that clinicians would not combine'. Dorothy Smith (1975) would disagree with both Gove and Tudor and Dohrenwend and Dohrenwend because of her view that available mental illness statistics are not a simple reflection of the experiences of wellness and illness in a population. Rather they indicate, in part, the distribution and availability of psychiatrists, beds in psychiatric hospitals, psychologists and other caregivers who have the power to label a caseload as either suffering from mental illness or not. She argues that the usual process of reasoning about mental illness goes something like the following: a situation causes stress; this leads to mental illness which then leads one to seek psychiatric assistance. This model assumes that mental illness is an objective social state which exists prior to treatment. She proposes a different model in which mental illness is not seen as a distinct disease or an entity. It is the last in a chain of events and results from a definition by the social control agencies involved.

Physical illness and gender

The problem is, of course, confounded when we remember that Smith is talking about a process whereby male psychiatrists control the behaviour of patients of different sexes on very different criteria. Definitional incommensurability is not only a characteristic, however, of the mental illness data but also of the physical illness data.

One distinction is between illness and illness behaviour. In this model researchers are concerned to differentiate between physical symptoms and the social behaviour which results from those symptoms. The primacy of the physical is felt to be irrefutable. Others would argue that this is a false dichotomy because human beings are social actors. As such they must continually construct social reality. The physical realm is not separate: it can only be known through social interpretation. From this viewpoint it does not make sense to speak of symptoms except as they are socially constructed. Illness behaviour and not illness *per se* as a physiological construct is the appropriate focus of analysis for the sociologist.

There are three strategies for measuring illness and illness behaviour. These include the self-perceptions of illness as indicated in an interview survey, an assessment made by a physician of the health of an individual and entered on medical records, and standardized clinical examinations (Mechanic, 1976). The first alternative gives an indication of the social experience of health and illness without necessary regard to its medical diagnosis or treatment. Self-report gives data on the meaning made of the experiences of health and illness in the everyday lives of respondents to the extent that this is possible within the constraints and limitations of social survey data. Physical assessment is based both on self-perception and on physiological complaints and, it appears, the biases of specific doctors. There is evidence, for instance, that physicians tend to do more extensive work-ups when men report symptoms than when women report the same symptoms (Armitage et al., 1979). As well, we know that people of different backgrounds (Zborowski, 1952) are more or less sensitive to the same symptoms, and thus present them differently to physicians. Perhaps the least vulnerable to social definition is the third technique for measuring illness, which involves direct physical measurements such as X-rays, blood pressure, blood and urine samples, electrocardiograms and so on.

However, in the same way that mortality rates are known to be affected by the biases of those who sign the death certificates, whether doctors, coroners, or others (Wilkins, 1970; Atkinson, 1971), it seems plausible to suppose that clinically defined measures of physiological characteristics and functioning are similarly in error. If records of an occurrence believed to be so objectively measurable as death are known to be susceptible to social construction it appears at least a possibility that other physiological measures and diagnoses are similarly fated to biases such as sexism.

In addition to the variability in the concept of illness which arises out of viewing it as a self-perceived, clinically diagnosed and/or laboratory-measured phenomenon, there are complex facets of illness within each of these three categories. Thus self-perceived illness itself differs in many respects, from non-existent or unnoticed symptomatology, to mild and transitory, to serious but acute and limited, to chronic and debilitating, to chronic and terminal. It varies in the degree of painfulness, in the extent to which the illness is believed to be stigmatizing; in the extent to which it interrupts the everyday life of the person in other ways; in its contagion and resultant isolation; in the amount of stress it engenders in the person, and his or her family and other relations; in its treatability; in its social meaning; and in its usefulness or message, among other things. In these, and undoubtedly in numerous other ways illness is multifaceted and to some extent experienced differently by different people and differently by the same people at different times.

Even when illness is considered to be that which the physician labels as illness, variations in meaning abound. Clinician's diagnosis involves presence or absence, the degree, the severity or the extensiveness of impairment and specific diagnostic categories among other things.

A standard source for information on the health of the population of the United States of America is the *National Health Survey* which is a repeated questionnaire survey of a stratified random sample of households all over the USA. The health indices included are the following:

> The incidence of acute conditions, number of acute conditions, restricted activity, bed disability and days lost from primary activity, direct acute conditions, overall days of bed disability, physician visits and discharges from shortstay hospitals.
>
> (Nathanson, 1975:57)

As Nathanson suggests, 'Illness, disability and use of health services represent conceptually distinct aspects of areas in which comparability is limited'. In another review Verbrugge (1976), relying essentially on the same data source, defines illness in a more exclusive manner. Here she includes only rates of acute conditions, and chronic conditions, restricted activity days and bed disability days and limitation of activity, and of mobility due to chronic conditions (1976:388). Furthermore, each of these definitions is more specifically defined (e.g. an acute condition is one which began sometime during the two weeks prior to the interview and which involved either medical attention or restricted activity). Verbrugge begins with these rather general, if exclusive, categories from the *National Health Survey*. She then examines particular diagnostic categories such as infective and parasitic diseases, respiratory conditions, digestive system conditions, injuries, and other acute conditions (1976:390). Elaborating then on sex differences with this complex of dependent variables indicating illness, Verbrugge is led to conclude 'that more females have a [chronic] condition but they are less severe than males' conditions', and, on the other hand, females are sicker from acute conditions because they stay in bed and restrict their activity more (p. 397). It seems, with these data at least, whether or not one finds a difference between men and women, and in what direction, depends on the diagnostic category (the definition of the dependent variable).[3]

Gove and Hughes (1979) attempt to examine sex differences in yet another version of illness, what they call 'real illness'. They attempt to deal with the supposition that the differences in male and female rates arise out of reporting (either to physicians or in survey research), not 'real' differences. Verbrugge (1976) and Mechanic (1976), for instance, have argued that the differences are not real but artifacts of the willingness of women to report illness. Verbrugge documents this assertion with some evidence (1977), as she finds that, disease by disease, the sex with the highest likelihood of morbidity is the sex with the highest rate of mortality. Unfortunately the data that Gove and Hughes bring to bear on this issue again define the dependent variable differently, i.e. the response to the question concerning overall general health, felt illness, inability to pursue normal activities and days in bed in the previous two weeks, and 'an index which combined indications of the different types of impairment that were weighed for severity and multiplied by the number of days of their occurrence' (1979:135). In addition, these authors distinguish between mental and physical illness and suggest that mental illness is causally prior to physical illness. To indicate mental illness, Gove and Hughes (1979) use a scale with some validity and reliability (according to two earlier studies in which Gove was involved). While they claim that they have chosen the particular items which were included in the scale so that it does 'not contain items that can be interpreted as physical symptoms of organic disorders', they have not documented this statement. It seems that in contradiction to what the authors believe, 'symptoms' described in the scale are often typical of the experiential component of an illness that is often manifest as physical illness (Benson, 1979). Thus their causal model is in serious jeopardy of suffering from the conceptual and operational overlap of the dependent and independent variables.

Confusions and contradictions abound amongst the concepts of the dependent variable. This is a serious drawback to the accumulation of knowledge. Illness is indicated by self-perceived symptoms presented verbally in a survey research study, by means of the medical records of clinical assessments by physicians who have been approached by lay people because they have seen themselves as ill and in need of treatment, or by physical assessment of specific physiological mechanisms such as blood pressure, galvanic skin response, vision, cholesterol counts, and so on. Rather arbitrary distinctions are made between physical and mental illness. Physical illness is believed to be indicated by days in bed while mental illness is said to be suggested by a series of questions of mood state, or by (psychiatric) diagnosis. These distinctions may not be this clear, however. It seems that when people stay in bed they may be malingering, feeling symptoms of physical illness or those of mental illness such as depression.

Illness is clearly not a unitary concept. To treat it as if there is a clear referent is premature. We do not know enough about the social meaning of illness nor its aetiology accurately to differentiate physical from mental illness. Nor do we know enough about the sense in which days of bed disability, for instance, relate to hospital discharge rate to include them in the same category and call them both by the same name – illness. Additional problems need to be examined when we add other variables in the attempt to explain morbidity rates. It may be that rates of illness are different for men and for women not because men and women have a different proclivity for this 'objective' phenomenon but rather because illness means something quite different to the members of each sex. Days of disability and hospital discharge data could, for instance, result from accidents rather than illness. But accidents might not be considered relevant to respondents who are asked about their chronic or acute ailments. From another perspective it might be argued that accidents, incarceration, alcoholism and cigarette addiction (in which male rates are far larger than female), while not illnesses in the sense that they may not be reported as symptoms in a survey research interview, are nevertheless 'illness' in the sense that they are immediately tied to physiological malfunctioning in the body and, as well, may lead to other more debilitating symptoms and even death. Indeed, illnesses resulting from these behaviours are among the major causes of death for men (Lalonde, 1974).

The larger conceptual issue regarding gender has to do with the validity and efficacy of asking questions about sex differences and explaining these differences in terms of social roles. The problem with this is akin to the story of the blind man who felt the toe of the elephant and exclaimed on the basis of its size and the hardness at its front that it must be a mouse. We are explaining a minuscule and contextless behaviour when the social-structural, cultural and economic forces which move persons dialectically are ignored. Questions about sex and illness are ambiguous unless the social construction of the categories of meaning associated with all of sex, gender and illness are explored in their full social, political and economic surroundings. Social-role hypotheses look at the ways in which women's roles, as domestic labourers, wives, mothers, employers, employees and so on, are associated with different sorts and levels of health and illness. The assumption is that these roles have the same meanings, first, to different women and, then, to women and men; or that the context and the content of domestic labour is comparable across classes, cultural/ethnic groups, educational levels and so on. As Oakley has shown so clearly, even in the sphere of one occupation – housework – this is not the case (Oakley, 1974:61–78). Moreover, this argument ignores the fundamental fact that 'the social situations of men and women today are structurally and ideologically discrepant, and the dominant value system of modern industrialized societies assigns greater importance and prestige to masculine than to feminine roles' (Oakley, 1974:2).

Indisputably, the field of illness research is fraught with innumerable difficulties as the result of the lack of conceptual clarity with regard to the dependent and independent variables.

Methodological issues in the study of illness

Most research in the field of gender roles and illness is positivistic in its orientation. That is, for the most part, research is modelled on the natural and physical sciences: the search for universal causal laws of the if x then y variety; the belief in the possibility of value freedom in empirical observation and analysis; the assumptions of objectivity, replicability, comparability and generalizability characterize this research. All of these are aspects of the methodology which typify epidemiological studies such as those discussed in this paper. Innumerable books and articles have already been written in both a critical and in an accepting vein. A general examination of the methodology is not at issue here. There are particular methodological problems, however, in this health/illness literature.

Biases in health survey research data arising out of the relationship between the interviewers and the respondents have been documented by the US National Centre for Health Statistics (Nathanson, 1977:20). Apparently most information in this routine, recurrent survey is proxy. Approximately 80 per cent of the respondents are women who then give information about themselves, and about the men in their lives. There is a consistent bias which results from the use of proxy respondents. Proxy interviews generally understate the morbidity of the absent person (Nathanson, 1977:20). This could be a serious source of difficulty in the literature, particularly as the hypotheses of interest focus on the comparative rates of illness for men and women. If women are more likely than men to respond in the survey interview and if people who respond tend to under-report the existence of a given phenomenon for those whom they are discussing, it follows that women will – simply as a result of the methodology employed – say that they suffer more illness than the men whose health they are reporting. Yet controls for this sort of bias are not generally forthcoming, nor are their effects widely understood.

The effects of the response characteristics of 'yeasaying' and 'naysaying' and 'social desirability' have also been tentatively explored in this literature (Selltiz et al., 1976). Phillips and Segal (1969) have argued that the reason that the rates of mental illness are generally higher for women is that it is much more acceptable or more socially desirable for women to acknowledge symptoms of weakness or stress. This argument has been applied to the literature on physical illness as well. In fact, one of the major explanatory hypotheses offered – one with a good deal of credibility – is that women are reportedly more likely to be ill because they are more willing to express their disease or distress. Mechanic (1976), however, has argued the point and suggested that men and women are not differentially likely to relate symptoms but rather they are likely to relate different symptoms. Women are more likely to experience distress in terms of physical symptomatology while men are more likely to express distress through 'acting out'. That is, men have been more likely to smoke cigarettes, to drink alcohol, to commit violent crimes and so on. Survey research, in that it does not allow for these sorts of distress symptoms, is sexist in its very definition of illness and illness behaviour.

There are other methodological problems. First, the specific questions which are asked and taken to reflect illness vary from study to study. At times, a general question is asked to indicate whether the respondent believes that his or her overall health is 'poor' or 'good' (see Gove and Hughes, 1979). At times health is viewed as measured by specific symptomatology. In the same study, Gove and Hughes asked respondents whether or not they had had to stay in bed, were unable to do the things that they normally did, or did not feel well during the past two weeks. Gove and Hughes did not equate this variable with the general health variables described above, however, but rather called it functional impairment, a distinct additional aspect of the whole illness experience. Woods (1979), in her reports of morbidity, utilized a description of symptom complexes rather than individual symptoms. A list of possible complaints was read to each subject, who was then asked to indicate which of these had been experienced over the last four weeks. Subjects were then asked to group the symptoms they perceived to be related. It was thought that the person's perceptions of which complaints were related in what was termed a 'symptom complex' would be more relevant to illness patterns and illness behaviour than isolated complaints. In this same study, illness behaviour was distinguished from illness and taken to refer to what subjects had done in response to the symptom complex, such as visiting a health professional, 'Putting down a usual activity, resting in bed, using nonprescription drugs, consulting the lay network, or visiting a health professional' (Woods, 1979). We have already discussed the definitions provided by Nathanson (1977) and Verbrugge (1976) in an earlier section of the paper. Muller defines health/illness exceedingly pragmatically. Health capital, as she terms it, should be based on a definition of health capital for women which is measured by reproductive efficiency and the experiences of women with regard to fertility, general health, employment and household responsibilities (1979:37). Questions range from single-item indicators to multiple-item indicators; from current health in the past two weeks to health in the past two months, to health in the last six months; from health/illness behaviour to health-care utilization rates, from acknowledgment of diagnostic categories, to no acknowledgment of diagnostic categories (cardiovascular and respiratory disease, scarlet fever, typhoid, smallpox, measles, whooping cough, and so on (Ortmeyer, 1979)).

It is difficult to know or to estimate the extent to which we can compare responses to questions which have been asked with such widely discrepant degrees of specificity. To what extent does chronic and/or acute illness refer to the same category of meaning? To what extent can a question of general health refer to the same social experience as a bout of influenza? To what extent do illness behaviours (what people do when they think they are sick) belong in the same reservoir of meaning as the feeling or acknowledgment of a symptom? To what extent do health-care utilization rates correspond to rates of experienced symptomology or to rates of experienced disability? All of these questions remain unanswered. The complexity that is involved in the measurement of physical illness is exacerbated in the realm of 'mental illness': in the first place, because a rather arbitrary distinction between mental and physical illness is made; second, because the measurements of mental illness also frequently vary markedly from study to study.

As was indicated earlier, most health data are gathered by women from women and this is the case whether or not the information is taken to be about men or not. Women have been interviewed out of convenience, since they are much more willing to be interviewed, easier to locate and thus less expensive (in terms of interviewing costs). Official rationales for interviewing wives only would point to the fact that wives know and understand the experiences of their husbands as readily as the husbands themselves. Wives are believed to be the chief caretakers of the well-being of their husbands and, in particular, in this culture are expected to be responsible for the most intimate of the details of the lives of their spouses (feeding, cleaning clothes, and so on). This is an unfortunate assumption because as literature in family sociology has demonstrated, husbands and wives live with very different understandings of the same situations (Bernard, 1972). Discrepant world views and discrepant information seem to be more characteristic of the lives of husbands and wives than not. Saffilios-Rothschild (1970) reviews literature which notes that the range of discrepant responses is from 15 per cent to 30 per cent in one study to 23 per cent to 64 per cent in another study. In particular, it appears that women tend to under-report the illnesses of their husbands. While this phenomenon is of interest in itself and might well tell us more about the construction of the illness experience and label in a marital relationship, wives' answers should not be considered to be valid indicators of the health of husbands.

In addition, the calculation of an overall health score is not unproblematic. Whether or not all types of illness, disability, and health-care utilization figures should be given equal weight remains an open question. It assumes that all of these are of equal value in this complex illness experience we are attempting to study. Further, whether or not illnesses of different diagnostic categorization should be given equal or different weights is also debatable.

Another difficulty with data which are based on available statistics such as hospital discharge rate, first admission to hospital and so on is that they do not take into consideration the proportion of the population of the specific sex in question. That is, we may indeed discover that women are more likely to be admitted to hospital than men. This comparison, however, is unfounded unless we compare the number of women who are hospitalized to the number of women who are not hospitalized and the number of men who are hospitalized to the number of men who are not hospitalized. The independent variable is taken to be sex in this literature and it is the way in which sex affects the probability of illness that is at issue. Thus the percentages or the ratios must be based on the total in the category of the independent variable. The problem is that the best explanation for the greater likelihood of female illness may be that there are more women in the population than men. This problem is particularly noteworthy when we consider the combined effects of age and sex. Older people are more likely to use health services than younger people (Crandall, 1980). There are more older women than older men because women live an average of approximately seven years longer than men (Crandall, 1980; Eshleman and Clarke, 1978). These two facts taken together would lead us to expect that simply by virtue of population sex ratios, older women would comprise a larger proportion of the sick population, not as a result of social factors but simply as the result of the population ratios.

The literature described must be evaluated from another perspective, as well. On the whole, it pays remarkably little attention to reproductive orders and disorders. Although hospital stays for delivery may be exempted when hospital bed and hospital discharge rates, for instance, are calculated, the ways in which the secondary effects of these medical experiences get counted in other health statistics are ignored. Moreover, it could be argued that the experiences of pregnancy, delivery and postpartum examinations sensitize women and indeed, iatrogenically induce in women illnesses (symptoms) which they might not otherwise experience. There is a way in which women's reproductive experiences contaminate the rest of the health experiences of women. There are other serious criticisms of the literature which has been reviewed here and these are epistemological and/or feminist in their orientation. All of the empirical literature criticized is positivist, or social factist (Ritzer, 1975). But as has been argued elsewhere (Clarke, 1981) reliance on positivism provides an inadequate and myopic view of the social world. Activism (Boughey, 1978) would provide us with a needed critical and radical examination of the social action of individuals, groups and societies. It assumes injustice and exploitation. It would include an analysis of the structural determinants of women's alienation, false consciousness, political and economic disenfranchisement and ill-health. The definitionist perspective would describe the subjective, everyday 'lived experience' (McBride and McBride, 1981). It would begin with a trust in the world views of women themselves as recorded by female sociologists.

To incorporate thoroughly the six principles of feminist analysis described by Millman and Kanter (1975) all three paradigms are necessary. They interweave to form a variegated mesh which is more complete because it is multi-faceted. Medical sociology has taken place in the existing society and has taken for granted the structures and values of the existing society. It has also meant that outside attempts at an objective analysis have been stressed at the expense of the subjective meaning to the social actors; that private worlds have been neglected in favour of public worlds; that the potential for a radically altered future has been dismissed in the face of the overwhelming reality of the present; that formal arrangement and structures have been described with the loss of the informal; that male language, models and methods have been utilized to the detriment of women and that sex has not often been taken into account as a factor in behaviour, (see Millman and Kanter (1975) for a fuller discussion of this phenomenon.)

Conclusion

As we have seen, illness is a multi-faceted, complex phenomenon which has been measured in a wide variety of ways in many different studies. Such variability limits severely our ability to generalize from study to study, to treat data as comparable or to establish firm conclusions. How can theory explain why one sex is more likely to be ill than the other when we are not at all sure what is meant by the very concept of illness? When we do not know whether men or women view the same things as symptoms of illness, when we do not know to what extent physicians diagnose the same symptoms differently in men and women, when we do not know about the differential effects on men and women of the hospital experience, how can we theorize about sex differences in illness? Nathanson has summarized the literature to find three possible theoretical explanations for the presumed differences in the morbidity rates of men and women. And yet, there is a way in which there can be no adequate, systematic theory-building as of yet because of the conceptual indeterminacy in the definition and problems in the measurement of illness and gender: that the explanations are to some extent contradictory is not surprising given the state of the research. To redress the imbalance, to turn the dubious conceptions of sex and illness which have been discussed herein on their heads, would demand significant reconceptualization and design in the empirical research in this area.

Notes

1 The following is a list of major studies published in this past decade: Chesler, 1972; Crane, 1975; Dohrenwend and Dohrenwend, 1976, 1977; Ehrenreich and English, 1981; Gove, 1972, 1973, 1980, 1981; Gove and Hughes, 1979; Gove and Tudor, 1974; Mechanic, 1976; Nathanson, 1975, 1977; Radloff, 1977; Renne, 1971; Smith, 1975; Verbrugge, 1976, 1977, 1979; Waldron, 1976; Muller, 1979; Ortmeyer, 1979; Wallen et al., 1979. The critical evaluation which I will offer here is based on these studies.
2 Gender and sex refer to different aspects 'masculine and feminine'. Classification by sex is based on physiologically based properties primarily while classification by gender refers to social dimensions of action as either male or female. For a more

complete discussion see (Tresemer, 1975, Eshleman and Clarke, 1978). From this point on the paper will use the term gender when referring to the research which is being reviewed as it is the more appropriate term.
3 When Dohrenwend and Dohrenwend (1976) re-analyse the trends in sex and mental illness rates first established by Gove and Tudor (1974), they too find correlation reversals with different definitions. Dorothy Smith, reanalysing the Gove and Tudor (1974) findings but using Canadian data and comparing the sex and mental illness rates with different definitions of mental illness, came up with the opposite results.

References

Armitage, Karen J., Schneiderman, L. J. and Bass, Robert A. (1979), 'Response of physicians to medical complaints in men and women', *Journal of the American Medical Association*, 241(20), (May): 2186–7.
Arms, Suzanne (1975), *Immaculate Deception*. Boston: Houghton Mifflin.
Atkinson, J. Maxwell (1971), 'Societal reactions to suicide: the role of coronors' definitions', in Stanley Cohen (ed.), *Images of Deviance*. Harmondsworth: Penguin, pp. 165–81.
Barret, M. and Roberts, H. (1978), 'Doctors and their patients: the social control of women in general practice', in Carol and Barry Smart (eds), *Women, Sexuality and Social Control*. London: Routledge and Kegan Paul.
Benson, Herbert (1979), *The Mind/Body Effect*. New York: Berkley Books.
Bernard, Jessie (1972), *The Future of Marriage*. New York: World.
Bornstein, P. E. et al. (1973), 'The depression of widowhood after thirteen months', *British Journal of Psychiatry*, 122:561–6.
Boughey, Howard (1978), *The Insights of Sociology: An Introduction*. Boston: Allyn & Bacon.
Brown, George W. and Harris, Tirril (1978), *The Social Origins of Depression*. Toronto: Tavistock.
Charmaz, Kathy (1980), *The Social Reality of Death*. Don Mills, Ontario: Addison-Wesley.
Chesler, Phyllis (1972), *Women and Madness*. New York: Avon.
Clarke, Juanne (1978) 'Sex differentiation and its future', *Journal of Comparative Studies*, 9(2), summer.
Clarke, Juanne (1981), 'A multiple paradigm approach to the sociology of medicine, health and illness', *Sociology of Health and Illness*, 3(1), March.
Cooperstock, Ruth, and Lennard, Henry L. (1979), 'Some social meanings of tranquilliser use', *Sociology of Health and Illness*, 1(3).
Corea, Gena (1977), *The Hidden Malpractice: How American Medicine Mistreats Women*, New York: Jove.
Crandall, Richard C. (1980), *Gerontology: A Behavioral Science Approach*. Reading, Mass. Addison-Wesley.
Crane, Diana (1975), *The Sanctity of Social Life: Physicians' Treatment of Critically Ill Patients*. New York: Russell Sage Foundation.
Dohrenwend, Barbara Snell and Dohrenwend, Bruce P. (1974), *Stressful Life Events: Their Nature and Effects*. New York: Wiley.
Dohrenwend, Barbara Snell and Dohrenwend, Bruce P. (1976), 'Sex differences in psychiatric disorders', *American Journal of Sociology*, 91:1447–59.

Dohrenwend, Barbara Snell and Dohrenwend, Bruce P. (1977), 'Reply to Gove and Tudor's comments on "Sex Differences in Psychiatric Disorders"', *American Journal of Sociology*, 82:1336–45.

Ehrenreich, Barbara and English, Deirdre (1972), *Witches, Midwives, and Nurses: A History of Women Healers*. Glass Mountain Pamphlet, no. 1, Old Westbury, New York: The Feminist Press.

Ehrenreich, Barbara and English, Deirdre (1973), *Complaints and Disorders: The Sexual Politics of Sickness*. Glass Mountain Pamphlet, no. 2. Old Westbury, New York: The Feminist Press.

Ehrenreich, Barbara and English, Deirdre (1978), *For Her Own Good: 150 Years of the Expert's Advice to Women*. New York: Anchor Press/Doubleday.

Ehrenreich, Barbara and English, Deirdre (1981), 'The sexual politics of sickness', in Peter Conrad and R. Kern (eds), *The Sociology of Health and Illness*. New York: St Martins.

Eshleman, J. Ross and Clarke, Juanne (1978), *Intimacy, Committments and Marriage; Development of Relationships*. Boston: Allyn & Bacon.

Fox, John W. (1980), 'Gove's specific sex role theory of mental illness: a research note', *Journal of Health and Social Behavior*, 21 (Sept.):260–7.

Gove, Walter R. (1972), 'Sex roles, marital roles and mental illness', *Social Forces*, 51:34–44.

Gove, Walter R. (1973), 'Sex, marital status and mortality', *American Journal of Sociology*, 79:45–67.

Gove, Walter R. and Geerken, Michel R. (1978), 'Response bias in surveys of mental health: an empirical investigation', *American Journal of Sociology*, 82(1), pp. 1289–317.

Gove, Walter R., Hughes, Michael (1979), 'Possible causes of the apparent sex differences in physical health: an empirical investigation', *American Sociological Review*, 44 (Feb.):126–46.

Gove, Walter R., and Hughes, Michael (1980), 'Reply to Mechanic and Verbrugge. Sex differences in physical health and how medical sociologists view illness', *American Sociological Review*, 45 (June):514.

Gove, Walter R., and Hughes, Michael (1981), 'Belief vs. data: more on the illness behavior of men and women', *American Sociological Review*, 46 (Feb.): 125–7.

Gove, Walter R., and Tudor, Jeanette (1974), 'Adult sex roles and mental illness', *American Journal of Sociology*, 78(4), 812–35.

Haire, Doris (1972), *The Cultural Warping of Childbirth*. Rochester, New York: International Childbirth Education Association, 1972).

Kemper, Theodore D. and Bologh, Roslyn Wallach (1981), 'What do you get when you fall in love? Some health status effects', *Sociology of Health and Illness*, 3(1) (March):72–88.

Krause, Elliott H. (1972), *Power and Illness: The Political Sociology of Health and Medical Care*. New York: Elsevier.

Lalonde, Marc (1974), *A New Perspective on the Health of Canadians: A Working Document*. Ottawa: Information Canada.

LaRocco, James M., House, James S. and French, John R. P. (1980), 'Social support, occupational stress – health', *Journal of Health and Social Behavior*, 2(1) (Sept):202–18.

Leeson, Joyce and Gray, Judith (1978), *Women and Medicine.* London: Tavistock Publications.

Lennane, K. Jeanne and Lennane, R. John (1973), 'Alleged psychogenic disorders in women – a possible manifestation of sexual prejudice', *New England Journal of Medicine*, 288.

McBride, Angela B. and McBride, William L. (1981), 'Theoretical Underpinnings for Women's Health', *Women and Health*, Vol 6 (1/2) Spring/Summer, pp. 37–55.

Maddison, David and Agnes, Viola (1968), 'The health of widows in the years following bereavement', *Journal of Psychosomatic Research*, 12:299–306.

Marcus, Alfred C. and Seeman, Teresa E. (1981a), 'Sex differences in health status: a reexamination of the nurturant role hypothesis', *American Sociological Review*, 46 (Feb.).119–23.

Marcus, Alfred C. and Seeman, Teresa E. (1981b), 'Sex differences in reports of illness and disability: a preliminary test of the "fixed role obligations" hypothesis', *Journal of Health and Social Behavior*, 22 (June):179–82.

Mechanic, David (1972), 'The concept of illness behavior', *Journal of Chronic Diseases*, 15:180–94.

Mechanic, David (1976), 'Sex, illness, behavior and the use of health services', *Journal of Human Stress* (Dec.):29–40.

Mechanic, David (1980), 'Comment on Gove and Hughes', *American Sociological Review*, 45 (June):513.

Miller, Jean Baker (1976), *Toward a New Psychology of Women.* Boston: Beacon Press, 1976.

Millman, M., and Kanter, R. M. (1975), *Another Voice: Feminist Perspectives on Social Life and Social Science.* Garden City, N.Y.: Anchor Press.

Muller, Charlotte (1979), 'Women and health statistics: Areas of deficient data collection and integration', *Women and Health*, 4(1) (Spring):37–59.

Nathanson, Constance A. (1975), 'Illness and the feminine role: A theoretical review', *Social Science & Medicine*, 9:57–62.

Nathanson, Constance A. (1977), 'Sex, illness and medical care: A review of data, theory and method', *Social Science & Medicine*, 11:13–25.

Navarro, Vincente (1975), 'Women in health care', *New England Journal of Medicine*, 292, 398–402.

Oakley, Ann (1974), *The Sociology of Housework.* London: Martin Robertson.

Oakley, Ann (1980), *Women Confined: Towards a Sociology of Childbirth.* Oxford: Martin Robertson.

Ortmeyer, Linda E. (1979), 'Female natural advantage? Or, the unhealthy environment of males? The status of sex mortality differentials', *Women and Health*, 4(2) (Summer):121–34.

Parker, D., Wolz, M., Parber, E. and Harford, T. (1980), 'Sex roles and alcohol consumption: A research note', *Journal of Health and Social Behavior*, 21 (March):43–8.

Phillips, D. L. and Segal, B. F. (1969), 'Sexual status and psychiatric symptoms', *American Sociological Review*, 34:58–72.

Radloff, L. (1977), 'Sex differences in depression: the effects of occupation and marital studies', *Sex Roles*, 1:249–65.

Renne, Karen (1971), 'Correlate of dissatisfaction in marriage', *Journal of Marriage and the Family*, 32:54–67.

Roberts, Helen (ed.) (1981), *Doing Feminist Research*. London: Routledge & Kegan Paul.

Reynolds, W. Jeff, Rushing, William and Mils, David (1974), 'The validation of functional status index', *Journal of Health and Social Behavior*, 21:43–8.

Ritzer, George (1975), *Sociology: A Multiple Paradigm Science*, Allyn & Bacon, Boston.

Rohrbaugh, Joanna Bunker (1979), *Women/Psychology's Puzzle*. New York: Basic Books.

Rosenfeld, Sarah (1980), 'Sex differences in depression', *Health and Social Behavior* (March), 21(1).33–42.

Rushing, William (1979), 'Marital status and mental disorder: Evidence in favour of a behavioral model', *Social Forces*, 58(2):540–55.

Saffilios-Rothschild, Constantine (1970), 'A study of family power structure: a review 1960–1969', *Journal of Marriage and the Family* (November):539–49.

Scully, Diana (1980), *Men Who Control Women's Health. The Miseducation of Obstetrician – Gynecologists*. Boston: Houghton Mifflin Company.

Scully, Diana and Bart, Pauline (1981), 'A Funny Thing Happened on the Way to the Orifice: Women in Gynecology Textbooks' in Peter Conrad and R. Kern, (eds), *The Sociology of Health and Illness*. New York: St Martins.

Seaman, Barbara (1972), *Free and Female*. New York: Howard, McCann & Geoghegan.

Selltiz, Claire, Wrightsman, L. S. and Cook, S. W. (1976), *Research Methods in Social Relations*. New York: Holt, Rinehart & Winston.

Singer, Eleanor, Robin Garfinkel, Steven Cohen and Leo Srole (1976), 'Mortality and mental health: evidence from the midtown Manhattan restudy', *Social Science & Medicine*, 10:517–25.

Smith, Dorothy (1974), 'Women's perspective as a radical critique of sociology', *Sociological Enquiry*, 1(1):7–13.

Smith, Dorothy (1975), 'The statistics on mental illness: what they will not tell us about women and why', in *Women Look at Psychiatry*. Vancouver: Press Gang Publishers, pp. 73–119.

Smith, Dorothy E. and David, Sara J. (eds) (1975), *Women Look at Psychiatry*. Vancouver: Press Gang Publishers.

Stellman, Jeanne M. (1971), *Women's work, women's health: Myths and realities*. New York: Pantheon Books.

Stellman, Jeanne M. (1971), *Retirement in American Society*. New York: Cornell University Press.

Sudnow, D. (1967), *Passing On: The Social Organization of Dying*. New York: Prentice Hall.

Tessler, R. and Mechanic, D. (1978), 'Psychological distress and perceived health status', *Journal of Health and Social Behavior*, 19:254–62.

Thoits, Peggy (1981), 'Undesirable life events and psychophysiological distress', *American Sociological Review*, 46(1) (Feb):97–110.

Tresemer, David (1975), 'Assumptions made about gender roles', in Millman and R. M. Kanter (eds), *Another Voice*. Garden City: Anchor Books, pp. 308–39.

Verbrugge, Lois M. (1976), 'Females and illness: Recent trends in sex differences in the United States', *Journal of Health and Social Behavior*, 17 (Dec.):387–403.

Verbrugge, Lois M. (1977), 'Sex differences in morbidity and mortality in the United States', *Journal of Health and Social Behavior*, 17:387:403.

Verbrugge, Lois M. (1977), 'Comment on Walter R. Gove and Michael Hughes', *American Sociological Review*, February. Possible Causes of the Apparent Sex Differences in Physical Health', *American Sociological Review*, 45 (June):507–13.

Verbrugge, Louis M. (1979), 'Female illness rates and illness behavior: Testing hypotheses about sex differences in health', *Women and Health*, 4(1) (Spring), pp. 61–80.

Waitzkin, Howard B. and Waterman, Barbara (1974), *The Exploitation of Illness in Capitalist Society*. Indianapolis: Bobbs-Merrill.

Waldron, Ingrid (1976), 'Why do women live longer than men?' *Social Science & Medicine*, 10:349–62.

Wallen, Jacqueline, Waitzkin, Howard and Stoeckle, John D. (1979), 'Physical stereotypes about female health and illness: A study of patient's sex and the informative process during medical interviews', *Women and Health*, 4(2) (Summer): 135–46.

Warheit, George J., Holzer, Charles, Bill, Roger and Prey, Sandra (1976), 'Sex, marital status, and mental health: A reappraisal', *Social Forces*, 55(2) (Dec.):459–71.

Weissman, Myrna M. and Klerman, Gerald L. (1977), 'Sex differences and the epidimology of depression', *Archives of General Psychiatry*, 34:98–111.

Wilkins, James L. (1970), 'Producing suicides', *American Behavioral Scientist*, 14:135–201.

Wilson, S. J. (1982), *Women, The Family and the Economy*. Toronto: McGraw-Hill, Ryerson.

Woods, Nancy Fugate (1979), 'Symptom reports and illness behavior and employed women and homemakers', *Journal of Community Health*, 5(1) (Fall):95–104.

Zborowski, M. (1952), 'Cultural component in responses to pain', *Journal of Social Issues*, 8:16–30.

Zola, Irving (1972), 'Medicine as an institution of social control', *Sociological Review*, 4.

8

WHAT IS GENDER?

Feminist theory and the sociology of human reproduction

Ellen Annandale and Judith Clark

Source: *Sociology of Health and Illness*, 18:1 (1996), 17–44.

Abstract

Feminist theory and research on the sociology of human reproduction have historically been bound together as each has developed. Yet recently sociologists of reproduction and 'women's health' have lost sight of core debates in feminist theory. They still tend to work with the assumption that feminism is an internally coherent body of thought, despite the emergence of significant internal divisions since the mid-1980s. In this paper we evaluate the challenge that feminist post-structuralism poses to prior conceptualisations of gender in the context of reproductive health through a critique of sociological work in this area from the 1970s and 1980s. We conclude with a critical exploration of the new insights that might emerge from a post-structuralist 'deconstruction' of gender in the context of human reproduction.

Introduction

Feminist scholarship has now been active in the field of medical sociology for well over twenty years. During this period it has mounted a significant challenge to the patriarchal visions of both the sociological and health care establishments. Issues of health and illness were virtually synonymous with the emergence of second wave feminism, yet recently the sociology of health and illness has drifted away from core debates in feminist theory. As previously marginalised theoretical positions become established they often undergo a process of *dissipation*; their conceptual foundations lose their currency as they are incorporated into, or co-opted by, the mainstream (Fine

1993). Much research in the sociology of health and illness now uses feminist theory only tacitly. This means that it is often *derivative* of a particular feminist perspective rather than a close application of its guiding ideas. As a consequence, interpretative frameworks are often more implicit than explicit and researchers tend to work from the assumption that feminism is an internally coherent body of thought. In reality, however, it is increasingly marked by internal divisions. Feminism is widely recognised to have undergone a major transformation during the late 1980s and early 1990s. As Michele Barrett has recently remarked,

> contemporary Western feminism, confident for several years about its 'sex-gender' distinction; analyses of 'patriarchy', or postulation of 'the male gaze' has found all these various categories radically undermined by the new 'deconstructive' emphasis on fluidity and contingency.
>
> (Barrett 1992:202)

Writers in the area of gender and health such as Lesley Doyal (1994) and Deborah Lupton (1994) have drawn our attention to emerging tensions within feminism, but their implications for the way in which we conceptualise the influence of patriarchy upon women's bodies and their health has not yet been fully appreciated. The recent challenge of feminist post-structuralism, in particular, invites us to re-evaluate the current state of gender-related research on reproductive health.

In this paper we reflect upon the contribution that second wave 'modernist feminism' has made to our understanding of gender and health and the challenge that is posed by post-structuralism. The field of gender and health is wide and, since we cannot do justice to the full range of concerns which might be raised in a short paper, we have chosen to focus upon issues in the sociology of reproduction. Reproduction could be viewed as a paradigmatic case since it may embody the contrasts between modernist and postmodernist perspectives in accentuated form. However, feminist work on reproduction has been at the centre of and informs sociological work on gender and health and has at some point been an overriding concern of most of the eminent writers in the field. Concerns with reproduction centre on birth but also encroach upon conceptualisations of health more broadly. Social, legal and medical discourse puts reproduction in the foreground in discussions of individuals' rights and responsibilities, and sociological conceptualisations of women's and men's health develop out of these debates (for example, in dividing lives into the public and the private, work and home *etc*).

The paper begins with a discussion of the post-structuralist critique of the modernist conceptualisations of gender that are embedded in research on the sociology of human reproduction. Particular attention is given to the negative consequences that can arise from feminist thinking which is premised upon a binary division between women and men, male and female, and sex and gender. These consequences include: the universalising and valorising of gender differences; a preoccupation with the abnormalities of women's reproductive health; and a focus on women to the neglect of gender (and men's health) which, it is argued, inhibits our ability truly to understand women's experience. The paper concludes with an exploratory reconceptualisation of gender and reproductive health through the lens of feminist post-structuralism.

Feminist theories, gender and health

The contemporary acceptance of gender as a legitimate area of study in the sociology of health and illness, belies a hard fought and ongoing battle for recognition. Early challenges to male hegemony emphasised women's invisibility (Clarke 1983). Oakley (1974), for example, wrote of women's concealment in academia and the consequent exclusion of areas of social life, such as the domestic world, from the vision of sociology. A distorted picture was created by malestream social theory as it attempted to fit women into pre-defined male-oriented categories. In retrospect, it is clear (Oakley 1985) that sexism in sociology cannot be overcome just by bringing women into the various subareas of the discipline (such as the sociology of work, deviance, the state, and so on), rather the various domains of sociology need restructuring. As second wave feminist theory gained momentum during the 1970s and 1980s, a range of contested approaches began to emerge.

Basic and common to *all* feminisms is the understanding that patriarchy privileges men by taking the male body as the 'standard' and fashioning upon it a range of valued characteristics (such as good health, mastery, reason and so on) and, through a comparison, viewing the female body as deficient, associated with illness, with lack of control and with intuitive rather than reasoned action. In associating 'deficiencies' of the female body with women's *reproductive* capacity, patriarchy conflates biological sex and social gender. The broad task of feminism has been to question this elision by showing that gender is socially constructed. Through this we can identify the social processes that construct the female body as inferior and that discriminate against women (and favour men). At the most general level, then, feminist theories of health, illness and health care have the same task in common: the attempt to show that women's experience of health is socially constructed rather than built directly upon biology or the materiality of the body.

However, there are significant differences in the particular way in which feminists theorise patriarchy and its relationship to health. Indeed, a broad appeal to the *socially constructed* nature of sex and gender itself conceals a range of different positions. For example, much second wave feminist writing refers to the way in which women's social experience (including her health and health care) is mediated by the institutions of patriarchy, usually in oppressive ways. There is the sense that we can lift the veil of the social and reveal the 'reality' beneath. Foucauldian social constructionism develops a quite different agenda. As Nettleton writes, it is an approach which is very 'different to the sociology of medical or scientific knowledge which aims to expose the social, technological or ideological interests which distort or contribute to the creation of certain types of knowledge' (1992:149). Rather, women's bodies and their experience are only *knowable* through the discourses that constitute them. In these terms 'the sexed body can no longer be conceived as the unproblematic biological and factual base upon which gender is inscribed, but must itself be recognised as constructed by discourses and practices that take the body as their target and as their vehicle of expression'. (Gatens, 1992:132).

Differences in the way in which various feminist theories conceptualise the relationship between sex and gender have a number of implications for the way in which we understand women's health. Undoubtedly, a number of objections can be raised against categorising feminist thought: it can obscure more than it reveals and can lead to the stereotyping of particular views (Stacey 1993). Clearly, there is a danger of artificially constructing a common position out of what is, in effect, a continuum of views. However, it is possible to suggest that there are feminists who hold more in common with each other than with other groups of thinkers, while also appreciating that heuristic groupings (such as liberal, radical, marxist, and post-structuralist feminisms) may conceal differences between individual writers.

Liberal feminists argue that there is no intrinsic relationship between sex/biology and gender. Emphasis is placed on women's access to positively valued 'male roles' and male experiences (see Wolf 1994) which are associated with good health. As a consequence of focusing on rational behaviour, the body is mute and passive (Jaggar 1983, Scott and Morgan 1993). Radical feminism takes a contrasting approach which endorses a strong connection between sex and gender. It attempts to undermine patriarchal privilege by positively valuing what is distinctive about the female, rather than the male body. The body is central to, and for some radical feminists effectively determinate of, women's experience. Control over the body is also central to marxist feminism, although many writers in this tradition are critical of what is seen as radical feminism's essentialism, arguing that while the 'biological base' is important, it is modified in different social contexts according to women's historical relationship to the means of production under patriarchy (Allen 1983, Barrett 1980). There are, then, important differences within second wave 'modernist' feminist thought. However, from the perspective of a post-structuralist critique they have much in common. It is to this perspective that we now turn.

Feminist post-structuralism

Some writers claim a particular affinity between feminism and post-structuralism (see Fraser and Nicholson 1990, Hekman 1990) notably in regard to the work of Foucault (Sawicki 1991, Weedon 1987) even though, as will be discussed later in the paper, this affinity is recognised not to be without tensions by many (see Diamond and Quinby 1988, McNay 1992). For some, such as Shilling (1993), feminism itself is an enabling condition (far too lightly acknowledged by male writers (Morris 1988)) for the development of post-structuralist discourses generally, and for particular areas such as the sociology of the body.

With its rejection of the 'grand narratives' of modernist thought, which guarantee some forms of knowledge as legitimate and morally 'right', post-structuralism has forced feminism to confront head-on a range of dilemmas that have been under review for some time. In particular, it is critical of Marxist/socialist and radical feminisms which are premised upon an ultimate 'cause of oppression' (be it patriarchy and/or the class structure) for all women, and which believe that the privileged reason carried by particular social groups, such as the proletariat or women (Haraway 1990, Sarup 1993), is the harbinger of liberation. The work of black feminists (which traverses the spectrum of feminist thought) has been particularly important in drawing attention to the oppressions that can result from the notion of 'sisterhood' (hooks 1984) with its implication that gender is the sole determinant of women's fate (Collins 1990).

It is difficult to provide a concise overview of the defining features of post-structuralist feminism, even speaking of *a* post-structuralism can be seen by some to run the risk of 'violating some of its central values – heterogeneity, multiplicity, and difference' (Flax 1990:188). Central, however, is a reconsideration of prior conceptualisations of the 'subject'. In modernist social thought the individual subject is the prime agent of social transformation. In post-structuralism this is inverted and the focus is on how subjectivity is shaped, not on how individuals shape the world (Linstead 1993). The rejection of any sense of an 'essential subject', coupled with a challenge to the search for original causes (Barrett 1992) and the rational pursuit of reason (Flax 1990), culminates in the view that knowledge (held by the individual, which includes the sociologist) is never authentic. Since we can never uncover 'reality' in pure form or find a guiding logic for social change, a social realist epistemology is clearly rejected (Fox 1993). There is no 'objective reality' out there in the social world to be discovered by the sociologist. Rather, the various 'truths' that seem to exist for us – such as, the existence of women and men, old and young people – are discursive categories created through the use of binary logic.

Jane Flax summarises the appeal of post-structuralism to feminism in the following way. Its focus, she writes, is on 'how to understand and (re)constitute the self, gender, knowledge, social relations, and culture without resorting to linear, holistic, or binary ways of thinking and being' (1990:29). The deconstructive method intends to reveal that gender differences are created textually: the privileged term depends on unconscious displacement or suppression of its opposite (Derrida 1982, Grosz 1990). Thus the category 'woman' depends for its existence on the 'opposite' category 'man'; one cannot be understood without the other. In creating this opposition we artificially, and inappropriately, divide people into two camps. Once we have done this we build a series of other characteristics on top of gender i.e. women are unhealthy, men are healthy; women are irrational, men are rational and so on. It is by this process that man is privileged. The aim in deconstruction is to show that real life experience is not like this; attributes and experiences like acting rationally or being healthy cross-cut gender and are not the province of men or women *as a group*. Central to post-structuralist feminism's political agenda is the aim 'to destabilise – challenge, subvert, reverse, [and] over-turn' (Barrett and Phillips 1992:1) these hierarchical oppositions by recognising commonalities across gender so that men can no longer be easily associated with all that is valued and women with all that is de-valued.

Such an approach is becoming increasingly evident in feminist work in anthropology, psychology and the natural sciences. By the 1980s feminist scientists, in particular biologists, had begun to raise questions not just about androcentricity but also about the dualistic thinking which has led to the construction of the scientific paradigm, which includes biomedicine, as masculine and anything outside it as necessarily feminine and unscientific, constraining our knowledge of the natural world and forcing it into organisations, which might not exist (Bleier 1984).

The biography of Barbara McClintock, a cytogeneticist (Fox Keller 1983), illustrates the way in which the 'masculine paradigm' with its 'male hierarchy' may be called into question. Her challenge to scientific and thus male authority came through a reconceptualisation of the relational order of the behaviour of molecules. Using 'feminine methods': feeling, intuition and ideas of relatedness; in her own terms 'a feeling for the organism', McClintock discovered that the molecules of which the cells are composed, rather than being directed by what Crick and Watson had called a 'master molecule' with its implicit hierarchical order, were controlled through their complex interaction. A similar challenge came from Fox Keller's (1985) account of the 'pacemaker concept' in theories of aggregation in cellular slime mould. Fox Keller was interested in the differentiation of cells from the same initial cell in morphogenic development. Cellular slime mould provided an interesting case since it has the 'property of existing alternatively as single cells or as a multicellular organism' (1985:151). In questioning the triggers for aggregation, Fox Keller found that what were later to be called pacemaker or founder cells, were not needed; aggregation could occur without prior differentiation. In much the same way that a 'master molecule' concept held sway in the McClintock story, Fox Keller reveals here that a monocausal 'governor understanding' cut out more 'global, interactive accounts' (1985:155) of cell diffusion until the 1980s.

Twentieth century science increasingly shows a tendency to abandon the certainty of Enlightenment ideas such as Newtonian physics. Although it would be inappropriate to call McClintock's or Fox Keller's work feminist, a number of feminist writers on science have addressed themes which are consistent with a postmodernist position in their call for a science which is 'de-centred, pluralistic, non-hierarchical and hermeneutic' (Hekman 1990:226). But, in broader terms, feminism has been reluctant to recognise this such that 'no major feminist critic of science has explicitly embraced postmodernism' (Hekman 1990:331). The advocacy of a distinctly feminist standpoint epistomology in particular takes us a long way from such a position. In this regard McClintock's acceptance into the 'male scientific community' justified through her award of a Nobel Prize, raises a number of issues. Does her work involve a reconceptualisation of science in which a new approach is legitimated and a multi-faceted scientific paradigm is the result? Or, might it represent a 'male take over', in which men incorporate 'feminine' methods into scientific practice, turning science once more into a gender-blind activity? Referring to Fox Keller's (1985) description of McClintock's style, Hekman quite appropriately warns that,

> to appeal to intuition as opposed to reason ... entails not a displacement of [the] gender-based dichotomy, but an attempt to move from one side of the hierarchy to its opposite, to privilege the disprivileged side. The advocacy of intuition involves reifying the distinction between reason and emotion, rationality and irrationality that is central to Enlightenment epistemology. What is needed is not a reliance on intuition to the exclusion of reason but a means of breaking down the distinction between the two modes of thought.
>
> (1990:132–3)

Though undoubtedly the complex of modern medicine comprises many paradigms, the extent to which dualism is embedded in our thinking may only be fully appreciated when investigating the healing systems of other societies. For example, Ngubane (1976) has illustrated the ways that concepts of health, illness and treatment among the Zulu are related to the whole person within the physical and social environment. Ots (1990) has confronted the problem of dualistic thought in his work in Chinese medicine, showing that whereas in the Western system of medicine, emotions and somatic function are separated, in Chinese thinking they are not. Emotional changes and specific somatic dysfunction are recognised but seen as corresponding and sometimes identical. Duality is collapsed thus making possible, for example, 'the melancholy spleen'. In contradistinction, recent therapies in the USA and Europe use the privileged status of the mind in the treatment of cancer (Delvecchio Good *et al.* 1990, Gordon 1990, Pandolphi 1990).

Hutheesing in 'Becoming a Lisu Woman' explains that, 'I needed the study of a minority group to understand my own Western assumptions of oppression and of the superimposition of male and female' (1993:99). In her explanation of the gender system, 'women were both "superior" and "inferior" depending on the context of the situation and the frame of reference of the observer'. In a study of motherhood, in many ways similar to that of Oakley (1980), Schrijvers (1993), a feminist anthropologist, has shown how her conceptualisations changed with the experience of resistance in the early 1970s to trying to combine motherhood with work, and the relative freedom she experienced in Sri Lanka where work and motherhood were the norm. Her conceptualisations changed as she 'confronted the different experiences and images of mothering both in herself and those subjects involved' (1993:156). This gave rise, in her own words, to a 'multivocal discourse' dependent upon its historical, local and personal location (1993:156).

In contradistinction to developments in feminist anthropology and feminist science, suggestions of ways to improve women's health and health care from the sociology of health and illness appear to retain the legacy of binary thinking making a basic distinction between men and women, reproduction and production, home and work, emotion and reason and so on. The *privileges* which inhere in the binaristic conceptualisations which gird health care are clearly criticised, but the *oppositions themselves* tend to go unchallenged. In these terms critique centres on the *consequences of dualisms* for women's health while failing to offer a thoroughgoing *criticism of them* in the context of gender. Ironically, this means that feminism can end up colluding with biomedicine as it engages and perpetuates the very modernist (*i.e.* binary) thinking which has historically sustained male hegemony. We turn now to an exploration of how this takes place.

The post-structuralist critique applied to the sociology of reproduction

From the perspective of feminist post-structuralism binaristic thinking has had a number of negative consequences for research on gender and health. These include: the universalising of women's health and health care experience and, in some cases, the valorisation of gender differences; a preoccupation with the abnormal and the pathologisation of women's health; the production of poorly drawn health care 'alternatives' and the homogenisation of the 'mainstream'; and, finally, a focus on women rather than gender (and a consequent lack of attention to men's health).

The universalising of women's experience and the valorisation of gender differences

In summarising the dilemma of 'modernist' feminism, Di Stefano (1990:73) writes that 'the choice seems to be one between a politics and epistemology of identity (sameness) or difference'. This is an ongoing debate among feminists, for example psychologists have struggled with the consequences of the substantiation of these positions through scientific evidence (Kitzinger, 1994). More broadly, in 'equality feminism' identified in early work (Beauvoir, Freidan etc.) and in contemporary liberal feminist work (especially in the USA; see Wolf, 1994) there is an appeal to gender-neutral humanism where a central place is given to the rational subject (Jaggar 1983, Tong 1992). Concern is with the particular roles and statuses that men and women inhabit. Explicitly or implicitly, women's circumstances (which includes her health) are problematic because she is excluded from the valued social positions held by men (for example, the world of paid employment). In the 1970s, political agendas centred quite appropriately upon identifying barriers (particularly legal and educational) to women's access to the public sphere. This body of thought has had a considerable influence upon research on the gendered patterning of illness (see Verbrugge 1985).[1] Yet here men are still the standard against which women are defined, a position which also holds for radical feminist work, even though the latter operates within an epistemology of difference rather than identity. Referring to the problems of assimilation for women, Di Stefano aptly characterises the counter-appeal of radical feminism; 'the critical activity and insight produced by the voice of the other [*i.e.* women] provides a visceral, tangible sense of alternatives' (1990:71). Yet, as she goes on to note, the 'choice' between improving women's conditions (and, in our terms, their health) by reference to either sameness (liberal feminism) *or* difference (radical feminism) is a pseudo-choice since it is a choice already framed by a 'gendered narrative of *us* and *them*' (1990:73).

Post-structuralist feminism 'stands on the back of' this previous work. Indeed, as Bordo notes, how 'could we now speak of the differences that inflect *gender* if gender had not first been shown to make a difference?' (1990:141). Aware of the need to keep in mind that radical feminism is not a unitary position (Hanmer 1990), we can nonetheless identify as a common theme the designation of patriarchy as the root of oppression militating against any possibility of 'equality on men's terms' (Rowland and Klein 1990). While it is clearly recognised in most of this work that women are located differently by geography, age, class and race, and may experience oppression differently, there is simultaneously the view that women form an inherent class.

Feminised difference is a project for the elimination of women's oppression which is, importantly for our concern with health, built around control of the body. Women's embodiment (as differentiated from that of men) is crucially anchored in reproduction and a given affinity with 'nature'. The extent to which this work is imbued with essentialism is a subject of quite heated debate in feminism. Essentialism can be defined as a belief in a true essence 'that is most irreducible, unchanging, and therefore constitutive of a given person or thing' (Fuss 1989:2). Here female/male can be seen as prior to the social experience mapped onto them. Essentialism has been argued to underpin much of radical feminism through the work of such writers as Mary Daly, Andrea Dworkin, Adrienne Rich and Susan Griffin all of whom have given attention to issues of women's health.

The term radical feminism, of course, covers a wide spectrum of thought. (Ramazanoglu (1989) identifies it as the feminism most difficult to define because of its diversity.) In its *strongest* form there is a celebration of women's bodies and the capacity to nurture and create (Gatens 1992), and motherhood is celebrated (Weedon 1987). There is a sense of a pure and original femininity, a female essence outside of the social and untainted by patriarchy (Fuss 1989). The work of Nancy Chodorow (1978) exemplifies this. For Chodorow, a distinct self is formed out of the process of mothering which creates women as different from men through the formation of an essentially *relational* form of interaction with others. In these terms, women must reclaim their bodies from men. The following quote from Lipshitz illustrates this perspective; 'women are witchlike in being able to give birth to live beings and are therefore possessors of an invisible internal substance that provokes fear because it links them to another world than that of male culture' (1978:39). Similarly, Rich summarises her views in the following way,

> I have come to believe ... that female biology ... has far more radical implications than we have yet come to appreciate. Patriarchal thought has limited female biology to its own narrow specifications. The feminist vision has recoiled from female biology for these reasons; it will, I believe, come to view our physicality as a resource, rather than a destiny. In order to live a fully human life we require not only control of our bodies ..., we must touch the unity and resonance of our physicality, our bond with the natural order, the corporeal ground of our intelligence.
>
> (1992:39)

Rich sees men as jealous and fearful of women's reproductive power. Mary Daly calls for women to discover a new identity founded on 'true' femaleness, based on women's biological nature: 'for we are rooted, as are animals and trees, wind and seas, in the Earth's substance. Our origins are in her elements' (Daly 1984:4). Aspects of femaleness are not open to men and here the '"true" female self is identified with wild, undomesticated nature' (Weedon 1987:134).

In the writing of some radical feminists' experience is valorised in gendered terms through the explicit claim of a superior female morality (Tong 1992, Segal 1987). Griffin exclaims – 'we are mothers ... the small body lying against our body vulnerable ... we love this body, because we are part of the body ... If men bore children, we imagine, they would burst from their heads ... and be fully grown, and dressed, and god-like, with no need to eat, no substance pouring from their substance' (1980:72–3). Here, then, men are different from women; even if they *could* give birth, that birth and their child would be very different to the child of woman; their experience would be very different, less 'real'.

Of course, not all radical feminists adhere to this 'strong' position. Even those who once appeared to do so have begun to re-think their earlier work. For example, in the 1970s edition of *Of Woman Born* Adrienne Rich wrote: 'the diffuse, intense sensuality radiating out from clitoris, breasts, uterus, vagina; the lunar cycles of menstruation; the gestation and fruition of life which can take place in the female body' (1970:39), has as yet unrealised radical implications. To live a fully human life, Rich wrote, women must realise their 'bond with the natural order.' In the new preface to the 1992 edition of the same book, she writes that she never intended her work to lend itself to sentimentalisation of women's nurturance, and that she would now no longer envisage patriarchy as a pure product (Rich 1992). Andrea Dworkin (1988), whose work is often singled out as essentialist, claims that the whole criticism of essentialism is misplaced. She writes that essentialism is biological determinism, virtually equivalent to Nazism and, as such, has no rightful place in feminism. The debate over feminist essentialism is, then, highly contested and unresolved. With its freight of reductivist determinism, 'essentialism' is likely to be a position that most feminists would want to avoid. Nonetheless, it does seem fair to say that the notion of a 'raw material' that women hold in common, often provides the starting point for the social construction of gender in radical feminism. For example, Rowland and Klein wish to avoid a determinist logic built around the body in favour of a constructivist position, but still remark that 'the fact that women belong to the social group which has the capacity for procreation and mothering, and the fact that men belong to the group that has the capacity to carry out, and does, acts of rape and violence against women, must intrude into the consciousness of being male and female (1990:297–8).

Within contemporary feminism the essentialist position which politicises the body through biological difference inherits some of the problems for which the natural science paradigm has been criticised. Classification, within this paradigm (Barnes 1982) proceeds on the basis of similarities and differences according to the particular properties which objects have. There is in this procedure a clear and precise ordering of data such that a future instance of a particular object has a predetermined classification. In consideration of the biological categorisation of sex, based upon chromosome composition, categoric distinctions may be made between male and female.

Critics have pointed to the tendency of feminist work which centres on difference to collapse a distinction between sex and gender. This occlusion continues in feminist work despite research which shows that markers for sex at birth are drawn from continuous data (Birke 1992, Shilling 1993). Between two and three per cent of individuals are born with inter-sexual characteristics. But, despite the fact that there is no absolute distinction between the sexes only 'variations on a continuum whose midpoints are less densely populated than its outer edges', 'there is great cultural pressure to erase these midpoints' (Epstein 1990:124). The experience of living on these boundaries and the pressure to 'chose sides' is poignantly demonstrated in the writings of Herculine Barbin (Foucault 1980). Physicians are under great cultural pressure to mark sex at birth and to use surgical and hormonal interventions to maintain binary gender as an absolute (Epstein 1990).

Hence, we can see biology as 'distorted' by socio-legal classification as gender differences are socially created (Delphy 1993) by the suppression of similarities and the exaggeration of differences (Connell 1987). A classification based on traits, and the search for a 'universally correct' position (Davis 1992) forces us into oversimplification and acceptance of a uni-dimensionality, dichotomies artificially drawn and the possible consequences of an essentialist picture of women which is false. The conventional use of a classification procedure of semantic differences and the structure of language may be seen at one and the same time as both conservative and oppressive. This is not to adopt an anti-essentialist stance, but only to point out that

> a danger underlies the strategy of difference, a danger that deploying commonalities *among* women unavoidably embeds such traits *within* women. Thus, feminist efforts to transform differences between women and men, differences we have assumed are socially constructed and therefore subject to change, may have the unwanted effect of perpetuating gender as an essential, irreducible part of identity.
>
> (Frug 1992:36)

While it is evident that social science work on gender, health and health care may not have explicitly adopted the perspectives that we have outlined, it is in many ways *derivative* of them and, because of this, it inherits their underlying dualistic and, arguably, essentialist thought where,

> what both feminists and phallocentrists see as hegemony based on masculine perceptions of domination, performance, hierarchy, abstraction, and rationality, finds its antipode in a woman's community proclaiming itself as naturally nurturant, receptive, cooperative, intimate, and exulting in the emotions ... [feminists] assume that

such principles exist and that they have been fixed and dichotomous since the dawn of patriarchal history. . . . *Thus it is that the dominant culture and the counterculture engage in a curious collusion in which . . . a rebellious feminism takes up its assigned position at the negative pole.*

(Cocks 1984:33, 34 our emphasis)

Central to the post-structuralist line of argument, then, is the point that duality can become more enslaving than liberating. Reproduction is centred in universal discourses in sociological work on health care; in reclaiming birth (from male obstetrics), it can become the province of all women. Eisenstein, referring to women and the law, expresses this well; she writes: when the "difference" of childbearing homogenises females as mothers, mothers are denied their individuality: all women become the same – mothers – which immediately characterises them as "different" from men' (1988:90). Thus in an attempt to create what we can term a 'reverse privilege', reproduction is still *centred* for women and put on the agenda as if it were central to all women's lives. This may serve to lock women *into* reproductive roles which may be politically problematic since the centrality of reproduction, contraception and childbirth to *biomedicine* is transferred to women's experiences. This *may be* the reality of their experience, but equally importantly, it may not. To a certain extent this may be seen as an unavoidable consequence of a critique which appears as if it must engage the dichotomies of biomedicine to develop its own narrative.

Pre-occupation with the abnormal: criticisms of obstetrics and the proposed midwifery alternative

In the area of reproduction, and more broadly, there is a pre-occupation with the *abnormal*. The critique (quite rightly) points to the iatrogenic properties of biomedicine but, unfortunately, this again centres on pathology. Ironically, it is almost as if women cannot be well any more (and, as discussed below, men cannot be ill) – witness the large number of books on women's health *problems* (with the emphasis on problems) within both the academic and more popular press. To a degree this serves to confirm women's disadvantaged cultural position through their (ill) health.

'Alternatives' to male-biomedicine were heavily valorised in research in the 1970s and 1980s. This was particularly evident in suggested alternatives to mainstream gynaecological and obstetric care. Sheila Kitzinger, for example, wrote that

the new midwifery has a vital part to play in the woman's movement and is at the very centre of the great creative upheaval which is taking place as we reclaim our bodies and come to learn about, understand and glory in them. This new midwifery gives vivid expression to the way in which women are discovering strength and sisterhood as we turn to help and support one another during the intense, exhilarating and powerful experience of childbirth.

(1988:18)

A clear line of demarcation tends to be drawn in the literature between obstetrics and midwifery: each is portrayed as a unitary and internally coherent body of thought and practice which is at odds with the other (see Oakley 1984, Graham and Oakley 1986, Rothman 1982). The 'alternative' female-midwifery is clearly put forward as the better model. The assumption that we can uncover a contraposition which is unitary has been pervasive in research on the conduct of birth. The fact that the alternative form of maternity care proposed in research in the 1970s and 1980s was not *explicitly stated* as a need *for all groups of women* (ethnic minorities, different social classes, ages etc.) and, instead, that potential different needs were silenced, only serves to underscore the universalistic assumptions of much of this research. The charge of elitism evidenced in the privileged white middle-class voice of much research, and the silence around differences between women, applies well to Barbara Katz Rothman's influential 1982 work *In Labour, Women and Power in the Birth Place* which ends with an implicit call for a home-based natural birth experience (in contrast to an earlier experience of giving birth in hospital). This is made in joyous terms with little recognition that many women may not be in the position to avail themselves of such an 'alternative' even if they wanted to. If we conceive of power as a fundamentally male preserve we are led to gloss over ways in which women may exert power over others (Flax 1990), including other women (Annandale 1988, hooks, 1984). In these terms, as recent institutional reforms stimulate community midwifery (Winterton Report, 1992 and responses to it) midwives may begin to consider the notion of affinity with women embedded in such concepts as 'continuity of care' (in historical and contemporary contexts) as masking the potential exploitation of midwives by their clients (Hardy 1993).

The demarcation between obstetrics and midwifery begins to explain why we have an extremely poorly drawn picture of 'alternatives' (be it in childbirth or any other area) – they exist in opposition to dominant practice 'A' (obstetrics) but they do not appear as 'B', but as 'not A'. Within this framework the lived experience of midwifery (for example) is revealed only as the largely unresearched antithesis of obstetrics. An alternative is called into existence in powerful and convincing terms, while at the same time its central precepts (such as 'women controlled', 'natural birth') are vaguely drawn and in practical terms carry little meaning. Thus feminist work tends to enter into complicity with male hegemonic culture by attributing to it the power which it gives itself. Cocks writes that the more feminism 'describes itself as all the established society is not, the more it shows itself an unwitting prisoner of the established conceptual schema, which delineates for it definition and counterdefinition, image and counterimage (1984:33). Power and control are conceptualised as oppositional and all encompassing; women become, in Sawicki's words, 'passive objects of medical surveillance and management', 'patriarchal models of thinking and behaving, and the technological instruments of patriarchy, become inherently dominating, controlling and objectifying' (1991:76, 73). Women can become victims.

There is an appeal to a return to what childbirth 'really is', yet as Treichler (1990) maintains, this is untenable since discourse *itself* is the site in which birth becomes knowable. 'Alternatives' (or forms of resistance) are poorly drawn precisely because their meaning is always constructed through a process of deferral (Derrida 1982, Fox 1992). We would argue that alternatives' such as 'natural birth' are *relational concepts* constituted *through* dialogue with biomedicine. Obstetrics and midwifery are self-referential: natural birth finds the conditions for its existence in its very critique of biomedicine (as, in much the same terms, obstetrics developed historically).

The frameworks of women, their partners and friends, midwives, nurses and obstetricians are unlikely to be opposed in an ontological sense but instead may elide and collide in response to local contexts. Thus the dominant discourse (of obstetrics, for example) *must* itself create the conditions, or discursive space, for a reverse or alternative form. Indeed, the very existence of the dominant form depends on points of resistance to act as a target and support (Burrell 1988). So power is a resource for action and it is possible (or, perhaps, even necessary) to recognise areas such as childbirth as a contested site in both contemporary and historical form. Such an approach moves away from a passive conceptualisation of women controlled by obstetrics (while still recognising the institutional power of dominant discourse), and presumes the co-presence of a contested voice.

Men's health

We turn now to a third consequence of binary thinking in feminist research on gender and health which is that there has been a focus on women rather than gender, and that men's health has been relatively ignored. Much of the feminist discourse on health and social experience centres on women and cuts out men. This can be problematic even in areas which have in recent traditions been reclaimed as female. As Eisenstein notes, this means that 'femininity and biological motherhood are one and the same; masculinity and fatherhood [can] have no similar biological relationship (1988:91). Christine Delphy has recently questioned what she terms 'the maternal demand' in the women's movement which sees the baby as 'automatically affiliated to the woman who brought it into the world' (1992:16). This, she writes, circumscribes women's identity to motherhood, assumes that only a parent can defend a child, and gives exorbitant rights to some groups (women) and not others (men).

Explanation for the invisibility of men in the reproductive process cannot rest with duality alone since cross culturally and historically childbirth has been and still is very largely the province of women, but the entrenchment of women in their reproductive role can leave men without one (Meerabeau 1991, Mason 1993). This lack of involvement, as a consequence, is particularly evident in the investigations and treatments of infertility where researchers (see McNeil *et al.* 1990) have quite rightly pointed to the pathologisation of women's reproductive systems and have significantly questioned the object of technologically assisted reproduction. Yet it is interesting to note that despite this invocation and the questioning of why men have not been the focus of *medicine*'s attention, sociologists have gone little way towards an understanding of aspects of male infertility themselves. Part of the reason for this may be that, once again, at one and the same time as they criticise *biomedicine*'s pathologisation of women, sociologists also engage its problematic as they replicate a focus on abnormalities of women's reproduction (although, see Tiefer, 1987). As Pfeffer states, 'implicit in the medical definitions and unchallenged by feminists, is the assumption that the male reproductive system is structurally efficient, and that its functions proceed smoothly' (1985:31). Just as biomedicine fractures social experience, so too can social science research on infertility, where social relations of gender (between men and women and between men and between women) are displaced as women and men are posed as opposites and attention is on individuals rather than the relations between them.

A further consequence of ignoring men and treating women as *a priori distinct* from men is that women's health is constructed as 'poor' against an implicit assumption that male health is 'good'. Ironically, man is privileged as unproblematic or is exempted from determination by gender roles (Flax 1990). In such a view women 'cannot' be well and, importantly at this point in our argument, men cannot be ill; they are 'needed' to be well to construe women as sick. Men's poor health remains invisible. This is a fundamental problem, not just because it is important to look at the social context of men's health, but that the assumption of absolute difference undermines our ability even to understand women's health (as different).

A growing body of both qualitative and quantitative research reveals that women either 'are' or perceive themselves to be more ill than men and make more use of health services (Kandrack *et al.* 1991, Verbrugge 1985). In some interpretations of quantitative data where men and women are distinguished, male health status is glossed over since it is relevant only to construct women's health as poor in relative terms. While data may indeed portray worse health among women (the factor which tends to be focused on in interpretation), they are also likely to show a residue of ill health among men to be worthy of study (see Blaxter 1990).

This ironic privileging of male bodies as healthy is also becoming apparent in theoretical work. For example, Shilling's (1993) recent study of the body and social theory contains a discussion of 'naturalistic views of the body' which focuses overwhelmingly on women's bodies. Where men are referred to, it is only to provide an unarticulated point of contrast for women. Thus feminist work on body size and shape (i.e. Chernin 1983, Orbach 1988) is discussed as problematic for its reliance on the essentialist premise that women's bodies have natural shapes and sizes which are distorted by society/patriarchy. Whatever the merits of this criticism in and of itself, Shilling's placing of it in the foreground to the neglect of any possible equivalent concerns among men, only serves to promote body shape and size as 'women's difficulty' and to demote any problems experienced by men. And, attendant upon this, body size and shape as an issue which might cross-cut gender is removed from discussion altogether.

As has been pointed out, the invisibility of the male body as an explicit research focus is 'constructed through and within a wider framework of male dominance' (Hearn and Morgan 1990:7) and this may serve to keep male activities hidden from critical scrutiny. There are, then, from a feminist perspective, a number of 'dangers' in treating the construction of masculinity in men as conceptually equivalent to that of femininity in women. If investigation of the social construction of male-masculinity centres on revealing the 'down side' of masculinity there can be problems if it is suggested that 'female' should be added to 'male' qualities (Ramazanoglu 1992). If this happens, 'the exploration of men's pain is then an area which needs very careful critical attention if men are not to emerge both as the dominant gender and as the "real" victims of masculinity' (Ramazanoglu 1992:346). Yet there is no reason why these concerns cannot be kept to the fore while we also remain cognizant of the possibility that 'patriarchal discourse need not be seen as homogeneous and uniformity oppressive' (Pringle and Watson 1992:130) for women or uniformly liberating and unproblematic for men, and that women do not need to be portrayed as inevitable victims and men as victors. Finally, in the context of health and health care, similarities between women and men and differences between women and between men can be made as pertinent as commonalities built on the elision of sex and gender (Annandale and Hunt, 1990).

Theorising gender in the context of reproductive health

Taking reproduction as a paradigmatic case, we have tried to illustrate one way in which a conventional understanding of the world and relations of power embedded in engendered difference has been reached. Implicit in the feminist post-structuralist critique has been the position that we might begin to explore gender and health in a different way; that we might dislodge the opposition between men and women and recognise the ground in between (Eisenstein 1988).

However, the movement towards such an approach is highly contested by many feminists. Central to their concern is the possibility that deconstruction will diffuse feminist politics. For example, Barrett and Phillips ask whether 'feminists can or should destabilise the binary opposition between men and women that gives the category woman its meaning' (1992:8) and question whether to do so might pull the rug from under the feminist struggle. Mascia-Lees et al. (1989) note the concern that post-structuralist feminism may *itself* be a metaphor for loss of ground felt by men in a period of change in global power relations. In these terms, post-structuralism might, in fact, operate in the service of white male knowledge/power (Bordo 1990). For some, the implicit androcentricity of the work of Derrida, Lacan, Foucault and others, renders their work an entirely inappropriate base for the development of feminism. Jackson voices her concern that in post-structuralism, '"women" are all being deconstructed out of existence, and "gender" is replacing women as the starting point of feminist analysis' (1992:31). In her view, 'the logical outcome of postmodernism is . . . postfeminism'. For these reasons many feminists are openly sceptical about any alliance with post-structuralism.

Clearly, these concerns deserve serious consideration. There is an understandable disquiet about relinquishing 'structures' which appear to embody an emancipatory capacity (Lovibond 1993) and which, it is felt, are the only form in which oppression can be signified. But post-structuralism does not inevitably eradicate a politics of gender. It does not deny poverty, racism and sexism, rather it rejects the ability of 'grand theories' to provide answers to these problems (Smart 1990). Recent commentaries have begun to suggest that by counterposing its own distinct epistemology against forms of 'modernist' thought, post-structuralist feminism ends up setting up a dichotomy itself, ironically undermining its own position by buying into the very duality which it seeks to undermine. This has led some (see Spivak 1989) to suggest that feminist politics can best proceed through a 'strategic' use of theory. In these terms the conditions of women's lived experience (including her health) can sometimes be improved by acting 'as if women are a category (Riley 1988) and sometimes by emphasising the plurality of experience (which may cross-cut gender).

In this last section we tentatively suggest some ways in which a reconceptualisation of gender might be achieved considering as we do the paradoxes and consequences that are integral to it. Pivotal to such a reconceptualisation is the necessary deconstruction of the culture/nature dualism, for although it has not always historically been the case that culture has been privileged over nature (Jordanova 1989), the critique of medical and scientific discourse, and in particular of childbirth in the decade 1970–1980, has illustrated and reaffirmed the association and affinity of women with nature and their cultural domination by men.

As well as disaggregating the elided dualisms of male/female, culture/nature, masculine/feminine, mind/body, and deconstructing each dualism itself, reconceptualisation also of necessity involves the destabilisation of existing theories, or at the very least, a preparedness to come to terms with the dilemmas posed by contradictory ideologies (Davis 1992, Frug 1992, Harding 1991). This process may be fraught with methodological problems as feminists try to avoid oversimplification and wrestle with the complexities of women's lives as they are bound up with social class, ethnicity, education and the social environment. The complexities of specific situations and contingency may be accommodated through the classificatory system which Barnes (1982) calls 'finitism', where concepts are developed through a procedure in which, rather than through their similarities and differences, objects or phenomena are assessed according to their contingent properties at one particular point in time. Such mutability of concepts allows the continuous data of sex, mentioned earlier, and the problem of their undecidability, to be taken care of. In theory, with situation and contingency accounted for, the possibility is opened up for sex and gender differences to be asserted, only when necessary or desired.

In practice, however, detachment from, or assertion of, a sex and gender identity may be difficult to achieve particularly at the lay-professional interface of the medical encounter, where the elision of dualisms is met head on. Patients see themselves and doctors see their patients in gendered terms. For the patients, the gendered view emerges from a holistic conception (Saltonstall 1993) of the 'lived body', while for doctors this may be overlaid with the dualism of the 'Cartesian model'. Whether perceived in a holistic or dualistic manner, the likely consequences in consultations which involve issues of contraception, fertility, pregnancy, childbirth and other conditions affecting the sex organs, would be affirmation and reinforcement of a sex and gender identity, thus inhibiting gender's strategic use.

However, paradoxically, through the use of high technology medicine (which can be viewed as an integral part of the 'Cartesian model'), medical specialists may assist men and women to overcome a gendered notion of their bodies. Foetal imagery and *in vitro* fertilisation and the accompanying medical language may present them with an ungendered if not dismembered view of themselves. Davis-Floyd's (1994) research in America into women's views about the use of technology in childbirth revealed that for some women 'technocratic control', as it has been characterised, was highly valued and provided an empowering experience for them. A similar conclusion has been reached by Evans' (1985) research in Britain. The discovery that women found the use of technology a liberating experience was a finding contradictory to the feminist researcher's view, yet, as Davis-Floyd (1994) points out, somehow the plurality of women's experiences has to be recognised. Here is an example of women, through their doctors, using technology to meet their own ends, and, by recognising that they did so, of an attempt by the feminist researcher to be reflexive about her advocacy of a particular stance in a particular situation (Davis 1992). What is emerging from this discussion is that whilst the body remains a source of political contention, women's liberation may arise from reconceptualisations of it.

Grosz refers to the use of 'hinge' terms as a means of reconceptualising dichotomies (1990:97). In Derrida's terms new concepts 'function as undecidibility, vacillating between both oppositional terms, occupying the ground of their "excluded' middle"' (Derrida 1982:9). For Grosz (1990) this provides a way for feminism to debate the place of patriarchy while not working within its binary logic. New terms are to serve crucially to disrupt and erode the power of 'normalizing discourses', to open up space for suppressed heterogeneity and differences (Flax 1990).

Applied in the context of gender and health, the body, as a hinge term constituted through social relations, is both culture and nature; 'only human bodies create culture and in the process transform themselves corporeally (as well as conceptually)' (Grosz quoted in Wiltshire 1992:17). In both creating and being transformed by culture, the body as culture and nature is by the same token both sex and gender. In the future, new creations of culture raise the possibility of the body, in concept and configuration, as neither sexed nor gendered. In the continuous data of sex, this process may already be in its early stages of development.

In providing a way through which the reproductive body and its processes may be perceived – for example, the nineteenth century notion of menstruation as 'menstrual economy' (Jalland and Hooper 1986), or the twentieth century medical textbook metaphor of 'signal response', or women's notion of 'hassle' (Martin 1987) – metaphorical language not only demonstrates its relevance to historical and cultural understanding, but also opens up the possibility of reconceptualisations and change. The construction of metaphors engages both empiricism and creativity, so it can be argued they unite reason and imagination (Lakoff and Johnson 1980) thus solving the problem which Hekman (1990) alerted us to in her discussion of the deconstruction of gender in feminist science (referred to on page 23). By requiring us to understand one concept through another, the use of paradoxical terms enables the metaphor to destabilise our conventional understandings (Clark and Williams 1992) and allows the generation of new meanings.

In relation to human reproduction, metaphors for the womb have fixed women historically and culturally, reflecting and constituting their notions of themselves and their connection to the foetus. As in Grosz's (1990) use of hinge terms mentioned above, the metaphors which women use also resolve the nature/culture dichotomy, through expressions which relate to the work that they do. Cooking metaphors, for example, date back to medieval Europe, where the foetus was dough baked in the oven (Gelis 1991) and are paralleled in the twentieth century by the notion of an empty womb as a plundered kitchen (Feldman-Savelsberg 1994), or the agrarian metaphor of a barren field, denoting infertility (Jeffrey *et al.* 1989). Clearly, while such metaphors help to break down the nature/culture dichotomy, this is achieved by 'fixing' gender in a binary way revealing that metaphorical thinking can be as oppressive as it is liberating. In the examples that have been given, female reproduction is fixed through domestic imagery, other metaphors annex male reproduction with instrumentality – firing blanks in the context of infertility, for example. However, the construction of *new* metaphors can serve a different purpose, helping us to dislodge gendered thinking in the context of fertility-infertility. For example, if we envisage the body as a 'network' we are pushed in the direction of seeing reproduction as an integrated system and fertility-infertility as the product of the *inter*-relation of bodies. The system metaphor traverses the feminised (domesticity) and masculinised (instrumentality) dichotomy refiguring the reproductive body in a new way.

In such terms sociologists of reproduction would be led away from focusing on 'women's problems' and the pathologisation of women's bodies that was discussed earlier in the paper. Interestingly, this would have an affinity with postmodern visions of the body which some have argued are becoming apparent in medicine. For example, Levin and Solomon (1990) suggest that the new scientific approach of the late twentieth century leads us to see the body in a qualitatively different way from the past. The old biomedical model, it is argued, has been replaced by a postmodern alternative which asks medical science to 'abandon its model of simple causes and work out a new model of multifactoral influence: a model for which the network, rather than the straight arrow, might be an appropriate heuristic symbol' (Levin and Solomon 1990:520). Levin and Solomon claim that this new postmodern vision of the workings of the body which attends to the complex bidirectional interactions between the central nervous system, the immune system and experience, increasingly dissolves 'the three long-standing dualisms of mind and body, body and environment, individual and population' (Levin and Solomon 1990:533).

Exegeses on the postmodern condition, taken alongside a concern with the metaphorical body, turn our attention to the possibility that attempts to create the space for new relations of gender (in the manner discussed above) may be stimulated by broader social changes. In the work of Lyotard (1986), Jameson (1984) and others, new forms of technology and information are seen as central to a shift from a social order built upon production to one centred on reproduction/consumption. Haraway refers to the move from an organic, industrial society to a 'polymorphous, information system' (1990:203). In such a context, the body comes to be seen as a project ripe for construction and reconstruction (Bordo 1993) as previously conceived boundaries (for example, between mind and body) blur. Shilling portrays the irony of this, while rationalization may have provided us with the potential to control our bodies more than ever before, and have them controlled by others, its double-edged nature has also reduced our certainty over what constitutes a body, and where one body finishes and another starts.

(1993:38)

Combining a focus on gender relations in postmodernity with a concern for overturning traditional gender dichotomies, Haraway refers to the 'informatics of domination' (1990:203). The new informatics refigure women in new ways,

the actual situation of women is their integration/exploitation into a world system of production/reproduction and communication called the informatics of domination. The home, work place, market, public arena, the body itself – all can be dispersed and interfaced in nearly infinite, polymorphous ways, with large consequences for women and others – consequences which are very different for different people and which make potent oppositional international movements difficult to image and essential for survival.

(Haraway 1990:205)

In such a context, Haraway argues, it is no longer possible to conceive of lives in terms of public/private, personal/political, market/home and so on. Machines, she claims, have made ambiguous the difference of natural and artificial, mind and body. To be sure, there are 'dangers' for women, but these cannot be seen as a product of masculinism-capitalism. Haraway employs a 'network image' in place of these dichotomies 'suggesting the profusion of spaces and identities and the permeability of boundaries in the personal body and in the body politic' (1990:212). In the school, work place, hospital, 'if we learn how to read . . . webs of power and social life, we might learn new couplings' (1990:212). She discusses new high-technology work in Silicon Valley, California recognising the problems that accrue from the restructuring of work (for example, the feminisation of poverty, high levels of male unemployment), but argues that high-technology (in the world of work and more broadly) challenges dualism since it is no longer 'clear who makes and who is made in the relation between human and machine. It is not clear what is mind and what is body in machines that resolve into coding practices' (1990:219). Haraway uses the image of the cyborg (a hybrid machine-organism), stating that 'insofar as we know ourselves in both formal discourse (*e.g.* biology) and in daily practice (*e.g.* the homework economy . . .), we find ourselves to be cyborgs, hybrids, mosaics, chimeras' (1990:219–20). Cyborg imagery is, then, another way in which to deconstruct duality and challenge the theoretical positions which construct science/technology (including that around birth) as 'simply' male demonology.

Concluding comment

Feminist theory is in the midst of significant change. The recent emergence of feminist post-structuralism has thrown long-standing debates over the notion of a 'sisterhood' among women, and the issue of essentialism into particular relief, generating heated debates that look set to run for some time to come.

Post-structuralism contests the binary conceptualisations of gender that have traditionally girded the sociology of human reproduction. It suggests that feminist thinking which is premised upon a binary division between women and men, male and female, and sex and gender reinforces women's oppression rather than emancipates them. Universalising discourses draw attention towards commonalities within women (and within men) and draw attention away from differences within men and women, and from commonalities that cross-cut gender. The method of deconstruction that is integral to feminist post-structuralism has a clear political agenda: it seeks to destabilise gender as a hierarchical binary opposition and find the ground in between (Eisenstein 1988) so that men can no longer be easily associated with all that is valued and women with all that is de-valued in society. In the context of the sociology of human reproduction this provides an added impetus to the reconceptualisation of fertility-infertility in inter-relational terms (rather than as 'women's difficulty'), and attempts to decouple the historical association of women with reproduction which has long sustained male hegemony.

Acknowledgments

We wish to thank two anonymous referees of the journal for their very helpful comments on an earlier version of this paper.

Note

1 Research on social roles and health tends to conceptualise women's and men's health in these terms, linking health to specific roles (such as paid worker, marital status and so on, Nathanson 1980). Here the adherence to normative dualism resonates of liberal feminist assumptions which underpin much of the research in this area. In survey research the differences that are assumed are often not even explored since until quite recently samples were often sex-specific and different questions about roles were asked of men and women.

References

Allen, J. (1983) Marxism and the man question. In Allen, J. and Patton, P. (eds) *Beyond Marxism*. Leichardt: Intervention Publishing.

Annandale, E. (1988) How midwives accomplish natural birth: managing risk and balancing expectations, *Social Problems*, 35, 95–110.

Annandale, E. and Hunt, K. (1990) Masculinity, femininity and sex: an exploration of their relative contribution to explaining gender differences in health, *Sociology of Health and Illness*, 12, 24–46.
Barnes, B. (1982) *T. S. Kuhn and Social Science*. London: Macmillan.
Barrett, M. (1980) *Women's Oppression Today*. New York: New Left Books.
Barrett, M. (1992) Words and things: materialism and method in contemporary feminist analysis. In Barrett, M. and Phillips, A. (eds) *Destabilizing Theory*. Cambridge: Polity Press.
Barrett, M. and Phillips, A. (1992) 'Introduction'. In Barrett, M. and Phillips, A. (eds) *Destabilizing Theory*. Cambridge: Polity Press.
Birke, L. (1992) 'In pursuit of difference: scientific studies of women and men.' In Kirkup, G. and Smith Keller, L. (eds) *Science, Technology and Gender*. Milton Keynes: Open University Press.
Blaxter, M. (1990) *Health and Lifestyles*. London: Routledge.
Bleier, R. (1984) *Science and Gender: A Critique of Biology and its Theories on Women*. Oxford: Pergamon Press.
Bordo, S. (1990) 'Feminism, postmodernism, and gender-scepticism.' In Nicholson, L. (ed) *Feminism/Postmodernism*. London: Routledge.
Bordo, S. (1993) *Unbearable Weight. Feminism, Western Culture and the Body*. London: University of California Press.
Burrell, G. (1988) Modernism, postmodernism and organisational analysis 2: the contribution of Michel Foucault, *Organisation Studies*, 9/2, 221–35.
Chernin, K. (1983) *Womansize. The Tyranny of Slenderness*. London: Woman's Press.
Chodorow, N. (1978) *The Reproduction of Mothering*. London: University of California Press.
Clark, J. and Williams, K. (1992) Meaning and Metaphor In *Jane Eyre. Warwick Working Papers in Sociology*, No. 19.
Clarke, J. (1983) Sexism, feminism and medicalisation: a decade review. *Sociology of Health & Illness*, 5, 62–81.
Cocks, J. (1984) Wordless emotions: some critical reflections on radical feminism. *Politics and Society*, 13, 27–58.
Collins, P. (1990) *Black Feminist Thought*. London: Harper Collins Academic.
Connell, R. (1987) *Gender and Power*. Cambridge: Polity.
Daly, M. (1984) *Pure Lust, Elemental Feminist Philosophy*. London: Women's Press.
Davis, K. (1992) Towards a feminist rhetoric: the Gilligan debate revisited, *Social Science & Medicine*, 15, 219–31.
Davis-Floyd, R. W. (1994) The technocratic body: American childbirth as cultural expression, *Social Science & Medicine*, 38, 1125–40.
Delphy, C. (1992) Mothers' Union?, *Trouble and Strife*, 24, 12–19.
Delphy, C. (1993) Rethinking sex and gender, *Women's Studies International Forum*, 16, 1–9.
Delvecchio Good, M. Good, B. J. Schaffer, C. and Lind, S. E. (1990) American oncology and the discourse of hope, *Culture, Medicine and Psychiatry*, 14, 59–79.
Derrida, J. (1982) *Margins of Philosophy*. London: Harvester Press.
Di Stefano, C. (1990) 'Dilemmas of difference: feminism, modernity, and post-modernism.' In Nicholson, L. (ed) *Feminism/Postmodernism*. London: Routledge.

Diamond, I. and Quinby, L. (1988) (eds) *Feminism and Foucault. Reflections on Resistance*. Boston: Northeastern University Press.

Doyal, L. (1994) 'Challenging medicine? Gender and the politics of health care.' In Gabe, J., Kelleher, D. and Williams, G. (eds) *Challenging Medicine*. London: Routledge.

Dworkin, A. (1988) Dangerous and deadly, *Trouble and Strife*, 14, 42–5.

Eisenstein, Z. R. (1988) *The Female Body and the Law*. London: University of California Press.

Epstein, J. (1990) Either/Or – Neither/Both: Sexual ambiguity and the ideology of gender, *Genders*, 7 (Spring), 99–142.

Evans, F. (1985) 'Managers and labourers: women's attitudes to reproductive technology.' In Faulkner, W. and Arnold, E. (eds) *Smothered by Invention*. London: Pluto Press.

Feldman-Savelsberg, P. (1994) Plundered kitchens and empty wombs: fear of infertility in the Cameroonian grassfields, *Social Science & Medicine*, 39, 463–74.

Fine, G. A. (1993) The sad demise, mysterious disappearance, and glorious triumph of symbolic interactionism, *Annual Review of Sociology*, 19, 61–87.

Flax, J. (1990) *Thinking Fragments: Psychoanalysis, Feminism, and Postmodernism in the Contemporary West*. Oxford: University of California Press.

Foucault, M. (1980) *Herculine Barbin, Being the Recently Discovered Memoirs of a Nineteenth Century French Hermaphrodite* (trans R. McDougall) New York: Pantheon.

Fox, N. (1992) Poststructuralism and the sociology of health and illness, *Medical Sociology News*, 18, 34–38.

Fox, N. (1993) *Postmodernism, Sociology and Health*. Buckingham: Open University Press.

Fox Keller, E. (1983) *A Feeling For the Organism*. New York: Freeman.

Fox Keller, E. (1985) *Reflections on Gender and Science*. Princeton: Yale University Press.

Fraser, N. and Nicholson, L. (1990) 'Social criticism without philosophy: an encounter between feminism and postmodernism'. In Nicholson, L. (ed) *Feminism/Postmodernism*. London: Routledge.

Frug, M. J. (1992) *Postmodern Legal Feminism*. London: Routledge.

Fuss, D. (1989) *Essentially Speaking*. London: Routledge.

Gatens, M. (1992) 'Power, bodies and difference.' In Barrett, M. and Phillips, A. (eds) *Destabilizing Theory*. Cambridge: Polity Press.

Gelis, J. (1991) *History of Childbirth: Fertility, Pregnancy and Birth in Early Modern Europe*. Cambridge: Polity Press.

Gordon, R. (1990) Embodying illness, embodying cancer, *Culture, Medicine and Psychiatry*, 14, 275–98.

Graham, H. and Oakley, A. (1986) 'Competing ideologies of reproduction: medical and maternal perspectives on pregnancy.' In Currer, C. and Stacey, M. (eds) *Concepts of Health, Illness and Disease*. Leamington Spa: Berg.

Griffin, S. (1980) *Women and Nature: The Roaring Inside Her*. New York: Harper and Row.

Grosz, E. (1990) 'Contemporary theories of power and subjectivity.' In Gunew, S. (ed) *Feminist Knowledge: Critique and Construct*. London: Routledge.

Hanmer, J. (1990) 'Men, power and the exploitation of women.' In Hearn, J. and Morgan, D. (eds) *Men, Masculinities and Social Theory*. London: Unwin Hyman.

Haraway, D. (1990) 'A manifesto for cyborgs: science, technology, and socialist feminism in the 1980s.' In Nicholson, L. (ed) *Feminism/Postmodernism*. London: Routledge.

Harding, S. (1991) *Whose Science, Whose Knowledge? Thinking From Women's Lives*. Milton Keynes: Open University Press.

Hardy, J. (1993) *Challenging Childbirth. How Should Midwives Respond?* Unpublished MA Thesis, Warwick University.

Hearn, J. and Morgan, D. (1990) 'Men, masculinities and social theory.' In Hearn, J. and Morgan, D. (eds) *Men, Masculinities and Social Theory*. London: Unwin Hyman.

Hekman, S. (1990) *Gender and Knowledge: Elements of a Postmodern Feminism*. Cambridge: Polity Press.

hooks, b. (1984) *Feminist Theory. From Margin to Centre*. Boston: South End Press.

Hutheesing, O. K. (1993) 'Facework of a female elder in a Lisu field, Thailand.' In Bell, D. Caplan, P. and Karim, W. J. (eds) *Gendered Fields. Women, Men and Ethnography*. London: Routledge.

Jackson, S. (1992) The amazing deconstructing woman, *Trouble and Strife*, 25 (winter), 25–31.

Jaggar, A. (1983) *Feminist Politics and Human Nature*. New Jersey: Roman and Allanheld.

Jalland, P. and Hooper, J. (1986) *Women From Birth to Death. The Female Life Cycle in Britain 1830–1914*. London: Harvester Press.

Jameson, F. (1984) Postmodernism, or the cultural logic of late capitalism, *New Left Review*, 146, 53–93.

Jeffrey, P. Jeffrey, R. and Lyon, A. (1989) *Labour Pains and Labour Power. Women and Childbearing in India*. London: Zed Books.

Jordanova, L. J. (1989) *Sexual Visions. Images of Gender in Science and Medicine Between the Eighteenth and Nineteenth Centuries*. London: Harvester Wheatsheaf.

Kandrack, M. Grant, K. and Segall, A. (1991) Gender differences in health related behaviour: some unanswered questions, *Social Science & Medicine*, 32, 579–90.

Kitzinger, C. (1994) Sex differences research: feminist perspectives, *Feminism and Psychology*, 4, 501–6.

Kitzinger, S. (ed) (1988) *The Midwife Challenge*. London: Pandora.

Lakoff, G. and Johnson, M. (1980) *Metaphors We Live By*. Chicago: Chicago University Press.

Levin, D. M. and Solomon, G. F. (1990) The discursive formation of the body in the history of medicine. *Journal of Medicine and Philosophy*, 15, 515–37.

Linstead, S. (1993) 'Deconstruction in the study of organisations.' In Hassard, J. and Parker, M. (eds) *Postmodernism and Organisations*. London: Sage.

Lipshitz, S. (1978) *Tearing the Veil, Essays on Femininity*. London: Routledge and Kegan Paul.

Lovibond, S. (1993) 'Feminism and postmodernism.' In Docherty, T. (ed) *Postmodernism: A Reader*. London: Harvester Wheatsheaf.

Lupton, D. (1994) *Medicine as Culture*. London: Sage.

Lyotard, J-F. (1986) *The Postmodern Condition: A Report on Knowledge*. Manchester: Manchester University Press.

McNay, L. (1992) *Foucault and Feminism*. Cambridge: Polity Press.
McNeil, M., Varcoe, I. and Yearley, S. (1990) *The New Reproductive Technologies*. Basingstoke: Macmillan.
Martin, E. (1987) *The Woman in the Body*. Milton Keynes: Open University Press.
Mascia-Lees, F., Sharpe, P. and Ballerino Cohen, C. (1989) The postmodern turn in Anthropology: cautions from a feminist perspective, *Signs*, 15, 7–33.
Mason, M-C. (1993) *Male Infertility – Men Talking*. London: Routledge.
Meerabeau, L. (1991) Husbands' participation in fertility treatment. They also serve who stand and wait, *Sociology of Health and Illness*, 13, 396–410.
Morris, M. (1988) *The Pirate's Fiancée. Feminism Reading Postmodernism*. London: Verso.
Nathanson, C. (1980) Social roles and health status among women: the significance of paid employment, *Social Science & Medicine*, 14a, 463–71.
Nettleton, S. (1992) *Power, Pain and Dentistry*. Buckingham: Open University Press.
Ngubane, H. (1976) 'Some aspects of treatment among the Zulu.' In London, J. B. (ed) *Social Anthropology and Medicine*. London: London University Press.
Oakley, A. (1974) *The Sociology of Housework*. New York: Pantheon.
Oakley, A. (1985) *The Sociology of Housework*. Oxford: Blackwell.
Oakley, A. (1984) *The Captured Womb*. Oxford: Blackwell.
Oakley, A. (1980) *Women Confined. Towards a Sociology of Childbirth*. New York: Schocken Books.
Orbach, S. (1988) *Fat is a Feminist Issue*. London: Arrow Books.
Ots, T. (1990) The angry liver, the anxious heart and the melancholy spleen. The phenomenology of perceptions in Chinese culture, *Culture, Medicine and Psychiatry*, 14, 21–58.
Pandolphi, M. (1990) Boundaries inside the body. Women's suffering in Southern peasant Italy, *Culture, Medicine and Psychiatry*, 14, 255–74.
Pringle, R. and Watson, S. (1992) 'Women's interests' and the post-structuralist state. In Barrett, M. and Phillips, A. (eds) *Destabilizing Theory. Contemporary Feminist Debates*. Cambridge: Polity.
Pfeffer, N. (1985) 'The hidden pathology of the male reproductive system.' In Homans, H. (ed) *The Sexual Politics of Reproduction*. Aldershot: Gower.
Ramazanoglu, C. (1989) *Feminism and the Contradictions of Oppression*. London: Routledge.
Ramazanoglu, C. (1992) 'What can you do with a man? Feminism and the critical appraisal of masculinity.' *Women's Studies International Forum*. 15, 339–50.
Rich, A. (1970) *Of Woman Born*. London: Virago.
Rich, A. (1992) *Of Woman Born*. London: Virago.
Riley, D. (1988) *'Am I that name?' Feminism and the Category of 'Women' in History*. Minneapolis: University of Minnesota Press.
Rothman, B. (1982) *In Labour. Women and Power in the Birth Place*. London: Junction Books.
Rowland, R. and Klein, R. D. (1990) 'Radical feminism: critique and construct.' In Gunew, S. (ed) *Feminist Knowledge: Critique and Construct*. London: Routledge.
Saltonstall, R. (1993) Healthy bodies, social bodies: men's and women's concepts and practices of health in everyday life, *Social Science & Medicine*, 36, 7–14.
Sarup, M. (1993) *An Introductory Guide to Post-structuralism and Postmodernism* (2nd edition). London: Harvester Wheatsheaf.

Sawicki, J. (1991) *Disciplining Foucault: Feminism, Power and the Body*. London: Routledge.
Schrijvers, J. (1993) 'Motherhood experienced and conceptualised: changing images in Sri Lanka and the Netherlands.' In Bell, D., Caplan, P. and Karim, W. J. (eds) *Gendered Fields. Women, Men and Ethnography*. London: Routledge.
Scott, S. and Morgan, D. (1993) (eds) *Body Matters*. London: Falmer Press.
Segal, L. (1987) *Is the Future Female?* London: Virago.
Shilling, C. (1993) *The Body and Social Theory*. London: Sage.
Smart, C. (1990) 'Feminist approaches to criminology or postmodern woman meets atavistic man.' In Gelsthorpe, L. and Morris, A. (eds) *Feminist Perspectives in Criminology*. Milton Keynes: Open University Press.
Spivak, G. (1989) with Ronney, E. 'In a word' Interview in *Differences*. 1, 124–56.
Stacey, J. (1993) 'Untangling feminist theory.' In Richardson, D. and Robinson, V. (eds) *Introducing Women's Studies*. London: Macmillan.
Tiefer, T. (1987) 'In pursuit of the perfect penis.' In Kimmel, M. S. (ed) *Changing Men*. London: Sage.
Tong, R. (1992) *Feminist Thought*. London: Routledge.
Treichler, P. A. (1990) 'Feminism, medicine and the meaning of childbirth.' In Jacobs, M., Fox Keller, E. and Shuttleworth, S. (eds) *Body/Politics. Women and the Discourse of Science*. London: Routledge.
Verbrugge, L. (1985) Gender and health: an update on hypotheses and evidence, *Journal of Health and Social Behavior*, 26, 156–82.
Weedon, C. (1987) *Feminist Practice and Poststructuralist Theory*. Oxford: Blackwell.
Wiltshire, J. (1992) *Jane Austen and the Body*. Cambridge: Cambridge University Press.
Winterton (1992) *Health Committee Report on Maternity Services*. London: H.M.S.O.
Wolf, N. (1994) *Fire With Fire*. London: Vintage Books.

9
WHO IS EPIDEMIOLOGICALLY FATHOMABLE IN THE HIV/AIDS EPIDEMIC?

Gender, sexuality, and intersectionality in public health

Shari L. Dworkin

Source: *Culture, Health and Sexuality*, 7:6 (2005), 615–23.

Abstract

This paper examines the shifting nature of contemporary epidemiological classifications in the HIV/AIDS epidemic. It first looks at assumptions that guide a discourse of vulnerability and circulate around risk categories. It then examines the underlying emphasis in public health on the popular frame of "vulnerable women" who acquire HIV through heterosexual transmission. Drawing on work on gender, sexuality, and intersectionality, the paper asks why a discourse of vulnerability is infused into discussions of heterosexually-active women's HIV risks but not those pertaining to heterosexually-active men's. The paper then moves to current surveillance categories that are hierarchically and differentially applied to women's and men's risks in the HIV epidemic. Here, the focus is on the way in which contemporary classifications allow for the emergence of the vulnerable heterosexually-active woman while simultaneously constituting lack of fathomability concerning bisexual and lesbian transmission risk. Lastly, theories of intersectionality, are used to examine current research on woman-to-woman transmission, and to suggest future more productive options.

She is the leading lady in the AIDS epidemic. She was under the surface, hidden, but finally emerged, rushed forward with newfound breath, born into existence with twin shoves: first, feminism; next epidemiological fathomability and visibility. She appeared in 1993 as vulnerable.

By the end of 1992, over 18,500 women in the United States had officially died of AIDS (Centers for Disease Control (CDC) 2002b). At the time, the AIDS case definition used by the US Centers for Disease Control did not include several disease manifestations common to women, including invasive cervical cancer and recurrent vaginal yeast infections (Hankins and Handley 1992). Following pressure from women's groups, a wealth of international data, and in conjunction with Council of State and Territorial Epidemiologists (CTSE), the CDC proposed an expansion of the AIDS surveillance case definition and solicited public comments in November 1991 (CDC 1992a). On September 2, 1992, the CDC held an open meeting in Atlanta to review information on the need for an expanded case definition (CDC 1992b). The AIDS case definition was formally expanded in 1993 (CDC 1992b, c).

And out she came. Officially via the tropes of heterosexuality and vulnerability. This is not to suggest that such a debut does not reflect a genuine trend in the epidemic at the time. Indeed, from 1987 to 1992, just prior to the CDC change, the number of AIDS cases for women in the USA increased by more than 1000%, with heterosexual contact reported to account for 60% of the identifiable risk for women (CDC 1993). However, once the case definition had changed, there was a veritable and discursive explosion, with reported cases of HIV in women increasing from 6,571 in 1992 to 16,824 in 1993 (Stine 2003).

Newfound visibility meant that women might be less likely to be excluded from drug trials and from studies of disease progression than they had been in the past (Fox-Tierney *et al.* 1999). At the juncture of a continually shifting base of medical knowledge, feminism, epidemiological classifications, sexual stratification systems, and the discursive realm, women were increasingly counted, and their attendant needs for care and prevention made more possible.

But who, precisely, was seen, and how, exactly, was she viewed and why? This paper critically examines the widely offered statement that women are especially vulnerable to HIV/AIDS in the USA and worldwide. It is not the goal to focus only on the *facts* of vulnerability among women and men of different races, sexualities, or regions; nor is it the intention to debate *whether* women or men (or certain women or men) are, in fact, "more" vulnerable. Rather, the goal is to examine the nature of epidemiological classifications and the discourse that surrounds these, to argue that such designations structure and limit current meanings, understandings, and the fathomability of gendered and sexualized vulnerability to HIV (Treichler 1999). The term fathomability here refers to the way in which particular social formations are constituted as identifiable, risky, or vulnerable, while others remain wholly unthinkable (Treichler 1999).

Vulnerable woman, invulnerable man: the (gendered) heterosexual couple

In 1994, heterosexual transmission surpassed injection drug use as the predominant route of transmission in US women with a diagnosis of AIDS (CDC 1995). Currently, heterosexual contact is said to account for approximately 60% of the identifiable risk in women, the largest category of identifiable risk in women (CDC 2002c). This trend is expected to continue, in part because heterosexual women are more likely to encounter an infected man than the reverse (Padian *et al.* 1997).

Within the global HIV literature, women are frequently deemed "more" or "especially" vulnerable to HIV infection than men due to an interaction between biological and social susceptibility factors. Due to genital physiology, gendered power relations, and the nature and pattern of relationships, studies generally suggest that male-to-female transmissibility is about twice that of female-to-male transmission (see, for example, Exner *et al.* 2003, Padian *et al.* 1997).

Numerous social, psychological, cultural, and institutional factors are cited as leading to women's greater vulnerability (Gupta 2002). There is strong evidence for a common sexual double standard, unequal economic and social status, and power differentials that affect safer sex negotiations. Women are often taught to be passive about bodily and sexual needs, and to put their needs aside in the interest of pleasing others (Reid 2000). Women are often most "at risk" with their current long-term male partner, where desires for trust, intimacy, and pleasure can lead to the erroneous assumption that a primary sexual relationship is safe (Simoni *et al.* 2000). Women are also viewed as especially vulnerable to HIV from the stance of much of the literature on sex work, and also in the literatures on rape and sexual violence (Wood and Jewkes 1997, Preston-Whyte *et al.* 2000).

All of the above "gendered" accounts leave heterosexual women hurt, disadvantaged or erased in sexual encounters and sexual safety. While there is a vast amount of evidence for these claims and heterosexual transmission as a risk category currently makes up a larger proportion of women's risk compared to men's risks in the USA (CDC 2002a), the question remains why is sexuality only gendered in the literature when describing women's vulnerability to HIV, when there are simultaneous or competing alternative explanations? How, after 30 years of interdisciplinary challenges to unitary notions of "sex" and "gender" that feature passive, powerless, vulnerable emphasized femininity and aggressive, powerful, violent hegemonic masculinity can this still be the *central* narrative surrounding HIV risk in the gender order (Connell 1987)?

The notion of a sex/gender system was introduced during the rise of second wave feminism, by writers such as Rubin (1975) in her classic essay 'The Traffic Of Women'. In it, heterosexuality was conceptualized as a specifically gendered and unequal material and social arrangement. The basis for women's oppression, Rubin argued, is the transformation of biological needs (sex) into a system of social relations (gender) through the kinship system. In such a system, women are transacted as gifts in the institution of marriage and it is the exchange partners, men, who are the beneficiaries. This exchange enables men to establish their dominance over women, and constrains women's sexuality into being responsive to men's needs. Furthermore, widely varying cultural valuations of women's and men's tasks fuel gender inequality and make it economically difficult for women to achieve independence on their own without heterosexual relations.

Two main assumptions support the sex/gender system described above. The same two assumptions have worked their way into the literature on HIV and "heterosexual transmission". First, heterosexual women are conceptualized as categorically oppressed and vulnerable, while heterosexual men are viewed as categorically powerful/invulnerable. Second, there is the assumption that a sex/gender system is constituted by biological women who have one gender role known as femininity (and are hurt by it in the HIV epidemic), while biological men have one gender role known as masculinity (and tend to hurt women with it).

Researchers interested in women's vulnerability to HIV/AIDS privilege the above assumptions that are contained in the logic of a sex/gender system not only when studying women, femininity, and HIV/AIDS, but also when studying men, masculinity, and HIV/AIDS. Here, men are frequently deemed to have greater decision-making or absolute power in the initiation, pace, and orchestration of sexual activity, sexual practices, and safer sex decisions (Exner *et al.* 1997). Furthermore, narrow cultural definitions of masculinity are said to normalize sex as a competitive, hierarchical win in which "scoring" is defined as a bodily right of access to and pleasure from multiple women's bodies in the sexual double standard (Seal and Ehrhardt 2003). In short, "traditional male gender roles" as these are socialized, and structural inequities in gendered power, are seen to influence risky sexual behavior.

Given that men are conceived of as so masculine, aggressive, unconcerned with partner needs, unable or unwilling to control their bodily needs amidst unwieldy power, needing multiple partners or are viewed as violent, it remains somewhat curious that the term "especially vulnerable" is not taken up more frequently in discussion of men and heterosexual transmission. In reality, men are positioned in quite variable positions within social structures and relationships, experience widely varying benefits of patriarchy, are frequently involved in migration and population movements and are also raped, sexually assaulted, and increasingly need to use sex work for material survival (Preston-Whyte *et al.* 2000). These facts are not frequently considered in a discourse of male vulnerability to HIV. Omitting a discourse of heterosexual men's vulnerability is even more alarming when thinking epidemiologically. That is, women cannot be put at risk via sexual transmission with a heterosexually active male partner unless that male partner is already infected and hence clearly vulnerable and at risk. More adequate analyses of gender in relation to HIV/AIDS need to consider women's and men's simultaneous privileges and inequalities in a triad made up of (1) different groups of women; (2) dominant male groups; and (3) subordinated men, such as marginalized racialized, classed, and sexualized men (Messner 1997, Connell 1995). Can we begin to break down the limitations of the logic of current work that often conceives of passive emphasized femininity and aggressive hegemonic masculinity as the key to understanding inequality in the gender order?

Several possibilities suggest themselves, first, there has been much theoretical challenge offered to concepts of "gendered oppression", which suggest that power is categorically owned by men and is used to oppress and dominate women. Not only is the assumption that "women" and "men" are unified or homogeneous categories flawed, but also the by structural realities, where both disenfranchised women *and* men in many societies now face massive economic and social destabilization domestically and globally (Parker *et al.* 2000). Class and race also play a large role in structuring the specificities of risk (Zierler and Kreiger 1997).

Second, a similar nuancing is needed for heterosexually-active men's risks. For example, in the USA, men of color in particular have lost tremendous economic ground over the last 30 years due to de-industrialization (Wilson 1996). Worldwide, research has also underscored how women migrants and not simply male migrants have, at times, been those forced to leave and return home for work, some of whom return home HIV positive to infect their HIV negative male partners (Lurie *et al.* 2003). It remains important, therefore, to uncover the ways in which women and men gain or lose ground in given economies and what impact this has on power, negotiations, and risk in relationships.

Concepts of intersectionality (race, class, gender, and sexuality) may be useful in this context (Collins 1999). Individuals do not have singular identities or experiences within social structures that expand or limit social practices, but rather, intersecting ones. It is evident, for example, that the epidemic in the USA has had disproportionate impact on the poorest and most marginalized women, predominantly women of color living in the inner cities of the northeastern seaboard (Kamb and Wortley 2000, CDC 2002a). Moreover, while overall numbers of women and men with HIV are approximately equal, in young people ages 13–19, a much greater proportion of HIV infections occur among females (CDC 2002a). Thus, the epidemic clearly traverses the fault lines of intersectionality, and transmission and infection (whether by sex or drugs) is linked to social and economic relations of inequality (Zierler and Kreiger 1997).

Despite this, surveillance categories do not currently rely on the intersection of several identities or behaviors and therefore do not facilitate easy analysis of the contextual factors that shape risk aside from "heterosexual transmission", "injecting drug use" or "men who have sex with men" (Young and Meyer in press).

Hierarchical inclusion, heterosexual transmission, and the queer disappearance of queer

In her later work, Rubin (1999) challenged her earlier notion of a sex/gender system when she argued that women do not simply face gendered but also sexual stratification. She challenges researchers to reconsider the automatic use of gender analysis to capture the state of sexuality for women. By extension, it is important to reflect not only on what is inside the frame of the discourse on vulnerability to HIV, but what is excluded or silenced (Lutzen 1995). When the CDC first recognized women's symptomology, women came rushing out of the HIV/AIDS closet. They often did so under the category of heterosexual transmission. Unlike the official categorization of men, which includes injecting drug users (IDU), men who have sex with men, indefinable, and a separate transmission category for men who have sex with men *and* who also engage in injecting drug use, women are said to have the following risks: IDU, heterosexual, and undefinable (Campbell 1999, CDC 2002c). Women who have sex with an injection drug user are added together with women classified under Asex with men@ to create an overall concept of "heterosexual transmission" (CDC 2002c). It is important to examine the way in which women are classified, given that this provides the contemporary basis for the constitution of heterosexual transmission (and implicitly heterosexual identity), while erasing the possibility of bi/lesbian transmission (and therefore identity) (Young and Meyer in press).

Under existing classification systems, a woman who always has had long sessions of oral sex with multiple women but has had one episode of heterosexual contact is counted as having heterosexual risk. A bisexual female who does not use drugs will be counted as having a heterosexual transmission risk. A bisexual woman who has anal sex with a gay man will be classified as having heterosexual transmission risks. A woman who has sex with women and men, and is the partner of both a female and a male injecting drug user, will be categorized as having heterosexual transmission risks.

The need for greater intersectionality in surveillance categories and the discourse that surrounds current modes of risk hierarchicalization becomes even clearer when we look at current research trends. For example, comprehensive reviews have found that large numbers of female injecting drug users are women who have sex with women (WSW) (from 20 to 40% across samples) (Young *et al.* 2000). However, such women are classified as injecting drug users in terms of HIV risks, and sexuality plays little role in prevention work thus far (Friedman *et al.* 2003). Research has also found that WSW IDUs have higher HIV incidence and prevalence rates than heterosexuals IDUs and that WSW IDUs are more likely to engage in sex with MSMs (Friedman *et al.* 2003).

With respect to WSW more generally, it has been found that WSW are more likely than non-WSWs to report sexual contact with a homosexual or bisexual man (Fethers *et al.* 2000). Under present classification systems, these women will be counted as having "heterosexual" transmission risks and may be conceived of as benefiting from HIV prevention interventions that are likely to only take gender inequality into account (Lemp *et al.* 1995). Furthermore, WSW have also been found to have more oral-penile and more anal intercourse and less vaginal intercourse than heterosexual women (Bevier *et al.* 1995). Again, these women will be counted as having heterosexual transmission risks where the literature generally conceives of risk as related to gender inequality.

The current focus not only erases a wide variety of risky sexual practices and identities other than heterosexual, but also leaves many women in a position to not be able to assess their risk accurately (Morrow and Allsworth 2000, Young and Meyer 2005). Lesbians or bisexual women may not think they are at risk due to popular conceptions that woman to woman sex is a no-risk practice (Albert 2001). These are vital considerations when considering that the "first case" of female-to-female transmission of HIV is now documented, reported as being most likely through "the use of sex toys, used vigorously enough to cause exchange of blood-tinged bodily fluids" (Reeves 2003: 29). In this newest case, the HIV-positive partner reports that she was instructed by her physician to use protection only with her male partners.

In Los Angeles, research with "high risk" Latina women reveals widespread bisexual activity. Respondents reported "*Si, tenemos sexo con mujeres, pero no somos marimachas*" ("Sure, we have sex with women, but we're not lesbians") (Ramos 1997: 127). In this same study, we learn of Cristina who considers herself "queer", went through a "slut phase", attended S&M and leather scenes with women and men, never washed her dildos, used drugs, and had blood squirted on her during a nipple piercing ceremony. There was also the less "unusual" case of Lourdes, who liked to lick her partner when she had her period since "*Me gusta ver el sangrado*" ("I liked to see her blood") (Ramos 1997: 133). There were also reports of tribadism that occurred (and occur outside of this study), where women rub the wettest part of their genitals together until they explode in orgasm, soaking the sheets (Ramos 1997). There are also clinical cases of those women and men who have oral sex with women, fully adoring of the building moistness, but then are surprised when met with a stream of female ejaculate that squirts into their eyes, nose, and mouth (Darling *et al.* 1990).

The CDC does report that "vaginal secretions and menstrual blood are potentially infectious and that mucous membrane (e.g. oral, vaginal, penile) exposure to these secretions have the potential to lead to HIV infection" and yet "information on whether a woman had sex with women is missing in half of case reports, possibly because the physician did not elicit the information or the woman did not volunteer it" (CDC 2000). Clearly, so as to garner a fuller sense of women's (and men's) sexual health, it would help to tackle heterosexism and homophobia in public health and to instill a conception of the erotic and *sexual* and not simply *gendered* constitution of society (Dowsett 1996, Parker 1999).

Intersectionality that recognizes the simultaneity of behaviors and/or identities could be helpful in enabling researchers to make new inroads into communities of poor inner city queer women whose female partners must sell sex to men to make ends meet. It will also perhaps make better sense of the circumstances and experiences of women in India (Thadani 1999), Mexico (Mogrovejo 1999), in Native American cultures (Lang 1999), in West Sumatra (Blackwood 1999), in Zimbabwe (Aarmo 1999), and all over the world who have sex with women, or with both women and men. How do such women conceive of their risk—and what are their risks?

How will current theories of gender address the butch women who have been studied in Jakarta and Lima (Wieringa 1999) if they might have sex with femme women who have multiple boyfriends (or the reverse)? What are the risks to female partners who conceive of themselves worldwide as embracing "female masculinity" across sexuality categories (Halberstam 1998), and are these different from those who might embrace femme identity across the categories (Pratt 1995)? We simply do not know.

Current epidemiological markings of women require the simultaneous breathing of some women into diseased existence while pushing others into the realm of the unfathomable (Foucault 1978). Since all decisions to draw boundaries around surveillance categories are by definition shifting, problematic, and involve a politics of inclusion and exclusion by their very nature, researchers should think carefully about automatically privileging singular, hierarchicalized categories—or embracing any singular theory of risk that underpins current categories. Theories of intersectionality may not provide a total solution, but this conceptual turn could begin to place some populations, behaviors, and identities into the realm of existence while allowing for much needed contextual understandings and discursive conceptions of "at risk" and "vulnerable". The US CDC is already moving in this direction in terms of men's categories (e.g., by keeping track of multiple risk behaviors as these intersect), but the thoroughness of a parallel move for the women's categories has yet to be made (CDC 2002c).

While analyses of gender are vital and will continue to take place, pushing beyond the notion that there is a singular sex/gender system in which biological women are feminine, oppressed, and vulnerable and biological men are masculine, invulnerable oppressors will be vital to future progress in the HIV epidemic. Examining intersectionality and the simultaneity of race, class, and shifting gender relations for women and men remains vital. Classification systems that privilege singular categorizations and underlying theories of gender or sexuality to explain risk are likely to be of limited use both in the USA and world-wide.

Acknowledgments

This research was supported by a training grant from the National Institute of Mental Health (T32 MH19139 Behavioral Sciences Research in HIV Infection; Principal Investigator, Anke A. Ehrhardt). The author is grateful to Gary Dowsett, Susie Hoffman, Jodi O'Brien, Ilan Meyer, Kari Lerum, Theresa Exner, Rita Melendez, Anke A. Ehrhardt, Theo Sandfort, Gary Oppenheimer, Leslie Heywood, Michael A. Messner, Faye Linda Wachs, Pat Warne and Isabel Howe for careful, diligent reads and insightful suggestions.

References

Aarmo, M. (1999) How homosexuality became 'UnAfrican': The case of Zimbabwe. In E. Blackwood and S. E. Wieringa (eds.) *Same Sex Relations and Female Desires: Transgender Practices Across Cultures* (New York: Columbia University Press), pp. 255–280.

Albert, S. (2001) Many Lesbian and Bisexual Women Unaware of Risks. *Gay Health*. Available at: http://www.gayhealth.com/iowa-robot/sex/?record'407.

Bevier, P. J., Chiasson, M. A., Heffernan, R. T. and Castro, K. G. (1995) Women at a sexually transmitted disease clinic: their HIV seroprevalance and risk behaviors. *American Journal of Public Health*, 85, 1366–1376.

Blackwood, E. (1999) Tombois in West Sumatra: Constructing Masculinity and Erotic Desire. In E. Blackwood and S. E. Wieringa (eds.) *Same Sex Relations and Female Desires: Transgender Practices Across Cultures* (New York: Columbia University Press), pp. 181–205.

Campbell, C. (1999) *Women, Families, and HIV/AIDS* (New York: Cambridge University Press).

Centers for Disease Control (1992a) Announcement of Meeting About Revising the AIDS Surveillance Case Definition. *Morbidity Mortality Weekly Report*, 41, 594–595.

Centers for Disease Control (1992b) 1993 Revised classification system for HIV infection and expanded surveillance case definition for AIDS among adolescents and adults. *Morbidity Mortality Weekly Report*, 41, 17.

Centers for Disease Control (1992c) Revision of the Proposed Expansion of the AIDS Surveillance Case Definition. *Morbidity Mortality Weekly Report*, 41, 829–830.

Centers for Disease Control (1993) *National HIV Serosurveillance Summary: Results through 1992* (Atlanta: US Department of Health and Human Services, Public Health Service).

Centers for Disease Control (1995) Update: AIDS Among Women in the United States, 1994. *Morbidity Mortality Weekly Report*, 44, 81–84.

Centers for Disease Control (2000) HIV/AIDS and US Women Who Have Sex with Women (WSW). Available at: http://www.cdc.gov/hiv/pubs/facts/wsw.htm.

Centers for Disease Control (2002a) AIDS Cases in Adolescents and Adults by Age: United States, 1994–2000. *HIV/AIDS Surveillance Supplemental Report*, 9(1).

Centers for Disease Control (2002b) Deaths among persons with AIDS through December 2000. *HIV/AIDS Surveillance Supplemental Report*, 8(1).

Centers for Disease Control (2002c) Cases of HIV Infection and AIDS in the United States, 2002. *Surveillance Report*. Volume 14.

Collins, P. H. (1999) Moving Beyond Gender: Intersectionality and Scientific Knowledge. In M. M. Feree, J. Lorber and B. B. Hess (eds.) *Revisioning Gender* (Thousand Oaks: Sage), pp. 261–284.

Connell, R. W. (1987) *Gender and Power* (Stanford, CA: Stanford University Press).

Connell, R. W. (1995) *Masculinities* (Berkeley, CA: University of California Press).

Darling, C. A., Davidson, J. K. Sr. and Conway-Welch, C. (1990) Female Ejaculation, Perceived Origins, the Grafenberg Spot/Area, and Sexual Responsiveness. *Archives of Sexual Behavior*, 19, 29–47.

Dowsett, G. (1996) *Practicing Desire: Homosexual Sex in the Era of AIDS* (Stanford, CA: Stanford University Press).

Exner, T. M., Hoffman, S., Dworkin, S. and Ehrhardt, A. A. (2003) Beyond the Male Condom: The Evolution of Gender-Specific HIV Interventions for Women. *Annual Review of Sex Research*, 14, 114–136.

Exner, T. M., Seal, D. W. and Ehrhardt, A. A. (1997) A Review of HIV Interventions for At-Risk Women. *AIDS and Behavior*, 2, 93–124.

Fethers, K., Marks, C., Mindel, A. and Estcourt, C. S. (2000) Sexually transmitted infections and risk behaviors in women who have sex with women. *Sexually Transmitted Infections*, 76, 345–349.

Foucault, M. (1978) *The History of Sexuality* (New York: Vintage Books).

Fox-Tierney, R. A., Ickovics, J. R., Cerrata, C. and Ethier, K. A. (1999) Potential sex differences remain understudied: A case study of inclusion of women in HIV/AIDS-related neuropsychological research. *Review of General Psychology*, 3, 44–54.

Friedman, S. R., Ompad, D. C., Maslow, C., Young, R., Case, P., Hudson, S., Diaz, T., Morse, E., Bailey, S., Des Jarlais, D. C., Perlis, T., Holligaugh, A. and Garfein, R. S. (2003) HIV Prevalence, Risk Behaviors, and High-Risk Sexual and Injection Networks Among Young Women Injectors Who Have Sex With Women. *American Journal of Public Health*, 93, 902–906.

Gupta, G. R. (2002) Gender, sexuality and HIV/AIDS: The what, the why, and the how. *SIECUS Reports*, 29(5), 6–12.

Halberstam, J. (1998) *Female Masculinity* (Durham, NY: Duke University Press).

Hankins, C. A. and Handley, M. A. (1992) HIV disease and AIDS in women: Current knowledge and a research agenda. *Journal of Acquired Immune Deficiency Syndromes*, 5, 957–971.

Kamb, M. L. and Wortley, P. M. (2000) Human Immunodeficiency Virus and AIDS in women. In M. Goldman and M. Hatch (eds.) *Women and Health* (San Diego, CA: Academic Press).

Lang, S. (1999) Lesbians, Men-Women, and Two-Spirits: Homosexuality and Gender in Native American Cultures. In E. Blackwood and S. E. Wieringa (eds.) *Same Sex Relations and Female Desires: Transgender Practices Across Cultures* (New York: Columbia University Press), pp. 91–118.

Lemp, G. F., Kellog, M., Nieri, T. A. and Giuliano, N. *et al.* (1995) HIV Seroprevalence and risk behaviors among lesbians and bisexual women in San Francisco and Berkeley, California. *American Journal of Public Health*, 85, 1549–1557.

Lurie, M. N., Williams, B. G., Zuma, K., Mkaya-Mwamburi, D., Garnett, G. P., Sweat, M. D., Gittelson, J. and Abdool Karim, S. S. (2003) Who Infects Whom: HIV-1 Concordance among Migrant and Non-Migrant Couples In South Africa. *AIDS*, 17, 2245–2252.

Lutzen, K. (1995) La mise en discours and Silences in Research on the History of Sexuality. In R. Parker and J. Gagnon (eds.) *Conceiving Sexuality: Approaches to Sex Research in a Postmodern World* (London: Routledge), pp. 19–32.

Messner, M. A. (1997) *The Politics of Masculinity: Men In Movements* (Thousand Oaks, CA: Sage).

Mogrovejo, N. (1999) Sexual Preference, the Ugly Duckling of Feminist Demands: The Lesbian Movement in Mexico. In E. Blackwood and S. E. Wieringa (eds.) *Same Sex Relations and Female Desires: Transgender Practices Across Cultures* (New York: Columbia University Press), pp. 308–336.

Morrow, K. M. and Allsworth, J. E. (2000) Sexual Risk in Lesbians and Bisexual Women. *Journal and the Gay and Lesbian Medical Association*, 4, 159–165.

Padian, N., Shiboski, S., Glass, S. and Vittinghoff, E. (1997) Heterosexual Transmission of human immunodeficiency virus in northern California: results from a 10 year study. *American Journal of Epidemiology*, 146, 350–357.

Parker, R. (1999) "Within Four Walls': Brazilian Sexual Culture and HIV/AIDS. In R. Parker and P. Aggleton (eds.) *Culture, Society, and Sexuality: A Reader* (London: Taylor & Francis), pp. 253–266.

Parker, R., Easton, D. and Klein, C. H. (2000) Structural barriers and facilitators in HIV prevention: A Review of international research. *AIDS*, 14(S1), S22–S33.

Pratt, M. B. (1995) *S/he* (Ithaca, NY: Firebrand Books).

Preston-Whyte, E., Varga, C., Oosthuizen, H., Roberts, R. and Blose, F. (2000) Survival Sex and HIV/AIDS in an African City. In R. Parker, R. M. Barbosa and P. Aggleton (eds.) *Framing the Sexual Subject: The Politics of Gender, Sexuality, and Power* (Berkeley, CA: University of California Press), pp. 165–190.

Ramos, L. (1997) '*Si, Tenemos Sexo Xon Mujeres, Pero No Somos Marimachas*' (Sure, We Have Sex With Women, But We're Not Lesbians.): Sexual Diversity in the Los Angeles Latina Community-Ethnographic Findings, 1987–1995. In N. Goldstein and J. L. Manlowe (eds.) *The Gender Politics of HIV/AIDS in Women* (New York: New York University Press), pp. 127–154.

Reeves, T. (2003) Female to female transmission-seeking answers and challenging myths. *HIV Austrailia*, 2, 29–30.

Reid, P. T. (2000) Women, Ethnicity, and AIDS: What's Love Got to Do With It? *Sex Roles*, 42, 709–722.

Rubin, G. (1975) The Traffic In Women: Notes on the Political Economy of Sex. In R. Reiter (ed.) *Towards an Anthropology of Women* (New York: Monthly Review Press).

Rubin, G. (1999) Thinking Sex: Notes for a Radical Theory of the Politics of Sexuality. In R. Parker and P. Aggleton (eds.) *Culture, Society, and Sexuality: A Reader* (London: Taylor & Francis), pp. 143–178.

Seal, D. W. and Ehrhardt, A. A. (2003) Masculinity and urban men: Perceived scripts for courtship, romantic, and sexual interactions with women. *Culture, Health, and Sexuality*, 5, 295–319.

Simoni, J. M., Walters, K. L. and Nero, D. K. (2000) Safer sex among HIV+ women: the role of relationships. *Sex Roles*, 42, 691–708.

Stine, G. J. (2003) *Aids Update 2002: An Annual Overview of Acquired Immune Deficiency Syndrome* (Saddle River, NJ: Prentice Hall).

Thadani, G. (1999) The Politics of Identities and Languages: Lesbian Desire in Ancient and Modern India. In E. Blackwood and S. E. Wieringa (eds.) *Same Sex Relations and Female Desires: Transgender Practices Across Cultures* (New York: Columbia University Press), pp. 67–90.

Treichler, P. (1999) AIDS, Homophobia, and Biomedical Discourse: An Epidemic of Signification. In R. Parker and P. Aggleton (eds.) *Culture, Society, and Sexuality: A Reader* (London: Taylor & Francis), pp. 190–266.

Wieringa, S. E. (1999) Desiring Bodies or Defiant Cultures: Butch-Femme Lesbians in Jakarta and Lima. In E. Blackwood and S. E. Wieringa (eds.) *Same Sex Relations and Female Desires: Transgender Practices Across Cultures* (New York: Columbia University Press), pp. 206–229.

Wilson, W. J. (1996) *When Work Disappears: The World of the New Urban Poor* (New York: Vintage Books).

Wood, K. and Jewkes, R. (1997) Violence, Rape, and Sexual Coercion: Everyday Love in a South African Township. *Gender and Development*, 5, 41–46.

Young, R. M. and Meyer, I. (2005) The Trouble With 'MSM' and 'WSW': Erasure of the Sexual Minority Person in Public Health Discourse. *American Journal of Public Health*, 95, 1144–1149.

Young, R. M., Friedman, S. R., Case, P. L., Ascencio, M. W. and Clatts, M. C. (2000) Women injection drug users who have sex with women exhibit increased HIV infection and risk behaviors. *Journal of Drug Issues*, 30, 499–524.

Zierler, S. and Krieger, N. (1997) Reframing Women's Risk: Social Inequalities and HIV Infection. *Annual Review of Public Health*, 18, 401–436.

10

HEGEMONIC MASCULINITY

Rethinking the concept

R. W. Connell and James W. Messerschmidt

Source: *Gender and Society*, 19:6 (2005), 829–59.

The concept of hegemonic masculinity has influenced gender studies across many academic fields but has also attracted serious criticism. The authors trace the origin of the concept in a convergence of ideas in the early 1980s and map the ways it was applied when research on men and masculinities expanded. Evaluating the principal criticisms, the authors defend the underlying concept of masculinity, which in most research use is neither reified nor essentialist. However, the criticism of trait models of gender and rigid typologies is sound. The treatment of the subject in research on hegemonic masculinity can he improved with the aid of recent psychological models, although limits to discursive flexibility must be recognized. The concept of hegemonic masculinity does not equate to a model of social reproduction; we need to recognize social struggles in which subordinated masculinities influence dominant forms. Finally, the authors review what has been confirmed from early formulations (the idea of multiple masculinities, the concept of hegemony, and the emphasis on change) and what needs to be discarded (one-dimensional treatment of hierarchy and trait conceptions of gender). The authors suggest reformulation of the concept in four areas: a more complex model of gender hierarchy, emphasizing the agency of women; explicit recognition of the geography of masculinities, emphasizing the interplay among local, regional, and global levels; a more specific treatment of embodiment in contexts of privilege and power; and a stronger emphasis on the dynamics of hegemonic masculinity, recognizing internal contradictions and the possibilities of movement toward gender democracy.

The concept of hegemonic masculinity, formulated two decades ago, has considerably influenced recent thinking about men, gender, and social hierarchy. It has provided a link between the growing research field of men's studies (also known as masculinity studies and critical studies of men), popular anxieties about men and boys, feminist accounts of patriarchy, and sociological models of gender. It has found uses in applied fields ranging from education and antiviolence work to health and counseling.

Database searches reveal more than 200 papers that use the exact term "hegemonic masculinity" in their titles or abstracts. Papers that use a variant, or refer to "hegemonic masculinity" in the text, run to many hundreds. Continuing interest is shown by conferences. In early May 2005, a conference, "Hegemonic Masculinities and International Politics," was held at the University of Manchester, England; in 2004, an interdisciplinary conference in Stuttgart was devoted to the topic "Hegemoniale Männlichkeiten" (Dinges, Ründal, and Bauer 2004).

The concept has also attracted serious criticism from several directions: sociological, psychological, poststructuralist, and materialist (e.g., Demetriou 2001; Wetherell and Edley 1999). Outside the academic world, it has been attacked as—to quote a recent Internet backlash posting—"an invention of New Age psychologists" determined to prove that men are too macho.

This is a contested concept. Yet the issues it names are very much at stake in contemporary struggles about power and political leadership, public and private violence, and changes in families and sexuality. A comprehensive reexamination of the concept of hegemonic masculinity seems worthwhile. If the concept proves still useful, it must be reformulated in contemporary terms. We attempt both tasks in this article.

Origin, formulation, and application

Origin

The concept of hegemonic masculinity was first proposed in reports from a field study of social inequality in Australian high schools (Kessler et al. 1982); in a related conceptual discussion of the making of masculinities and the experience of men's bodies (Connell 1983); and in a debate over the role of men in Australian labor politics (Connell 1982). The high school project provided empirical evidence of multiple hierarchies—in gender as well as in class terms—interwoven with active projects of gender construction (Connell et al. 1982).

These beginnings were systematized in an article, "Towards a New Sociology of Masculinity" (Carrigan, Connell, and Lee 1985), which extensively critiqued the "male sex role" literature and proposed a model of multiple masculinities and power relations. In turn, this model was integrated into a systematic sociological theory of gender. The resulting six pages in *Gender and Power* (Connell 1987) on "hegemonic masculinity and emphasized femininity" became the most cited source for the concept of hegemonic masculinity.

The concept articulated by the research groups in Australia represented a synthesis of ideas and evidence from apparently disparate sources. But the convergence of ideas was not accidental. Closely related issues were being addressed by researchers and activists in other countries too; the time was, in a sense, ripe for a synthesis of this kind.

The most basic sources were feminist theories of patriarchy and the related debates over the role of men in transforming patriarchy (Goode 1982; Snodgrass 1977). Some men in the New Left had tried to organize in support of feminism, and the attempt had drawn attention to class differences in the expression of masculinity (Tolson 1977). Moreover, women of color—such as Maxine Baca Zinn (1982), Angela Davis (1983), and bell hooks (1984)—criticized the race bias that occurs when power is solely conceptualized in terms of sex difference, thus laying the groundwork for questioning any universalizing claims about the category of men.

The Gramscian term "hegemony" was current at the time in attempts to understand the stabilization of class relations (Connell 1977). In the context of dual systems theory (Eisenstein 1979), the idea was easily transferred to the parallel problem about gender relations. This risked a significant misunderstanding. Gramsci's writing focuses on the dynamics of structural change involving the mobilization and demobilization of whole classes. Without a very clear focus on this issue of historical change, the idea of hegemony would be reduced to a simple model of cultural control. And in a great deal of the debate about gender, large-scale historical change is not in focus. Here is one of the sources of later difficulties with the concept of hegemonic masculinity.

Even before the women's liberation movement, a literature in social psychology and sociology about the "male sex role" had recognized the social nature of masculinity and the possibilities of change in men's conduct (Hacker 1957). During the 1970s, there was an explosion of writing about "the male role," sharply criticizing role norms as the source of oppressive behavior by men (Brannon 1976). Critical role theory provided the main conceptual basis for the early antisexist men's movement. The weaknesses of sex role theory were, however, increasingly recognized (Kimmel 1987; Pleck 1981). They included the blurring of behavior and norm, the homogenizing effect of the role concept, and its difficulties in accounting for power.

Power and difference were, on the other hand, core concepts in the gay liberation movement, which developed a sophisticated analysis of the oppression of men as well as oppression by men (Altman 1972). Some theorists saw gay liberation as bound up with an assault on gender stereotypes (Mieli 1980). The idea of a hierarchy of masculinities grew directly out of homosexual men's experience with violence and prejudice from straight men.

The concept of homophobia originated in the 1970s and was already being attributed to the conventional male role (Morin and Garfinkle 1978). Theorists developed increasingly sophisticated accounts of gay men's ambivalent relationships to patriarchy and conventional masculinity (Broker 1976; Plummer 1981).

An equally important source was empirical social research. A growing body of field studies was documenting local gender hierarchies and local cultures of masculinity in schools (Willis 1977), in male-dominated workplaces (Cockburn 1983), and in village communities (Herdt 1981; Hunt 1980). These studies added the ethnographic realism that the sex-role literature lacked, confirmed the plurality of masculinities and the complexities of gender construction for men, and gave evidence of the active struggle for dominance that is implicit in the Gramscian concept of hegemony.

Finally, the concept was influenced by psychoanalysis. Freud himself produced the first analytic biographies of men and, in the "Wolf Man" case history, showed how adult personality was a system under tension, with countercurrents repressed but not obliterated (Freud [1917] 1955). The psychoanalyst Stoller (1968) popularized the concept of "gender identity" and mapped its variations in boys' development, most famously those leading to transsexualism. Others influenced by psychoanalysis picked up the themes of men's power, the range of possibilities in gender development, and the tension and contradiction within conventional masculinities (Friedman and Lerner 1986; Zaretsky 1975).

Formulation

What emerged from this matrix in the mid-1980s was an analogue, in gender terms, of power structure research in political sociology—focusing the spotlight on a dominant group. Hegemonic masculinity was understood as the pattern of practice (i.e., things done, not just a set of role expectations or an identity) that allowed men's dominance over women to continue.

Hegemonic masculinity was distinguished from other masculinities, especially subordinated masculinities. Hegemonic masculinity was not assumed to be normal in the statistical sense; only a minority of men might enact it. But it was certainly normative. It embodied the currently most honored way of being a man, it required all other men to position themselves in relation to it, and it ideologically legitimated the global subordination of women to men.

Men who received the benefits of patriarchy without enacting a strong version of masculine dominance could be regarded as showing a complicit masculinity. It was in relation to this group, and to compliance among heterosexual women, that the concept of hegemony was most powerful. Hegemony did not mean violence, although it could be supported by force; it meant ascendancy achieved through culture, institutions, and persuasion.

These concepts were abstract rather than descriptive, defined in terms of the logic of a patriarchal gender system. They assumed that gender relations were historical, so gender hierarchies were subject to change. Hegemonic masculinities therefore came into existence in specific circumstances and were open to historical change. More precisely, there could be a struggle for hegemony, and older forms of masculinity might be displaced by new ones. This was the element of optimism in an otherwise rather bleak theory. It was perhaps possible that a more humane, less oppressive, means of being a man might become hegemonic, as part of a process leading toward an abolition of gender hierarchies.

Application

The concept of hegemonic masculinity, formulated in these terms, found prompt use. In the late 1980s and early 1990s, research on men and masculinity was being consolidated as an academic field, supported by a string of conferences, the publication of textbooks (e.g., Brod 1987) and several journals, and a rapidly expanding research agenda across the social sciences and humanities.

The concept of hegemonic masculinity was used in education studies to understand the dynamics of classroom life, including patterns of resistance and bullying among boys. It was used to explore relations to the curriculum and the difficulties in gender-neutral pedagogy (Martino 1995). It was used to understand teacher strategies and teacher identities among such groups as physical education instructors (Skelton 1993).

The concept also had influence in criminology. All data reflect that men and boys perpetrate more of the conventional crimes—and the more serious of these crimes—than do women and girls. Moreover, men hold a virtual monopoly on the commission of syndicated and white-collar forms of crime. The concept of hegemonic masculinity helped in theorizing the relationship among masculinities and among a variety of crimes (Messerschmidt 1993) and was also used in studies on specific crimes by boys and men, such as rape in Switzerland, murder in Australia, football "hooliganism" and white-collar crime in England, and assaultive violence in the United States (Newburn and Stanko 1994).

The concept was also employed in studying media representations of men, for instance, the interplay of sports and war imagery (Jansen and Sabo 1994). Because the concept of hegemony helped to make sense of both the diversity and the selectiveness of images in mass media, media researchers began mapping the relations between representations of different masculinities (Hanke 1992). Commercial sports are a focus of media representations of masculinity, and the developing field of sports sociology also found significant use for the concept of hegemonic masculinity (Messner 1992). It was deployed in understanding the popularity of body-contact confrontational sports—which function as an endlessly renewed symbol of masculinity—and in understanding the violence and homophobia frequently found in sporting milieus (Messner and Sabo 1990).

The social determinants of men's health had been raised earlier, but the sex role concept was too diffuse to be very useful. The concepts of multiple masculinities and hegemonic masculinity were increasingly used to understand men's health practices, such as "playing hurt" and risk-taking sexual behavior (Sabo and Gordon 1995). The concepts of hegemonic and subordinated masculinities helped in understanding not only men's exposure to risk but also men's difficulties in responding to disability and injury (Gerschick and Miller 1994).

The concept of hegemonic masculinity also proved significant in organization studies, as the gendered character of bureaucracies and workplaces was increasingly recognized. Ethnographic and interview studies traced the institutionalization of hegemonic masculinities in specific organizations (Cheng 1996; Cockburn 1991) and their role in organizational decision making (Messerschmidt 1995). A particular focus of this research was the military, where specific patterns of hegemonic masculinity had been entrenched but were becoming increasingly problematic (Barrett 1996).

Discussions of professional practice concerned with men and boys also found the concept helpful. Such practices include psychotherapy with men (Kupers 1993), violence-prevention programs for youth (Denborough 1996), and emotional education programs for boys (Salisbury and Jackson 1996).

These are the primary fields where the concept of hegemonic masculinity was applied in the decade following its formulation. But there was also a wider range of application, for instance, in discussions of art (Belton 1995), in academic disciplines such as geography (Berg 1994) and law (Thornton 1989), and in general discussions of men's gender politics and relation to feminism (Segal 1990). We may reasonably conclude that the analysis of multiple masculinities and the concept of hegemonic masculinity served as a framework for much of the developing research effort on men and masculinity, replacing sex-role theory and categorical models of patriarchy.

Eventually, the growing research effort tended to expand the concept itself. The picture was fleshed out in four main ways: by documenting the consequences and costs of hegemony, by uncovering mechanisms of hegemony, by showing greater diversity in masculinities, and by tracing changes in hegemonic masculinities.

Regarding costs and consequences, research in criminology showed how particular patterns of aggression were linked with hegemonic masculinity, not as a mechanical effect for which hegemonic masculinity was a cause, but through the pursuit of hegemony (Bufkin 1999; Messerschmidt 1997). Moreover, the pioneering research of Messner (1992) showed that the enactment of hegemonic masculinity in professional sports, while reproducing steep hierarchies, also comes at considerable cost to the victors in terms of emotional and physical damage.

Research has been fruitful in revealing mechanisms of hegemony. Some are highly visible, such as the "pageantry" of masculinity in television sports broadcasts (Sabo and Jansen 1992) as well as the social mechanisms Roberts (1993) calls "censure" directed at subordinated groups—ranging from informal name calling by children to the criminalization of homosexual conduct. Yet other mechanisms of hegemony operate by invisibility, removing a dominant form of masculinity from the possibility of censure (Brown 1999). Consalvo (2003), examining media reporting of the Columbine High School massacre, notes how the issue of masculinity was withdrawn from scrutiny, leaving the media with no way of representing the shooters except as "monsters."

International research has strongly confirmed the initial insight that gender orders construct multiple masculinities. Valdés and Olavarría (1998) show that even in a culturally homogeneous country such as Chile, there is no unitary masculinity, since patterns vary by class and generation. In another famously homogeneous country, Japan, Ishii-Kuntz (2003) traces the "emergence of diverse masculinities" in recent social history, with changes in child care practices a key development. Diversity of masculinities is also found in particular institutions, such as the military (Higate 2003).

Gutmann (1996), in the most beautifully observed modern ethnography of masculinity, studied a case where there is a well-defined public masculine identity—Mexican "machismo." Gutmann shows how the imagery of machismo developed historically and was interwoven with the development of Mexican nationalism, masking enormous complexity in the actual lives of Mexican men. Gutmann teases out four patterns of masculinity in the working-class urban settlement he studies, insisting that even these four are crosscut by other social divisions and are constantly renegotiated in everyday life.

Finally, a considerable body of research shows that masculinities are not simply different but also subject to change. Challenges to hegemony are common, and so are adjustments in the face of these challenges. Morrell (1998) assembles the evidence about gender transformations in southern Africa associated with the end of Apartheid, a system of segregated and competing patriarchies. Ferguson (2001) traces the decline of long-standing ideals of masculinity in Ireland—the celibate priest and the hardworking family man—and their replacement by more modernized and market-oriented models. Dasgupta (2000) traces tensions in the Japanese "salaryman" model of masculinity, especially after the "bubble economy" of the 1980s: A cultural figure of the "salaryman escaping" has appeared. Taga (2003) documents diverse responses to change among young middle-class men in Japan, including new options for domestic partnership with women. Meuser (2003) traces generational change in Germany, partly driven by men's responses to changes among women. Many (although not all) young men, now expecting women to reject patriarchal social relations, are crafting a "pragmatic egalitarianism" of their own. Morris and Evans (2001), studying images of rural masculinity and femininity in Britain, finds a slower pace of change but an increasing subtlety and fragmentation in the representation of hegemonic masculinity.

From the mid-1980s to the early 2000s, the concept of hegemonic masculinity thus passed from a conceptual model with a fairly narrow empirical base to a widely used framework for research and debate about men and masculinities. The concept was applied in diverse cultural contexts and to a considerable range of practical issues. It is not surprising, then, that the concept has attracted criticism, and to this we now turn.

Critiques

Five principal criticisms have been advanced since debate about the concept began in the early 1990s. In this section, we evaluate each criticism in turn, hoping to discover what is worth retaining from the original conception of hegemonic masculinity and what now needs reformulating.

The underlying concept of masculinity

That the underlying concept of masculinity is flawed has been argued from two different points of view, realist and poststructuralist. To Collinson and Hearn (1994) and Hearn (1996, 2004), the concept of masculinity is blurred, is uncertain in its meaning, and tends to deemphasize issues of power and domination. It is ultimately unnecessary to the task of understanding and contesting the power of men. The concept of multiple masculinities tends to produce a static typology.

To Petersen (1998, 2003), Collier (1998), and MacInnes (1998), the concept of masculinity is flawed because it essentializes the character of men or imposes a false unity on a fluid and contradictory reality. Some versions of this argument criticize masculinity research because it has not adopted a specific poststructuralist tool kit—which would, for instance, emphasize the discursive construction of identities (Whitehead 2002). The concept of masculinity is criticized for being framed within a heteronormative conception of gender that essentializes male-female difference and ignores difference and exclusion within the gender categories. The concept of masculinity is said to rest logically on a dichotomization of sex (biological) versus gender (cultural) and thus marginalizes or naturalizes the body.

No responsible mind can deny that in the huge literature concerned with masculinity, there is a great deal of conceptual confusion as well as a great deal of essentializing. This certainly is common in accounts of masculinity in pop psychology, in the mythopoetic men's movement, and in journalistic interpretations of biological sex-difference research. It is another matter, however, to claim that the concept of masculinity must be confused or essentialist or even that researchers' use of the concept typically is.

We would argue that social science and humanities research on masculinities has flourished during the past 20 years precisely because the underlying concept employed is not reified or essentialist. The notion that the concept of masculinity essentializes or homogenizes is quite difficult to reconcile with the tremendous multiplicity of social constructions that ethnographers and historians have documented with the aid of this concept (Connell 2003). Even further removed from essentialism is the fact that researchers have explored masculinities enacted by people with female bodies (Halberstam 1998; Messerschmidt 2004). Masculinity is not a fixed entity embedded in the body or personality traits of individuals. Masculinities are configurations of practice that are accomplished in social action and, therefore, can differ according to the gender relations in a particular social setting.

The idea that a recognition of multiple masculinities necessarily turns into a static typology is likewise not borne out by the development of research. A paradigmatic example is Gutmann's (1996) Mexican ethnography, already mentioned. Gutmann is able to tease out different categories of masculinity—for example, the macho and the *mandilón*—while recognizing, and showing in detail, that these are not monadic identities but always are relational and constantly are crosscut by other divisions and projects. Warren's (1997) observations in a British elementary school provide another example. Different constructions of masculinity are found, which generate effects in classroom life, even though many boys do not fit exactly into the major categories; indeed, the boys demonstrate complex relations of attachment and rejection to those categories.

Although the idea that the concept of gender embeds heteronormativity is now a familiar criticism (Hawkesworth 1997), it is a contested criticism (Scott 1997). While it correctly identifies a problem in categorical models of gender, it is not a valid criticism of relational models of gender (e.g., Connell 2002; Walby 1997) nor of historical approaches where the construction of gender categories is the object of inquiry. In the development of the concept of hegemonic masculinity, divisions among men—especially the exclusion and subordination of homosexual men—were quite central issues (Carrigan, Connell, and Lee 1985). The policing of heterosexuality has been a major theme in discussions of hegemonic masculinity since then.

The idea that the concept of masculinity marginalizes or naturalizes the body (because it is supposed to rest on a sex-gender dichotomy) is perhaps the most startling of the claims in this critique. Startling, because the interplay between bodies and social processes has been one of the central themes of masculinity research from its beginning. One of the first and most influential research programs in the new paradigm was Messner's (1992) account of the masculinity of professional athletes, in which the use of "bodies as weapons" and the long-term damage to men's bodies were examined. The construction of masculinity in a context of disability (Gerschick and Miller 1994), the laboring bodies of working-class men (Donaldson 1991), men's health and illness (Sabo and Gordon 1995), and boys' interpersonal violence (Messerschmidt 2000) are among the themes in research showing how bodies are affected by social processes. Theoretical discussion has explored the relevance of the "new sociology of the body" to the construction of masculinity (e.g., Connell 1995, chap. 2).

Critiques of the concept of masculinity make better sense when they point to a tendency, in research as well as in popular literature, to dichotomize the experiences of men and women. As Brod (1994) accurately observes, there is a tendency in the men's studies field to presume "separate spheres," to proceed as if women were not a relevant part of the analysis, and therefore to analyze masculinities by looking only at men and relations among men. As Brod also argues, this is not inevitable. The cure lies in taking a consistently relational approach to gender—not in abandoning the concepts of gender or masculinity.

Ambiguity and overlap

Early criticisms of the concept raised the question of who actually represents hegemonic masculinity. It is familiar that many men who hold great social power do not embody an ideal masculinity. On the other hand, Donaldson (1993) remarks that there did not seem to be much masculine substance to those men identified by researchers as hegemonic models. He discusses the case of the Australian "iron man" surf-sports champion described by Connell (1990), a popular exemplar of hegemonic masculinity. But the young man's regional hegemonic status actually prevents him doing the things his local peer group defines as masculine—going wild, showing off, driving drunk, getting into fights, and defending his own prestige.

Martin (1998) criticizes the concept for leading to inconsistent applications, sometimes referring to a fixed type of masculinity and on other occasions referring to whatever type is dominant at a particular time and place. Similarly, Wetherell and Edley (1999) contend that the concept fails to specify what conformity to hegemonic masculinity actually looks like in practice. And Whitehead (1998, 58; 2002, 93) suggests there is confusion over who actually is a hegemonically masculine man—"Is it John Wayne or Leonardo DiCaprio; Mike Tyson or Pele? Or maybe, at different times, all of them?"—and also about who can enact hegemonic practices.

We think the critics have correctly pointed to ambiguities in usage. It is desirable to eliminate any usage of hegemonic masculinity as a fixed, transhistorical model. This usage violates the historicity of gender and ignores the massive evidence of change in social definitions of masculinity.

But in other respects, ambiguity in gender processes may be important to recognize as a mechanism of hegemony. Consider how an idealized definition of masculinity is constituted in social process. At a society-wide level (which we will call "regional" in the framework below), there is a circulation of models of admired masculine conduct, which may be exalted by churches, narrated by mass media, or celebrated by the state. Such models refer to, but also in various ways distort, the everyday realities of social practice. A classic example is the Soviet regime's celebration of the *Stakhanovite* industrial worker, named for the coal miner Aleksandr Stakhanov who in 1935 hewed a world record 102 tons of coal in a single day, triggering a scramble to beat the record. Part of the distortion here was that the famous "shock workers" achieved their numbers with a great deal of unacknowledged help from coworkers.

Thus, hegemonic masculinities can be constructed that do not correspond closely to the lives of any actual men. Yet these models do, in various ways, express widespread ideals, fantasies, and desires. They provide models of relations with women and solutions to problems of gender relations. Furthermore, they articulate loosely with the practical constitution of masculinities as ways of living in everyday local circumstances. To the extent they do this, they contribute to hegemony in the society-wide gender order as a whole. It is not surprising that men who function as exemplars at the regional level, such as the "iron man" discussed by Donaldson (1993), exhibit contradictions.

At the local level, hegemonic patterns of masculinity are embedded in specific social environments, such as formal organizations. There are, for instance, well-defined patterns of managerial masculinity in the British corporations studied by Roper (1994) and Wajcman (1999). Socially legitimated hegemonic models of masculinity are also in play in families. For instance, men's gender strategies shape negotiations around housework and the "second shift" in the U.S. families studied by Hochschild (1989). Hegemonic patterns of masculinity are both engaged with and contested as children grow up. Gender is made in schools and neighborhoods through peer group structure, control of school space, dating patterns, homophobic speech, and harassment (Mac an Ghaill 1994; Thorne 1993). In none of these cases would we expect hegemonic masculinity to stand out as a sharply defined pattern separate from all others. A degree of overlap or blurring between hegemonic and complicit masculinities is extremely likely if hegemony is effective.

The overlap between masculinities can also be seen in terms of the social agents constructing masculinities. Cavender (1999) shows how hegemonic masculine models were constructed differently in feature films in the 1940s compared with the 1980s. This is not just a matter of the characters written into the scripts. Practice at the local level—that is, the actual face-to-face interaction of shooting the film as an actor—ultimately constructs hegemonic masculine fantasy models (in this case, "detectives") at the society-wide or regional level. (We will explore this question of the relations between levels in the Reformulation section of the article.)

The problem of reification

That the concept of hegemonic masculinity reduces, in practice, to a reification of power or toxicity has also been argued from different points of view. Holter (1997, 2003), in the most conceptually sophisticated of all critiques, argues that the concept constructs masculine power from the direct experience of women rather than from the structural basis of women's subordination. Holter believes that we must distinguish between "patriarchy," the long-term structure of the subordination of women, and "gender," a specific system of exchange that arose in the context of modern capitalism. It is a mistake to treat a hierarchy of masculinities constructed within gender relations as logically continuous with the patriarchal subordination of women. Holter (1997) tellingly points to Norwegian survey evidence showing that the gender identities of men do not map directly onto such equality-related practices as attitudes toward violence.

Holter (1997, 2003) certainly is correct that it is a mistake to deduce relations among masculinities from the direct exercise of personal power by men over women. At the least, we also must factor in the institutionalization of gender inequalities, the role of cultural constructions, and the interplay of gender dynamics with race, class, and region.

It is, indeed, research on these issues that shows the concept of hegemonic masculinity is not trapped in reification. Among the fruitful studies of institutional masculinities are those that reveal quite subtle variations, for instance, between the different branches of a single military force, the U.S. Navy (Barrett 1996). There are studies of locally specific hegemonic masculinities constructed in spaces such as a New Zealand country pub, which show the interweaving of masculinity with rural identity (Campbell 2000). Other research, especially studies of school classrooms (Martino 1995; Warren 1997), shows the fine-grained production and negotiation of masculinities (and femininities) as configurations of practice.

Collier (1998) criticizes the concept of hegemonic masculinity through its typical use in accounting for violence and crime. In the "masculinity turn" in criminology, Collier suggests, hegemonic masculinity came to be associated solely with negative characteristics that depict men as unemotional, independent, non-nurturing, aggressive, and dispassionate—which are seen as the causes of criminal behavior. Martin (1998, 473) similarly observes a drift toward a view of hegemonic masculinity not just as a type but as a negative type, for instance, in "saying that defending gun ownership is a defense of hegemonic masculinity."

This criticism has force. It draws on McMahon's (1993) accurate analysis of the psychologism in many discussions of men and masculinity. Men's behavior is reified in a concept of masculinity that then, in a circular argument, becomes the explanation (and the excuse) for the behavior. This can be seen in many discussions of men's health and problems of boys' education—indeed, any of the contemporary troubles assembled under the banner of a "crisis in masculinity." In pop psychology, the invention of new character types is endemic (the alpha male, the sensitive new-age guy, the hairy man, the new lad, the "rat boy," etc.). In this environment, hegemonic masculinity can become a scientific-sounding synonym for a type of rigid, domineering, sexist, "macho" man (in the Anglo usage, e.g., Mosher and Tomkins 1988).

Because the concept of hegemonic masculinity is based on practice that permits men's collective dominance over women to continue, it is not surprising that in some contexts, hegemonic masculinity actually does refer to men's engaging in toxic practices—including physical violence—that stabilize gender dominance in a particular setting. However, violence and other noxious practices are not always the defining characteristics, since hegemony has numerous configurations. Indeed, as Wetherell and Edley (1999) ironically observe, one of the most effective ways of "being a man" in certain local contexts may be to demonstrate one's distance from a regional hegemonic masculinity.

Collier (1998) sees as a crucial defect in the concept of hegemonic masculinity that it excludes "positive" behavior on the part of men—that is, behavior that might serve the interests or desires of women. This hardly is a problem once we get beyond a rigid trait theory of personality. Most accounts of hegemonic masculinity do include such "positive" actions as bringing home a wage, sustaining a sexual relationship, and being a father. Indeed it is difficult to see how the concept of hegemony would be relevant if the only characteristics of the dominant group were violence, aggression, and self-centeredness. Such characteristics may mean domination but hardly would constitute hegemony—an idea that embeds certain notions of consent and participation by the subaltern groups.

Collier (1998, 21) is right in remarking that what actually is being discussed in many accounts of hegemonic masculinity and crime (and, we may add, health and education) is "a range of popular ideologies of what constitute ideal or actual characteristics of 'being a man.'" What Collier misses, however, is that sophisticated research consistently goes on to explore the relationship of those ideologies to the daily lives of boys and men—including the mismatches, the tensions, and the resistances.

It is men's and boys' practical relationships to collective images or models of masculinity, rather than simple reflections of them, that is central to understanding gendered consequences in violence, health, and education. This has been evident since Messerschmidt's (1993) formulation of the idea that different crimes are used by different men in the construction of masculinities. Collier finds this idea unacceptable, either tautological and universalizing, or too multitudinous in what it explains. But there is nothing surprising about the idea of diverse practices' being generated from common cultural templates; there is nothing conceptually universalizing in the idea of hegemonic masculinity. Coordination and regulation occur in the live social practices of collectivities, institutions, and whole societies. The concept of hegemonic masculinity is not intended as a catchall nor as a prime cause; it is a means of grasping a certain dynamic within the social process.

The masculine subject

Several authors have argued that the concept of hegemonic masculinity is based on an unsatisfactory theory of the subject. Wetherell and Edley (1999) develop this critique from the standpoint of discursive psychology, arguing that hegemonic masculinity cannot be understood as the settled character structure of any group of men. We must question "how men conform to an ideal and turn themselves into complicit or resistant types, without anyone ever managing to exactly embody that ideal" (p. 337).

Wetherell and Edley (1999) suggest we should understand hegemonic norms as defining a subject position in discourse that is taken up strategically by men in particular circumstances. Hegemonic masculinity has multiple meanings—a point that some authors have offered as a criticism but that Wetherell and Edley take as a positive point of departure. Men can dodge among multiple meanings according to their interactional needs. Men can adopt hegemonic masculinity when it is desirable; but the same men can distance themselves strategically from hegemonic masculinity at other moments. Consequently, "masculinity" represents not a certain type of man but, rather, a way that men position themselves through discursive practices.

Whitehead (2002, 93) argues that the concept of hegemonic masculinity can "see" only structure, making the subject invisible: "The individual is lost within, or, in Althusserian terms, subjected to, an ideological apparatus and an innate drive for power." To Whitehead, the concept fails to specify how and why some heterosexual men legitimate, reproduce, and generate their dominance and do so as a social minority vis-à-vis women and other men. Consequently, use of the concept results "in obfuscation, in the conflation of fluid masculinities with overarching structure and, ultimately, in 'abstract structural dynamics'" (Whitehead 2002, 93–94). For Whitehead, it is preferable to concentrate on discourse as the means by which men come to know themselves, to practice "identity work," and to exercise gender power and resistance.

A related criticism derives from psychoanalysis. According to this view, the model of hegemonic masculinity presumes a unitary subject; but depth psychology reveals a multilayered or divided subject (Collier 1998; Jefferson 1994). Jefferson (2002) criticizes the "over-socialized view of the male subject" in studies of masculinity, which has resulted in a lack of attention to how men actually relate psychologically to hegemonic masculinity. Given multiple masculinities, Jefferson argues that researchers should ask "how actual men, with their unique biographies and particular psychic formations, relate to these various masculinities" (p. 73). Jefferson suggests that boys and men choose those discursive positions that help them ward off anxiety and avoid feelings of powerlessness.

The argument from discursive psychology is well taken and is well integrated with a fruitful research approach. A good example is Lea and Auburn's (2001) study of the story told by a convicted rapist in a sex-offender program, which shows how the narrating offender moves between conflicting ideologies of sexual interaction in a way that reduces his responsibility for the rape. Another example is Archer's (2001) exploration of the identity talk of young Muslim men in Britain, showing how they use a specific model of hegemonic masculinity ("powerful, patriarchal") to position themselves in relation to Afro-Caribbean men, white men, and Muslim women. From this work, we can learn not only how masculinities are constructed in discourse but also how they are used in discourse. Specifically, we learn how a locally hegemonic version of masculinity can be used to promote self-respect in the face of discredit, for instance, from racist denigration.

Discursive perspectives emphasize the symbolic dimension, whereas the concept of hegemonic masculinity was formulated within a multidimensional understanding of gender. Although any specification of hegemonic masculinity typically involves the formulation of cultural ideals, it should not be regarded only as a cultural norm. Gender relations also are constituted through nondiscursive practices, including wage labor, violence, sexuality, domestic labor, and child care as well as through unreflective routinized actions.

Recognizing the nondiscursive and unreflective dimensions of gender gives us some sense of the limits to discursive flexibility. That there are such limits is a point powerfully made in Rubin's (2003) study of female-to-male transsexual men. One is not free to adopt any gender position in interaction simply as a discursive or reflexive move. The possibilities are constrained massively by embodiment, by institutional histories, by economic forces, and by personal and family relationships. The costs of making certain discursive choices can be extremely high—as shown by the rate of suicide among people involved in transsexual moves.

Constraint also may arise from within the person. Rubin's (2003) respondents act as they do, and face the costs, because of an unshakeable conviction of being men—despite starting out with female bodies and being brought up as girls. They are convinced of being unitary subjects, although they live a contradiction that seems to exemplify Jefferson's (1994, 2002) argument for the divided subject. We agree with Jefferson that psychoanalytic practice and theory are important resources for understanding the complex subject of gender practice. However, Jefferson's particular psychoanalytic approach is not without problems (Messerschmidt 2005), and it is important to recognize the diversity and wealth of the psychoanalytic tradition. Approaches such as Sartre's existential psychoanalysis are helpful for understanding masculinities as projects and a masculine identity as always being a provisional accomplishment within a life course. Adlerian psychoanalysis, with its emphasis on the emotional consequences of gendered power relations in childhood, gave rise to the idea of the "masculine protest," which still resonates with contemporary discussions of marginalized youth.

The concept of hegemonic masculinity originally was formulated with a strong awareness of psychoanalytic arguments about the layered and contradictory character of personality, the everyday contestation in social life, and the mixture of strategies necessary in any attempt to sustain hegemony (Carrigan, Connell, and Lee 1985; Connell 1987). It is somewhat ironic that the concept is criticized for oversimplifying the subject, but it is, of course, true that the concept often has been employed in simplified forms.

Does the concept necessarily erase the subject? We flatly disagree with Whitehead's (2002) claim that the concept of hegemonic masculinity reduces to structural determinism. Masculinity is defined as a configuration of practice organized in relation to the structure of gender relations. Human social practice creates gender relations in history. The concept of hegemonic masculinity embeds a historically dynamic view of gender in which it is impossible to erase the subject. This is why life-history studies have become a characteristic genre of work on hegemonic masculinity.

The concept homogenizes the subject only if it is reduced to a single dimension of gender relations (usually the symbolic) and if it is treated as the specification of a norm. As soon as one recognizes the multidimensionality of gender relations (Connell 2002) and the occurrence of crisis tendencies within gender relations (Connell 1995), it is impossible to regard the subject constituted within those relations as unitary. There are, of course, different ways of representing the incoherence of the subject. The conceptual language of poststructuralism is only one way of doing that; psychoanalysis and the model of agency within contradictory social structures provide others.

The pattern of gender relations

In social theories of gender, there has often been a tendency toward functionalism—that is, seeing gender relations as a self-contained, self-reproducing system and explaining every element in terms of its function in reproducing the whole. Hawkesworth (1997) detects this tendency in most modern theories of gender, and Bourdieu's (2001) late intervention to explain masculine domination has given a new lease on life to functionalism in gender analysis.

The dominance of men and the subordination of women constitute a historical process, not a self-reproducing system. "Masculine domination" is open to challenge and requires considerable effort to maintain. Although this point was made in early statements on the hegemonic masculinity concept, it is not just a theoretical idea. There is detailed work that shows the tactics of maintenance through the exclusion of women, ranging from Bird's (1996) work on homosociality to the organizational research by Collinson, Knights, and Collinson (1990), Cockburn (1991), and Martin (2001).

There exists considerable evidence that hegemonic masculinity is not a self-reproducing form, whether through habitus or any other mechanism. To sustain a given pattern of hegemony requires the policing of men as well as the exclusion or discrediting of women. Evidence of such mechanisms ranges from the discrediting of "soft" options in the "hard" world of international relations, security threats, and war (Hooper 2001), to homophobic assaults and murders (Tomsen 2002), all the way to the teasing of boys in school for "sissiness" (Kimmel and Mahler 2003; Messerschmidt 2000).

In Demetriou's (2001) careful critique of the concept of hegemonic masculinity, the historicity of gender is acknowledged. Demetriou, however, suggests that another kind of simplification has occurred. He identifies two forms of hegemony, internal and external. "External hegemony" refers to the institutionalization of men's dominance over women; "internal hegemony" refers to the social ascendancy of one group of men over all other men. Demetriou argues that the relationship between the two forms is unclear in the original formulation of the concept and unspecified in current usages. Moreover, internal hegemony typically has been understood in an "elitist" way. That is, subordinate and marginalized masculinities are seen as having no impact on the construction of hegemonic masculinity. Nonhegemonic masculinities exist in tension with, but never penetrate or impact, the hegemonic masculinity. There is, then, a dualistic representation of masculinities.

Such a conceptualization, Demetriou (2001) argues, misses the "dialectical pragmatism" of internal hegemony, by which hegemonic masculinity appropriates from other masculinities whatever appears to be pragmatically useful for continued domination. The result of this dialectic is not a unitary pattern of hegemonic masculinity but a "historic bloc" involving a weaving together of multiple patterns, whose hybridity is the best possible strategy for external hegemony. A constant process of negotiation, translation, and reconfiguration occurs.

This conceptualization leads to a different view of historical change in masculinities. Hegemonic masculinity does not simply adapt to changing historical conditions. Rather, the hegemonic masculine bloc is a hybridization whose appropriation of diverse elements makes it "capable of reconfiguring itself and adapting to the specificities of new historical conjunctures" (Demetriou 2001, 355). As an example of this process, Demetriou (2001) discusses the increasing cultural visibility of gay masculinity in Western societies. This has made it possible for certain heterosexual men to appropriate "bits and pieces" of gay men's styles and practices and construct a new hybrid configuration of gender practice. Such an appropriation blurs gender difference but does not undermine patriarchy.

Demetriou's (2001) conceptualization of dialectical pragmatism in "internal hegemony" is useful, and he makes a convincing case that certain representations of masculinity, and some heterosexual men's everyday gender practices, have appropriated aspects of gay masculinities. Clearly, specific masculine practices may be appropriated into other masculinities, creating a hybrid (such as the hip-hop style and language adopted by some working-class white teenage boys and the unique composite style of gay "clones"). Yet we are not convinced that the hybridization Demetriou (2001) describes is hegemonic, at least beyond a local sense. Although gay masculinity and sexuality are increasingly visible in Western societies—witness the fascination with the gay male characters in the television programs *Six Feet Under*, *Will and Grace*, and *Queer Eye for the Straight Guy*—there is little reason to think that hybridization has become hegemonic at the regional or global level.

The concept of a hegemonic bloc brings into focus the issue of multiple hegemonic masculinities. Jefferson (2002, 71) and others have criticized the tendency to speak of just one pattern—"hegemonic masculinity is always used in the singular." There is a paradox here. Because every ethnography discovers a distinctive gender culture, every life-history study uncovers unique trajectories of men's lives, and every structural analysis defines new intersections of race, class, gender, and generation, it is logically possible to define "a thousand and one" variations of masculinity (Meuser and Behnke 1998). This surely is also true of claimants to hegemony. The point is strongly supported by Messner's (1997) mapping of masculinity politics in the United States, which revealed a range of movements with contrasting agendas. Yet when examined closely, most of these movements present a claim to be *the* way for men to think and live. Whatever the empirical diversity of masculinities, the contestation for hegemony implies that gender hierarchy does not have multiple niches at the top. We will return to this issue, which is important for understanding gender politics.

Review and reformulation

We now draw these threads together to suggest how the concept of hegemonic masculinity should be reshaped. We will indicate those features of the original concept that have held up well in the light of research and criticism, those features that should be discarded, and (in greater detail) those areas where the concept is in need of contemporary reformulation.

What should be retained

The fundamental feature of the concept remains the combination of the plurality of masculinities and the hierarchy of masculinities. This basic idea has stood up well in 20 years of research experience. Multiple patterns of masculinity have been identified in many studies, in a variety of countries, and in different institutional and cultural settings. It is also a widespread research finding that certain masculinities are more socially central, or more associated with authority and social power, than others. The concept of hegemonic masculinity presumes the subordination of nonhegemonic masculinities, and this is a process that has now been documented in many settings, internationally.

Also well supported is the idea that the hierarchy of masculinities is a pattern of hegemony, not a pattern of simple domination based on force. Cultural consent, discursive centrality, institutionalization, and the marginalization or delegitimation of alternatives are widely documented features of socially dominant masculinities. Also well supported is the original idea that hegemonic masculinity need not be the commonest pattern in the everyday lives of boys and men. Rather, hegemony works in part through the production of exemplars of masculinity (e.g., professional sports stars), symbols that have authority despite the fact that most men and boys do not fully live up to them.

The original formulations laid some emphasis on the possibility of change in gender relations, on the idea that a dominant pattern of masculinity was open to challenge—from women's resistance to patriarchy, and from men as bearers of alternative masculinities. Research has very fully confirmed the idea of the historical construction and reconstruction of hegemonic masculinities. Both at a local and a broad societal level, the situations in which masculinities were formed change over time. These changes call forth new strategies in gender relations (e.g., companionate marriage) and result in redefinitions of socially admired masculinity (e.g., the domestic partner rather than the Victorian patriarch).

What should be rejected

Two features of early formulations about hegemonic masculinity have not stood up to criticism and should be discarded. The first is a too-simple model of the social relations surrounding hegemonic masculinities. The formulation in *Gender and Power* attempted to locate all masculinities (and all femininities) in terms of a single pattern of power, the "global dominance" of men over women (Connell 1987, 183). While this was useful at the time in preventing the idea of multiple masculinities from collapsing into an array of competing lifestyles, it is now clearly inadequate to our understanding of relations among groups of men and forms of masculinity and of women's relations with dominant masculinities. For instance, dominance in gender relations involves an interplay of costs and benefits, challenges to hegemonic masculinity arise from the "protest masculinities" of marginalized ethnic groups, and bourgeois women may appropriate aspects of hegemonic masculinity in constructing corporate or professional careers. Clearly, better ways of understanding gender hierarchy are required.

Despite the critique of trait psychology in *Gender and Power*, and the appeal to psychoanalytic ideas about unconscious motivation, early statements about hegemonic masculinity, when they attempted to characterize the actual content of different configurations of masculinity, often fell back on trait terminology—or at best failed to offer an alternative to it. The notion of masculinity as an assemblage of traits opened the path to that treatment of hegemonic masculinity as a fixed character type that has given so much trouble and is rightly criticized in recent psychological writing. Not only the essentialist concept of masculinity but also, more generally, the trait approach to gender need to be thoroughly transcended.

What should be reformulated

In light of the research and critiques discussed above, we argue that the concept of hegemonic masculinity is in need of reformulation in four main areas: the nature of gender hierarchy, the geography of masculine configurations, the process of social embodiment, and the dynamics of masculinities. In the following subsections, we offer a line of thought, and some research suggestions, about each of these issues.

Gender hierarchy

Compared with original formulations of the concept, contemporary research has shown the complexity of the relationships among different constructions of masculinity. The recent research in discursive psychology indicates how different constructions of masculinity at the local level may serve as tactical alternatives. Structured relations among masculinities exist in all local settings, motivation toward a specific hegemonic version varies by local context, and such local versions inevitably differ somewhat from each other. Demetriou's (2001) notion of dialectical pragmatism captures the reciprocal influence of masculinities on each other; hegemonic masculine patterns may change by incorporating elements from the others.

Analyses of relations among masculinities now more clearly recognize the agency of subordinated and marginalized groups—often conditioned by their specific location (as discussed below). "Protest masculinity" (Poynting, Noble, and Tabar 2003) can be understood in this sense: a pattern of masculinity constructed in local working-class settings, sometimes among ethnically marginalized men, which embodies the claim to power typical of regional hegemonic masculinities in Western countries, but which lacks the economic resources and institutional authority that underpins the regional and global patterns.

Research has also documented the durability or survivability of nonhegemonic patterns of masculinity, which may represent well-crafted responses to race/ethnic marginalization, physical disability, class inequality, or stigmatized sexuality. Hegemony may be accomplished by the incorporation of such masculinities into a functioning gender order rather than by active oppression in the form of discredit or violence. In practice, both incorporation and oppression can occur together. This is, for instance, the contemporary position of gay masculinities in Western urban centers, where gay communities have a spectrum of experience ranging from homophobic violence and cultural denigration to toleration and even cultural celebration and political representation. Similar processes of incorporation and oppression may occur among girls and women who construct masculinities (Messerschmidt 2004).

The concept of hegemonic masculinity was originally formulated in tandem with a concept of hegemonic femininity—soon renamed "emphasized femininity" to acknowledge the asymmetrical position of masculinities and femininities in a patriarchal gender order. In the development of research on men and masculinities, this relationship has dropped out of focus. This is regrettable for more than one reason. Gender is always relational, and patterns of masculinity are socially defined in contradistinction from some model (whether real or imaginary) of femininity.

Perhaps more important, focusing only on the activities of men occludes the practices of women in the construction of gender among men. As is well shown by life-history research, women are central in many of the processes constructing masculinities—as mothers; as schoolmates; as girlfriends, sexual partners, and wives; as workers in the gender division of labor; and so forth. The concept of emphasized femininity focused on compliance to patriarchy, and this is still highly relevant in contemporary mass culture. Yet gender hierarchies are also affected by new configurations of women's identity and practice, especially among younger women—which are increasingly acknowledged by younger men. We consider that research on hegemonic masculinity now needs to give much closer attention to the practices of women and to the historical interplay of femininities and masculinities.

We suggest, therefore, that our understanding of hegemonic masculinity needs to incorporate a more holistic understanding of gender hierarchy, recognizing the agency of subordinated groups as much as the power of dominant groups and the mutual conditioning of gender dynamics and other social dynamics. We think this will tend, over time, to reduce the isolation of men's studies and will emphasize the relevance of gender dynamics to the problems—ranging from effects of globalization to issues of violence and peacemaking—being explored in other fields of social science.

The geography of masculinities

Change in locally specific constructions of hegemonic masculinity has been a theme of research for the past two decades. But with growing attention to globalization, the significance of transnational arenas for the construction of masculinity has also been argued. Hooper (1998, 2000) describes the deployment of hegemonic and other masculinities in the arenas of international relations, and Connell (1998) proposed a model of "transnational business masculinity" among corporate executives that was connected with neoliberal agendas of globalization.

Whether, or how far, such processes override more local and regional gender dynamics is still being debated. Pease and Pringle (2001), in a recent international collection, argue for a continued focus on understanding masculinities regionally and comparatively. At the least, we must understand that regional and local constructions of hegemonic masculinity are shaped by the articulation of these gender systems with global processes. In this vein, Kimmel (2005) has recently examined how the effects of a global hegemonic masculinity are embedded in the emergence of regional (white supremacists in the United States and Sweden) and global (al Qaeda from the Middle East) "protest" masculinities.

We consider these issues are now unavoidable for studies of masculinity and suggest the following simple framework. Empirically existing hegemonic masculinities can be analyzed at three levels:

1. Local: constructed in the arenas of face-to-face interaction of families, organizations, and immediate communities, as typically found in ethnographic and life-history research;
2. Regional: constructed at the level of the culture or the nation-state, as typically found in discursive, political, and demographic research; and
3. Global: constructed in transnational arenas such as world politics and transnational business and media, as studied in the emerging research on masculinities and globalization.

Not only do links between these levels exist; they can be important in gender politics. Global institutions pressure regional and local gender orders; while regional gender orders provide cultural materials adopted or reworked in global arenas and provide models of masculinity that may be important in local gender dynamics.

Let us consider specifically the relation between regional and local masculinities. Hegemonic masculinity at the regional level is symbolically represented through the interplay of specific local masculine practices that have regional significance, such as those constructed by feature film actors, professional athletes, and politicians. The exact content of these practices varies over time and across societies. Yet regional hegemonic masculinity shapes a society-wide sense of masculine reality and, therefore, operates in the cultural domain as on-hand material to be actualized, altered, or challenged through practice in a range of different local circumstances. A regional hegemonic masculinity, then, provides a cultural framework that may be materialized in daily practices and interactions.

As an illustration of this interplay between regional and local hegemonic masculinities, consider the example of sport. In Western societies, practice at the local level—such as engaging in professional sporting events—constructs hegemonic masculine models (e.g., "star athletes") at the regional level, which in turn affect other local settings. Research on secondary schooling provides a paradigmatic example, indicating that successful participation in sport often is a salient hegemonic masculine practice in this particular local setting (Messner 2002). For example, Light and Kirk (2000) examine an elite Australian high school, finding that a clear structure of masculinities existed at this school in which a specific hegemonic form was shaped through the embodied practice of rugby football—a code that is, of course, not confined to this school—centering on domination, aggression, ruthless competitiveness, and giving all for the school. (Compare the similar findings of Burgess, Edwards, and Skinner 2003.) Thus, regionally significant exemplary masculine models influence—although they do not wholly determine—the construction of gender relations and hegemonic masculinities at the local level.

It is tempting to assume a simple hierarchy of power or authority, running from global to regional to local, but this could be misleading. In discussions of globalization, the determining power of the "global" is often overestimated, while the resistance and capacity of what we are calling the "regional" goes unrecognized (Mittelman 2004). The limited research that has so far been done on masculinities in global arenas (e.g., Connell and Wood 2005; Hooper 2001) does not suggest a powerful formation with the capacity to overwhelm regional or local masculinities. Yet the evidence on global dynamics in gender is growing, and it is clear that processes such as economic restructuring, long-distance migration, and the turbulence of "development" agendas have the power to reshape local patterns of masculinity and femininity (Connell 2005; Morrell and Swart 2005). There is every reason to think that interactions involving global masculinities will become of more importance in gender politics, and this is a key arena for future research on hegemony.

Adopting an analytical framework that distinguishes local, regional, and global masculinities (and the same point applies to femininities) allows us to recognize the importance of place without falling into a monadic world of totally independent cultures or discourses. It also casts some light on the problem of multiple hegemonic masculinities, raised above. Although local models of hegemonic masculinity may differ from each other, they generally overlap. The interplay with society-wide gender dynamics is part of the explanation. Furthermore, hegemonic masculinities are, as we have just argued, to a significant degree constituted in men's interaction with women; therefore, the commonalities in women's gender practices also produce convergence. Accordingly, local constructions of hegemonic masculinity have a certain "family resemblance," to use Wittgenstein's term, rather than logical identity. In this sense, local plurality is compatible with singularity of hegemonic masculinity at the regional or society-wide level. The "family resemblance" among local variants is likely to be represented by one symbolic model at the regional level, not by multiple models.

Social embodiment

That hegemonic masculinity is related to particular ways of representing and using men's bodies has been recognized from the earliest formulations of the concept. Yet the pattern of embodiment involved in hegemony has not been convincingly theorized.

The importance of masculine embodiment for identity and behavior emerges in many contexts. In youth, skilled bodily activity becomes a prime indicator of masculinity, as we have already seen with sport. This is a key way that heterosexuality and masculinity become linked in Western culture, with prestige conferred on boys with heterosexual partners and sexual learning imagined as exploration and conquest. Body practices such as eating meat and taking risks on the road also become linked with masculine identities. This logically results in health promotion strategies that work by degendering —contesting hegemonic masculinity, or moving men in a more androgynous direction. But the difficulties of degendering strategies also are partly based in embodiment, for instance, in the commitment to risk-taking practices as means of establishing masculine reputation in a peer group context.

The common social scientific reading of bodies as objects of a process of social construction is now widely considered to be inadequate. Bodies are involved more actively, more intimately, and more intricately in social processes than theory has usually allowed. Bodies participate in social action by delineating courses of social conduct—the body is a participant in generating social practice. It is important not only that masculinities be understood as embodied but also that the interweaving of embodiment and social context be addressed.

The need for a more sophisticated treatment of embodiment in hegemonic masculinity is made particularly clear by the issue of transgender practices, which are difficult to understand within a simple model of social construction. This issue has been reframed by the rise of queer theory, which has treated gender crossing as a subversion of the gender order or at least as a demonstration of its vulnerability. Sharp debates over transsexualism have arisen, with some psychiatrists' questioning the very possibility of gender change. It is therefore not easy to be confident about the implications of transgender practice for hegemony. With Rubin (2003) and Namaste (2000), we consider that the masculinities constructed in female-to-male transsexuals' life courses are not inherently counterhegemonic. "Self-made men" can pursue gender equality or oppose it, just like nontranssexual men. What the transsexual experience highlights is modernity's treatment of the body as the "medium through which selves interact with each other" (Rubin 2003, 180).

To understand embodiment and hegemony, we need to understand that bodies are both objects of social practice and agents in social practice (Connell 2002). There are circuits of social practice linking bodily processes and social structures—many such circuits, which add up to the historical process in which society is embodied. These circuits of social embodiment may be very direct and simple, or they may be long and complex, passing through institutions, economic relations, cultural symbols, and so forth —without ceasing to involve material bodies. This can readily be illustrated by thinking about the gender patterns in health, illness, and medical treatment.

Among dominant groups of men, the circuits of social embodiment constantly involve the institutions on which their privileges rest. This is dramatically shown in a pioneering study by Donaldson and Poynting (2004) of the daily lives of ruling-class men. This study shows, for instance, how their characteristic sports, leisure, and eating practices deploy their wealth and establish relations of distance and dominance over other men's bodies. A rich field of research opens up here, especially when we consider how expensive technologies—computer systems, global air travel, secure communications—amplify the physical powers of elite men's bodies.

The dynamics of masculinities

Although long acknowledged, the internal complexity of masculinities has only gradually come into focus as a research issue. As indicated by our earlier discussion of the subject in gender practice, we must now explicitly recognize the layering, the potential internal contradiction, within all practices that construct masculinities. Such practices cannot be read simply as expressing a unitary masculinity. They may, for instance, represent compromise formations between contradictory desires or emotions, or the results of uncertain calculations about the costs and benefits of different gender strategies.

Life-history research has pointed to another dynamic of masculinities, the structure of a project. Masculinities are configurations of practice that are constructed, unfold, and change through time. A small literature on masculinity and aging, and a larger one on childhood and youth, emphasize this issue. The careful analysis of life histories may detect contradictory commitments and institutional transitions that reflect different hegemonic masculinities and also hold seeds of change.

Hegemonic masculinities are likely to involve specific patterns of internal division and emotional conflict, precisely because of their association with gendered power. Relationships with fathers are one likely focus of tension, given the gender division of labor in child care, the "long hours culture" in professions and management, and the preoccupation of rich fathers with managing their wealth. Ambivalence toward projects of change on the part of women are likely to be another, leading to oscillating acceptance and rejection of gender equality by the same men. Any strategy for the maintenance of power is likely to involve a dehumanizing of other groups and a corresponding withering of empathy and emotional relatedness within the self (Schwalbe 1992). Without treating privileged men as objects of pity, we should recognize that hegemonic masculinity does not necessarily translate into a satisfying experience of life.

Change over time, while certainly shaped by contradictions within masculinities, may also be intentional. Children as well as adults have a capacity to deconstruct gender binaries and criticize hegemonic masculinity, and this capacity is the basis of many educational interventions and change programs. At the same time, bearers of hegemonic masculinity are not necessarily "cultural dopes"; they may actively attempt to modernize gender relations and to reshape masculinities as part of the deal. A good example is the "new public management" in public-sector organizations, which rejects old-style bureaucracy and believes in "flatter" organizations, equal opportunity, and family-friendly employment policies. Yet even the modernization of masculinities may not solve problems. This too, as Meuser (2001) argues, generates contradictions that may lead to further change.

Gender relations are always arenas of tension. A given pattern of hegemonic masculinity is hegemonic to the extent that it provides a solution to these tensions, tending to stabilize patriarchal power or reconstitute it in new conditions. A pattern of practice (i.e., a version of masculinity) that provided such a solution in past conditions but not in new conditions is open to challenge—is in fact certain to be challenged.

Such contestation occurs continuously, through the efforts of the women's movement (at the local, regional, and global levels), among generations in immigrant communities, between models of managerial masculinity, among rivals for political authority, among claimants for attention in the entertainment industry, and so on. The contestation is real, and gender theory does not predict which will prevail—the process is historically open. Accordingly, hegemony may fail. The concept of hegemonic masculinity does not rely on a theory of social reproduction.

Put another way, the conceptualization of hegemonic masculinity should explicitly acknowledge the possibility of democratizing gender relations, of abolishing power differentials, not just of reproducing hierarchy. A transitional move in this direction requires an attempt to establish as hegemonic among men ("internal hegemony" in Demetriou's [2001] sense) a version of masculinity open to equality with women. In this sense, it is possible to define a hegemonic masculinity that is thoroughly "positive" (in Collier's [1998] sense). Recent history has shown the difficulty of doing this in practice. A positive hegemony remains, nevertheless, a key strategy for contemporary efforts at reform.

Conclusion

Concepts in the social sciences arise in response to specific intellectual and practical problems, and they are formulated in specific languages and intellectual styles. But they also have a capacity to travel and may acquire new meanings as they do. This has certainly happened with the concept of hegemonic masculinity, which has been taken up in fields ranging from education and psychotherapy to violence prevention and international relations. Some of the ambiguities that annoy critics stem from the varied uses that the concept has found and the ways it has been inflected in response to new contexts.

This is perhaps a general problem about conceptualization in the social sciences and humanities. As a theoretical formulation finds application in other settings and by other hands, the concept must mutate—and it may mutate in different directions in different environments. A specific concept may thus transform into a general way of talking, a style of analysis, or a characteristic figure in argument. There is nothing wrong with this process in itself—it is a common way that knowledge in the social sciences and humanities develops. But it means that new usages must also be open to critique and may lack some of the substance or justification of the original.

Thus, while we welcome most of the applications and modifications of the hegemonic masculinity concept as contributions to the understanding of gender dynamics, we reject those usages that imply a fixed character type, or an assemblage of toxic traits. These usages are not trivial—they are trying to name significant issues about gender, such as the persistence of violence or the consequences of domination. But they do so in a way that conflicts with the analysis of hegemony in gender relations and is therefore incompatible with (not just a variation on) both the initial statements and the main developments of this concept.

A renovated analysis of hegemonic masculinities, of the kind suggested above, has a growing relevance in the present moment of gender politics. In the rich countries of the global metropole, the shift from neoliberalism (the radical market agenda formulated in the 1970s) to neoconservatism (adding populist appeals to religion, ethnocentrism, and security) has made gender reaction an important political and cultural issue. In the developing countries, the processes of globalization have opened regional and local gender orders to new pressures for transformation and have also opened the way to new coalitions among groups of powerful men. In the global arenas of transnational corporations, media, and security systems, new patterns of hegemony are being forged. The making and contestation of hegemony in historically changing gender orders is a process of enormous importance for which we continue to need conceptual tools.

Acknowledgements

The authors are grateful to the journal's reviewers, Pat Martin, Mike Messner, and Kirsten Dellinger, for extremely helpful comments on an earlier draft of this article. We also extend our thanks to John Fisher, whose patient and inventive searching of bibliographical databases provided essential support for this article.

References

Altman, D. 1972. *Homosexual: Oppression and liberation.* Sydney, Australia: Angus and Robertson.

Archer, L. 2001. Muslim brothers, Black lads, traditional Asians: British Muslim young men's constructions of race, religion and masculinity. *Feminism & Psychology* 11 (1): 79–105.

Baca Zinn, M. 1982. Chicano men and masculinity. *Journal of Ethnic Studies* 10 (2): 29–44.

Barrett, F. J. 1996. The organizational construction of hegemonic masculinity: The case of the U.S. Navy. *Gender, Work and Organization* 3 (3): 129–42.

Belton, R. J. 1995. *The beribboned bomb: The image of woman in male surrealist art.* Calgary, Canada: University of Calgary Press.

Berg, L. D. 1994. Masculinity, place and a binary discourse of "theory" and "empirical investigation" in the human geography of Aotearoa/New Zealand. *Gender, Place and Culture* 1 (2): 245–60.

Bird, S. R. 1996. Welcome to the men's club: Homosociality and the maintenance of hegemonic masculinity. *Gender & Society* 10 (2): 120–32.

Bourdieu, P. 2001. *Masculine domination.* Stanford, CA: Stanford University Press.

Brannon, R. 1976. The male sex role: Our culture's blueprint of manhood, and what it's done for us lately. In *The forty-nine percent majority: The male sex role*, edited by D. S. David and R. Brannon. Reading, MA: Addington-Wesley.

Brod, H. 1987. *The making of masculinities: The new men's studies.* Boston: Allen and Unwin.

———. 1994. Some thoughts on some histories of some masculinities: Jews and other others. In *Theorizing masculinities*, edited by D. S. David and R. Brannon. Thousand Oaks, CA: Sage.

Broker, M. 1976. "I may be a queer, but at least I am a man": Male hegemony and ascribed versus achieved gender. In *Sexual divisions and society*, edited by D. Leonard Barker and S. Allen. London: Tavistock.

Brown, D. 1999. Complicity and reproduction in teaching physical education. *Sport, Education and Society* 4 (2): 143–59.

Bufkin, J. L. 1999. Bias crime as gendered behavior. *Social Justice* 26 (1): 155–76.

Burgess, I., A. Edwards, and J. Skinner. 2003. Football culture in an Australian school setting: The construction of masculine identity. *Sport, Education and Society* 8 (2): 199–212.

Campbell, H. 2000. The glass phallus: Pub(lic) masculinity and drinking in rural New Zealand. *Rural Sociology* 65 (4): 562–81.

Carrigan, T., R. W. Connell, and J. Lee. 1985. Toward a new sociology of masculinity. *Theory and Society* 14 (5): 551–604.

Cavender, G. 1999. Detecting masculinity. In *Making trouble: Cultural constructions of crime, deviance and control*, edited by J. Ferrell and N. Websdale. New York: Aldine de Gruyter.

Cheng, C. 1996. "We choose not to compete": The "merit" discourse in the selection process, and Asian and Asian American men and their masculinity. In *Masculinities in organizations*, edited by C. Cheng. Thousand Oaks, CA: Sage.

Cockburn, C. 1983. *Brothers: Male dominance and technological change.* London: Pluto.

———. 1991. *In the way of men: Men's resistance to sex equality in organizations.* London: Macmillan.

Collier, R. 1998. *Masculinities, crime and criminology: Men, heterosexuality and the criminal(ised) other.* London: Sage.

Collinson, D., and J. Hearn. 1994. Naming men as men: Implications for work, organization and management. *Gender, Work and Organization* 1 (1): 2–22.

Collinson, D., D. Knights, and M. Collinson. 1990. *Managing to discriminate.* London: Routledge.

Connell, R. W. 1977. *Ruling class, ruling culture.* Cambridge, UK: Cambridge University Press.

———. 1982. Class, patriarchy, and Sartre's theory of practice. *Theory and Society* 11:305–20.

———. 1983. *Which way is up? Essays on sex, class and culture.* Sydney, Australia: Allen and Unwin.

———. 1987. *Gender and power.* Sydney, Australia: Allen and Unwin.

———. 1990. An iron man: The body and some contradictions of hegemonic masculinity. In *Sport, men and the gender order*, edited by M. Messner and D. Sabo. Champaign, IL: Human Kinetics Books.

———. 1995. *Masculinities.* Cambridge, UK: Polity Press.

———. 1998. Masculinities and globalization. *Men and Masculinities* 1 (1): 3–23.

———. 2002. *Gender.* Cambridge, UK: Polity Press.

———. 2003. Masculinities, change and conflict in global society: Thinking about the future of men's studies. *Journal of Men's Studies* 11 (3): 249–66.

———. 2005. Globalization, imperialism, and masculinities. In *Handbook of studies on men & masculinities*, edited by M. S. Kimmel, J. Hearn, and R. W. Connell. Thousand Oaks, CA: Sage.

Connell, R. W., D. J. Ashenden, S. Kessler, and G. W. Dowsett. 1982. *Making the difference: Schools, families and social division.* Sydney, Australia: Allen and Unwin.

Connell, R. W., and J. Wood. 2005. Globalization and business masculinities. *Men and Masculinities* 7 (4): 347–64.

Consalvo, M. 2003. The monsters next door: Media constructions of boys and masculinity. *Feminist Media Studies* 3 (1): 27–46.

Dasgupta, R. 2000. Performing masculinities? The "salaryman" at work and play. *Japanese Studies* 20 (2): 189–200.

Davis, A. 1983. *Women, race, and class.* New York: Vintage.

Demetriou, D. Z. 2001. Connell's concept of hegemonic masculinity: A critique. *Theory and Society* 30 (3): 337–61.

Denborough, D. 1996. Step by step: Developing respectful and effective ways of working with young men to reduce violence. In *Men's ways of being*, edited by C. McLean, M. Carey, and C. White. Boulder, CO: Westview.

Dinges, M., E. Ründal, and D. Bauer. 2004. Programm. Program for the Hegemoniale Männlichkeiten conference, Stuttgart, Germany, 24–26 June.
Donaldson, M. 1991. *Time of our lives: Labor and love in the working class*. Sydney, Australia: Allen and Unwin.
———. 1993. What is hegemonic masculinity? *Theory and Society* 22:643–57.
Donaldson, M., and S. Poynting. 2004. The time of their lives: Time, work and leisure in the daily lives of ruling-class men. In *Ruling Australia: The power, privilege & politics of the new ruling class*, edited by N. Hollier. Melbourne: Australian Scholarly.
Eisenstein, Z. R. 1979. *Capitalist patriarchy and the case for socialist feminism*. New York: Monthly Review Press.
Ferguson, H. 2001. Men and masculinities in late-modern Ireland. In *A man's world? Changing men's practices in a globalized world*, edited by B. Pease and K. Pringle. London: Zed Books.
Freud, Sigmund. [1917] 1955. *From the history of an infantile neurosis. Complete psychological works*. Standard ed., Vol. 17. London: Hogarth.
Friedman, R. M., and L. Lerner. 1986. Toward a new psychology of men: Psychoanalytic and social perspectives. Special issue, *Psychoanalytic Review* 73 (4).
Gerschick, T. J., and A. S. Miller. 1994. Gender identities at the crossroads of masculinity and physical disability. *Masculinities* 2 (1): 34–55.
Goode, W. 1982. Why men resist. In *Rethinking the family: Some feminist questions*, edited by B. Thorne and M. Yalom. New York: Longman.
Gutmann, M. C. 1996. *The meanings of macho: Being a man in Mexico City*. Berkeley: University of California Press.
Hacker, H. M. 1957. The new burdens of masculinity. *Marriage and Family Living* 19 (3): 227–33.
Halberstam, J. 1998. *Female masculinity*. Durham, NC: Duke University Press.
Hanke, R. 1992. Redesigning men: Hegemonic masculinity in transition. In *Men, masculinity, and the media*, edited by S. Craig. Newbury Park, CA: Sage.
Hawkesworth, M. 1997. Confounding gender. *Signs: Journal of Women in Culture and Society* 22 (3): 649–85.
Hearn, J. 1996. Is masculinity dead? A critique of the concept of masculinity/masculinities. In *Understanding masculinities: Social relations and cultural arenas*, edited by M. Mac an Ghaill. Buckingham, UK: Open University Press.
———. 2004. From hegemonic masculinity to the hegemony of men. *Feminist Theory* 5 (1): 49–72.
Herdt, G. H. 1981. *Guardians of the flutes: Idioms of masculinity*. New York: McGraw-Hill.
Higate, P. R. 2003. *Military masculinities: Identity and the state*. London: Praeger.
Hochschild, A. 1989. *The second shift: Working parents and the revolution at home*. New York: Viking.
Holter, Ø. G. 1997. *Gender, patriarchy and capitalism: A social forms analysis*. Oslo, Norway: University of Olso.
———. 2003. *Can men do it? Men and gender equality—The Nordic experience*. Copenhagen, Denmark: Nordic Council of Ministers.
hooks, b. 1984. *Feminist theory: From margin to center*. Boston: South End.
Hooper, C. 1998. Masculinist practices and gender politics: The operation of multiple masculinities in international relations. In *The "man" question in international relations*, edited by M. Zalewski and J. Parpart. Boulder, CO: Westview.

———. 2000. Masculinities in transition: The case of globalization. In *Gender and global restructuring*, edited by M. H. Marchand and A. S. Runyan. London: Routledge.
———. 2001. *Manly states: Masculinities, international relations, and gender politics.* New York: Columbia University Press.
Hunt, P. 1980. *Gender and class consciousness.* London: Macmillan.
Ishii-Kuntz, M. 2003. Balancing fatherhood and work: Emergence of diverse masculinities in contemporary Japan. In *Men and masculinities in contemporary Japan*, edited by J. E. Roberson and N. Suzuki. London: Routledge Curzon.
Jansen, S. C., and D. Sabo. 1994. The sport-war metaphor: Hegemonic masculinity, the Persian-Gulf war, and the new world order. *Sociology of Sport Journal* 11 (1): 1–17.
Jefferson, T. 1994. Theorizing masculine subjectivity. In *Just boys doing business? Men, masculinities and crime*, edited by T. Newburn and E. A. Stanko. London: Routledge.
———. 2002. Subordinating hegemonic masculinity. *Theoretical Criminology* 6 (1): 63–88.
Kessler, S. J., D. J. Ashenden, R. W. Connell, and G. W. Dowsett. 1982. *Ockers and disco-maniacs.* Sydney, Australia: Inner City Education Center.
Kimmel, M. S. 1987. Rethinking "masculinity": New directions in research. In *Changing men: New directions in research on men and masculinity*, edited by M. S. Kimmel. Newbury Park, CA: Sage.
———. 2005. Globalization and its mal(e)contents: The gendered moral and political economy of terrorism. In *Handbook of studies on men & masculinities*, edited by M. S. Kimmel, J. Hearn, and R. W. Connell. Thousand Oaks, CA: Sage.
Kimmel, M. S., and M. Mahler. 2003. Adolescent masculinity, homophobia, and violence: Random school shootings, 1982–2001. *American Behavioral Scientist* 46 (10): 1439–58.
Kupers, T. A. 1993. *Revisioning men's lives: Gender, intimacy, and power.* New York: Guilford.
Lea, S., and T. Auburn. 2001. The social construction of rape in the talk of a convicted rapist. *Feminism & Psychology* 11 (1): 11–33.
Light, R., and D. Kirk. 2000. High school rugby, the body and the reproduction of hegemonic masculinity. *Sport, Education and Society* 5 (2): 163–76.
Mac an Ghaill, M. 1994. *The making of men: Masculinities, sexualities and schooling.* Buckingham, UK: Open University Press.
MacInnes, J. 1998. *The end of masculinity: The confusion of sexual genesis and sexual difference in modern society.* Buckingham, UK: Open University Press.
Martin, P. Y. 1998. Why can't a man be more like a woman? Reflections on Connell's masculinities. *Gender & Society* 12 (4): 472–74.
———. 2001. "Mobilizing masculinities": Women's experiences of men at work. *Organizations* 8 (4): 587–618.
Martino, W. 1995. Boys and literacy: Exploring the construction of hegemonic masculinities and the formation of literate capacities for boys in the English classroom. *English in Australia* 112:11–24.
McMahon, A. 1993. Male readings of feminist theory: The psychologization of sexual politics in the masculinity literature. *Theory and Society* 22 (5): 675–95.
Messerschmidt, J. W. 1993. *Masculinities and crime: Critique and reconceptualization of theory.* Lanham, MD: Rowman & Littlefield.

Messerschmidt, J. W. 1995. Managing to kill: Masculinities and the space shuttle Challenger explosion. *Masculinities* 3 (4): 1–22.

———. 1997. *Crime as structured action: Gender, race, class and crime in the making.* Thousand Oaks, CA: Sage.

———. 2000. *Nine lives: Adolescent masculinities, the body, and violence.* Boulder, CO: Westview.

———. 2004. *Flesh & blood: Adolescent gender diversity and violence.* Lanham, MD: Rowman & Littlefield.

———. 2005. Men, masculinities, and crime. In *Handbook of studies on men & masculinities*, edited by M. S. Kimmel, J. Hearn, and R. W. Connell. Thousand Oaks, CA: Sage.

Messner, M. A. 1992. *Power at play: Sports and the problem of masculinity.* Boston: Beacon.

———. 1997. *Politics of masculinities: Men in movements.* Thousand Oaks, CA: Sage.

———. 2002. *Taking the field: Women, men, and sport.* Minneapolis: University of Minnesota Press.

Messner, M. A., and D. Sabo, eds. 1990. *Sport, men, and the gender order: Critical feminist perspectives.* Champaign, IL: Human Kinetics Books.

Meuser, M. 2001. "This doesn't really mean she's holding a whip": Transformation of the gender order and the contradictory modernization of masculinity. *Diskurs* 1:44–50.

———. 2003. Modernized masculinities? Continuities, challenges and changes in men's lives. In *Among men: Moulding masculinities*, edited by S. Ervø and T. Johannson. Aldershot, UK: Ashgate.

Meuser, M., and C. Behnke. 1998. Tausendundeine Männlichkeit? Männlichkeitsmuster und socialstrukturelle Einbindungen. *Widersprüche* 67:7–25.

Mieli, M. 1980. *Homosexuality and liberation: Elements of a gay critique*, translated by D. Fernbach. London: Gay Men's Press.

Mittelman, J. H. 2004. *Whither globalization? The vortex of knowledge and ideology.* London: Routledge.

Morin, S. F., and E. M. Garfinkle. 1978. Male homophobia. *Journal of Social Issues* 34 (1): 29–47.

Morrell, R. 1998. Of boys and men: Masculinity and gender in southern African studies. *Journal of Southern African Studies* 24 (4): 605–30.

Morrell, R., and S. Swart. 2005. Men in the Third World: Postcolonial perspectives on masculinity. In *Handbook of studies on men & masculinities*, edited by M. S. Kimmel, J. Hearn, and R. W. Connell. Thousand Oaks, CA: Sage.

Morris, C., and N. Evans. 2001. "Cheese makers are always women": Gendered representations of farm life in the agricultural press. *Gender, Place and Culture* 8 (4): 375–90.

Mosher, D. L., and S. S. Tomkins. 1988. Scripting the macho man: Hypermasculine socialization and enculturation. *Journal of Sex Research* 25 (1): 60–84.

Namaste, V. K. 2000. *Invisible lives: The erasure of transsexual and transgendered people.* Chicago: University of Chicago Press.

Newburn, T., and E. A. Stanko. 1994. *Just boys doing business? Men, masculinities, and crime.* New York: Routledge.

Pease, B., and K. Pringle, eds. 2001. *A man's world? Changing men's practices in a globalized world.* London: Zed Books.

Petersen, A. 1998. *Unmasking the masculine: "Men" and "identity" in a sceptical age.* London: Sage.

———. 2003. Research on men and masculinities: Some implications of recent theory for future work. *Men and Masculinities* 6 (1): 54–69.

Pleck, J. 1981. *The myth of masculinity.* Cambridge, MA: MIT Press.

Plummer, K., ed. 1981. *The making of the modern homosexual.* London: Macmillan.

Poynting, S., G. Noble, and P. Tabar. 2003. "Intersections" of masculinity and ethnicity: A study of male Lebanese immigrant youth in Western Sydney. Unpublished manuscript, University of Western Sydney.

Roberts, P. 1993. Social control and the censure(s) of sex. *Crime, Law and Social Change* 19 (2): 171–86.

Roper, M. 1994. *Masculinity and the British organization man since 1945.* Oxford, UK: Oxford University Press.

Rubin, H. 2003. *Self-made men: Identity and embodiment among transsexual men.* Nashville, TN: Vanderbilt University Press.

Sabo, D., and D. F. Gordon, eds. 1995. *Men's health and illness: Gender, power and the body.* Thousand Oaks, CA: Sage.

Sabo, D., and S. C. Jansen. 1992. Images of men in sport media: The social reproduction of gender order. In *Men, masculinity, and the media*, edited by S. Craig. Newbury Park, CA: Sage.

Salisbury, J., and D. Jackson. 1996. *Challenging macho values: Practical ways of working with adolescent boys.* Washington, DC: Falmer.

Schwalbe, M. 1992. Male supremacy and the narrowing of the moral self. *Berkeley Journal of Sociology* 37:29–54.

Scott, J. W. 1997. Comment on Hawkesworth's "confounding gender." *Signs: Journal of Women in Culture and Society* 22 (3): 697–702.

Segal, L. 1990. *Slow motion: Changing masculinities, changing men.* London: Virago.

Skelton, A. 1993. On becoming a male physical education teacher: The informal culture of students and the construction of hegemonic masculinity. *Gender and Education* 5 (3): 289–303.

Snodgrass, J., ed. 1977. *For men against sexism: A book of readings.* Albion, CA: Times Change Press.

Stoller, R. J. 1968. *Sex and gender: On the development of masculinity and femininity.* New York: Science House.

Taga, F. 2003. Rethinking male socialization: Life histories of Japanese male youth. In *Asian masculinities*, edited by K. Louie and M. Low. London: Routledge Curzon.

Thorne, B. 1993. *Gender play.* New Brunswick, NJ: Rutgers University Press.

Thornton, M. 1989. Hegemonic masculinity and the academy. *International Journal of the Sociology of Law* 17:115–30.

Tolson, A. 1977. *The limits of masculinity.* London: Tavistock.

Tomsen, S. 2002. *Hatred, murder and male honour: Anti-homosexual homicides in New South Wales, 1980–2000.* Vol. 43. Canberra: Australian Institute of Criminology.

Valdés, T., and J. Olavarría. 1998. Ser hombre en Santiago de Chile: A pesar de todo, un mismo modelo. In *Masculinidades y equidad de género en América Latina*, edited by T. Valdés and J. Olavarría. Santiago, Chile: FLACSO/UNFPA.

Wajcman, J. 1999. *Managing like a man: Women and men in corporate management.* Sydney, Australia: Allen and Unwin.

Walby, S. 1997. *Gender transformations*. London: Routledge.

Warren, S. 1997. Who do these boys think they are? An investigation into the construction of masculinities in a primary classroom. *International Journal of Inclusive Education* 1 (2): 207–22.

Wetherell, M., and N. Edley. 1999. Negotiating hegemonic masculinity: Imaginary positions and psycho-discursive practices. *Feminism and Psychology* 9 (3): 335–56.

Whitehead, S. M. 1998. Hegemonic masculinity revisited. *Gender, Work, and Organization* 6 (1): 58–62.

———. 2002. *Men and masculinities: Key themes and new directions*. Cambridge, UK: Polity.

Willis, P. 1977. *Learning to labor: How working class kids get working class jobs*. Farnborough, UK: Saxon House.

Zaretsky, E. 1975. Male supremacy and the unconscious. *Socialist Revolution* 4:7–55.

11

THE 'FEMINISATION' OF HEALTH

Ellie Lee and Elizabeth Frayn

Source: D. Wainwright (ed.), *A Sociology of Health*, London: Sage, 2008, pp. 115–33.

- The past 20 years have seen the emergence of a new discourse of health, at the centre of which is the idea that 'prevention is better than cure'.
- Contemporary health concerns are often 'gendered'. The emergence of campaigns about 'men's health' is a notable development of recent years.
- There is a striking contrast between feminist constructions of the problem of women's health in the 1970s, and the contemporary problem of gender and health.
- In the context of the new discourse of health, 'masculinity' has come to be defined as a barrier to health, 'feminine' attitudes such as a willingness to consider oneself vulnerable and 'at risk', and to seek help have, in turn, been validated as desirable characteristics for both men and women.
- Contemporary gendered health concerns have much less to do with evidence-based developments in science and medicine, than with developments in the spheres of politics and society.
- The practical outcome of the feminization of health is that men as well as women may become more anxious and worried about their health, for little discernable benefit.

Masculinity is among the more significant risk factors associated with men's illness. [It] is not only a risk factor in disease etiology but it is also among the most significant barriers to men developing a consciousness about health and illness.

Michael Kimmel, 1995

A cursory examination of contemporary health concerns suggests that gender is significant for their construction. The idea set out above, for example, that 'masculinity' is a key 'risk factor' associated with ill health, is now widely held. The notion that a 'male' outlook on life is 'unhealthy', and is likely associated with the development of disease, has become commonplace.

It is not only the specialist and academic literature that discusses the significance of gender for ill health in this way. Cultural support is offered to the notion that 'masculine' attitudes and behaviours are unhealthy and undesirable, and by implication 'feminine' ones preferable. 'Binge drinking' for example, is often typified in the media by images of drunk, young women staggering through town centres. Headlines draw attention to the idea that a part of this problem of alcohol consumption today is the way in which young women are 'copying' the 'masculine', 'risky' behaviour typical of young men. An unfortunate outcome of greater sex equality, this approach suggests, is that women are becoming more 'unhealthy', as they are prone to behave in a way that is more 'male' than that of women in the past.

What should we make of this way of thinking about health and illness? How and why has 'masculinity' come to be stigmatised as unhealthy? It is useful to think of the 'gendering' of health concerns as part of the overall process this volume seeks to investigate. This is the emergence of what has been termed the 'new paradigm' of health and health care,[1] or, the new discourse of health (See chapters 1 and 5), and it draws upon the following set of related precepts:

- *Ill health is caused by attitudinal and behavioural factors.* Disease in contemporary society, it is claimed, results from the way society is organised, and in 'unhealthy' behaviour and attitudes that emerge as a result.
- *The emphasis of health care should shift from cure to prevention.* Health care, it is argued, needs to become more focused on health promotion programmes that encourage people who are not yet ill to be alert to the need to 'choose health' and modify their behaviour accordingly.
- *The meaning of 'health' should be redefined.* 'Health', it is suggested, should no longer be an assumed state of normality, and become instead a state of being that all apparently healthy individuals should ideally actively pursue in the course of their everyday life, through changing their behaviour.
- *Illness is best considered less an occasional aberration from normality to be addressed when it occurs, more a constant risk facing everybody.* It is suggested that an awareness of the risk of becoming ill is a useful outlook for people to have, since this requires us to engage as a matter of course in minimising our likelihood of becoming ill.

In sociological terms, this approach to health and illness can be thought of as one that makes *identity* central to definitions of health and ill health, as the following extract explains:

> Rather than simply being told how to act, or being treated by medical interventions when ill, people are being increasingly induced to monitor their own health and are being instilled with healthy attitudes. The control of health must therefore come from *within* the person.[2]

The new discourse of health brings with it an important socio-cultural process. It is *the life inside* the individual that is deemed in need of modification, since in order for health to be attained, change must take place *within the person*. In other words, it is *attitudes and emotions*, how individuals *think and feel*, that become the focus for the pursuit of health; or in the words of Kimmel, it is a 'consciousness of health and illness' that is considered to be the ideal mindset, and those who seek to improve health must find ways to develop this consciousness in others.[3]

In contemporary society, the means through which modification of behaviour, attitudes and feelings is now enacted is legion. There are many different ways in which people are being encouraged to monitor and control health from 'within the person'. Confronting and changing 'masculinity' can be considered one of them, however, and the primary purpose of this chapter is to explore this aspect of the new discourse of health.

To do so, we discuss gender and health in three ways. First, we consider how the problem of women's health has been defined in the past, to draw attention to some differences with today. Second, we detail some of the main features of the contemporary problem of men's health. Finally, we use the case study of campaigns about cancer screening, to illustrate the nature of, and problems with, this aspect of the new discourse of health.

The problem of 'women's health'

In contemporary society, attitudes and behaviours – in particular those considered to be associated with 'masculinity' – have come to be defined as 'unhealthy'. The construction of health concerns in terms of gender is a fairly recent phenomenon. The gendering of health is a development inextricably linked to the second-wave feminist movement, a movement that made the relationship between women, medicine and society a matter of significant public debate and contest. The development of the term 'medicalisation' – defined sociologically as the process through which experiences come to be understood in medical terms – is strongly associated with this historical development.[4] Employed to explore a range of experiences it is aspects of women's lives that have been particularly subject to analysis through use of this term by feminists.[5]

Feminist literature from the 1970s and 1980s 'emphasized the breadth of the medicalization of women's lives', notes Conrad.[6] Where women's lives were described and analysed as subject to medicalisation, at this time it tended to be the *problematic* effects of this process that were emphasised. As Reismann put it in her oft-quoted contribution on the subject, women were viewed as the 'main targets' of the medicalisation processes, indicating that the definition of women's experiences in terms of illness was considered to be negative. 'A plethora of female conditions has come to be . . . reconceptualized as illnesses' she wrote, citing as examples sexual dysfunctions, pregnancy care, fertility, menopause, ageing, teenage pregnancy and wife battering, premenstrual syndrome, and weight gain.[7]

Why did feminists respond to illness definitions in this way? One objection to medicalised accounts of women's experiences is that they *naturalise* demeaning and degrading ideas about women, a point made in one of the founding feminist statements about the problem of medicalisation, by Barbara Ehrenreich and Diedre English:

> The medical system is strategic for women's liberation . . . It holds the promise of freedom from hundreds of unspoken fears and complaints that have handicapped women throughout history . . . But the medical system is also strategic to women's oppression. Medical science has been one of the most powerful sources of sexist ideology in our culture. Justifications for sexual discrimination – in education, in jobs, in public, life – must ultimately rest on one thing that differentiates women from men: their bodies. Theories of male superiority ultimately rest on biology.[8]

Medicalised explanations for women's experience 'reduce women to their biology' it was argued, by explaining sex differences in society with reference to reproductive organs and hormones. In turn explanations of this sort continually draw attention to the idea that women are ill. 'Medicine's prime contribution to sexist ideology has been to describe women as sick, and as potentially sickening to men', stated Ehrenreich and English. Women throughout history have been considered 'the weaker sex' and excluded from major areas of social life on these grounds, they claimed, an outcome they described through discussion of nineteenth-century '"sick" women of the upper classes', made hypochondriac and hysterical through a life of enforced leisure, and the 'sickening women of the working classes', deemed a threat to social order in general and to children in particular. Medicine in this framework was viewed as one, very powerful, aspect, of an overall 'sexist ideology', and concepts such as 'hysteria' and 'pre-menstrual syndrome' were contested and objected to for this reason.

Another important theme in the discussion of medicalisation emphasised that medical interventions can *disempower* women. While medicine promised 'liberation and freedom' through, for example, enabling women to effectively regulate their fertility by using contraception and abortion, women's experience in practice was very different, argued some. An outlook of protest regarding medical interventions emerged as a result, described in 1976 by the feminist sociologist Ann Oakley:

> These protests cover such topics as the undue use of surgical abortion techniques ... the overuse of radical as opposed to constructive surgery for breast and reproductive tract diseases ... and perhaps, most central of alt, the modern, male-controlled, hospitalised and increasingly technological pattern of childbirth management.[9]

Medical care for women, it was claimed, failed to reflect women's needs and interests, a problem most clearly apparent when women experienced childbirth. Through the modern profession of obstetrics and the development of hospital-based childbirth, feminist critics claimed pregnant women had come to be construed as patients, with healthy women treated as if they were sick, and women's pregnancy and childbirth experiences consequently controlled by the medical profession.[10] Women's own control over their bodies and reproductive experience was for this reason diminished and childbirth emerged as probably the key area for criticism of medicalisation.

Some saw alternative health care as a solution, and they set up their own health care provision. The best-known project of this kind was the Boston Women's Health Collective which advocated self-help for women, rather than reliance on doctors, and whose manual *Our Bodies Ourselves* first published in 1972 rapidly made an international impact. In the Preface it states, of the women who set up the Collective:

> We had all experienced similar feelings of frustration and anger towards specific doctors and the medical maze in general, and initially we wanted to do something about those doctors who were condescending, paternalistic, judgemental, and non-informative ... [over time] we realised we really were capable of collecting, understanding and evaluating medical information.[11]

Exemplifying the spirit of defiance informing this approach was the Chicago-based underground abortion service 'Jane'. Set up when abortion was still illegal in the USA by women who believed abortion to be a basic precondition of women's equality, 'Jane' was staffed by a group of women who, first under the guidance of a doctor, trained themselves to perform abortion, and eventually carried out around 11,000 safe and successful abortion procedures during the early 1970s.[12] Such initiatives were more prominent in the USA and Australia, although there were attempts by British feminists to provide alternatives to mainstream medicine.[13]

There has been much debate about these feminist criticisms of modern medicine. One area of dispute concerns historical accuracy. Some feminist representations of modern medical care have implied there was once a 'golden age' of woman-centred 'natural childbirth', but little evidence has been presented to substantiate this claim. Such claims also run counter to evidence of a somewhat barbaric experience that led *women* to *demand* precisely the interventions subsequently represented as part of the unwelcome medicalisation of childbirth – for example drug-based pain relief.[14] Indeed, 'the movement for "natural" childbirth only arose when medical advances had freed women from these fears [of the pain of childbirth]', argued Strong.[15] In turn it has been suggested that there is no good reason to assume that female-dominated midwifery is 'good' for women, and high-tech reproductive medicine 'bad'.[16]

The 1980s and 1990s saw the emergence of arguments that approached the problem of 'women's health' in a way that departed from that of the 1970s.[17] Some have revised the original feminist formulation of the problem of medicalisation, in order to emphasise the possibility of women benefiting from and taking advantage of modern medicine. Attention has been drawn to the diversity of women's experiences of healthcare; women can and do benefit from mainstream medical treatment and are not passive recipients of it, it has been argued.[18] 'It is now difficult to identify a single feminist critique of medicine. Instead a variety of feminist approaches to health and health care have emerged', concludes Doyal of these developments.[19]

In relation to the main subject area of this chapter – the rise of concern about men's health – a third difference between feminist definitions of the problem of women's health in the 1970s, and more recent claims about this social problem are important. The former, as we have emphasised, articulated suspicion about female acquiescence to medical authority and intervention, and some on this basis made bold attempts to provide alternatives to mainstream medicine. In contrast, the problem of women's health is today often defined quite differently. It tends to be the *absence* of official, medical intervention that is bemoaned, and the need for *more* professional help is advocated. As we will go on to argue, it is this sort of approach, rather than that apparent in earlier decades, that has crossed the gender divide, and underpins the approach of those who argue that more needs to be done about men's health.

Take, for example, post-natal depression (PND). This psychiatric category was rejected at one time by many feminists for medicalising maternal experience and misrepresenting its nature.[20] More recently, in contrast, the category PND has come to be widely embraced as a useful term to describe how new mothers feel. A burgeoning body of literature emerged through the 1990s, including titles such as *Surviving Post-natal Depression* and *The New*

Mother Syndrome: Coping with Postpartum Stress and Depression. The overriding message of these books is that women have been left by doctors to 'suffer in silence', and it is vital that society, and in particular the medical profession, does more to recognise and diagnose PND and encourage women to seek medical help. The project of the authors of such books is to *generalise* the incidence of PND, so that most mothers come to be defined as victims of it. Thus the writer Kate Figes, in her widely read advice book for new mothers, argues, 'It [PND] is a sliding scale, starting with the "baby blues" affecting 80 per cent of women, and ending with puerperal psychosis . . . The vast majority of women sit somewhere on this scale'.[21] Interestingly, some feminists share this approach. American feminist Naomi Wolf for example claims that 400,000 American mothers each year are affected by depression after they have a baby, and she highlights what she sees as 'medical complacency in the face of women's suffering', because routine screening for post-natal depression is not normally provided in the USA by doctors.[22]

Post-natal Depression has thus come to be represented as common in one form or another to all mothers, and in turn most mothers are deemed in need of medical diagnosis and treatment. The demand is for *more diagnosis not less*, and this demand is not restricted to PND. Many illness categories, including pre-menstrual syndrome and post-traumatic stress disorder are discussed as 'hidden epidemics' that need to be more widely diagnosed in women by doctors. In recent years new categories of illness including Battered Women's Syndrome, Rape Trauma Syndrome and Childbirth Trauma Syndrome have been 'named' and their medical diagnosis promoted by some.[23] Some campaigners also argue that women need more screening of the cervix and breast, and more advice and guidance from doctors about issues including weight gain, weight loss, exercise, and pregnancy.

If in the past the problem of women's health was shaped by a feminist approach that comprised in part at least the defiant rejection of official illness categories, this suggests that other definitions of health and illness are now ascendant. The forthright message that women should resist the unwelcome foisting of medical labels and treatments upon them has waned, and the stronger tendency has been towards the emergence of the contrasting notion that *too little* is done by society to allow women to recognise their health problems. One implication of this redefinition of the problem of women's health is a shift in emphasis regarding the value of the 'feminine' and the 'masculine'.

Agnes Miles has explained this point, with reference to the work of the feminist critic of psychiatry, Philys Chesler. Chesler explained, in her account of why objections should be raised regarding 'the feminine' in the context of health and medicine, that 'women are socialized and pressed into accepting the feminine role, which is compatible with the position of a submissive and dependent help-seeker'. The role of help-seeker is a 'dependent and submissive one', she thus explained. For Chesler, in other words, 'help-seeking' was an outlook bound up with 'feminine' attitudes of passivity and submission which women were socialised to adopt.[24]

This point was made by Chesler as part of an account of why women were more likely to feel ill and visit doctors than men, and her emphasis was on the connection between 'help-seeking' and a damaging and negative socio-cultural context for women. The now widespread advocacy of the *positive* value of help-seeking draws attention to the extent to which a new validation of 'the feminine' has emerged. As we now detail, it is this development above all that is made manifest by campaigns about 'men's health'.

Men's health and the problem of 'masculinity'

> Within twenty years the feminist campaign to seize control over women's health from the medical profession has given way to a state-sponsored, doctor-led system of vaginal examination and cervical surveillance. It is doubly ironic that within the same period, male resistance to medical regulation was replaced by the demand, under the banner of 'men's health', for invasive screening tests analogous to cervical smears.[25]

The problem of 'men's health' has, as Fitzpatrick acerbically indicates, rapidly gained visibility and recognition. Twenty years ago, there was no such problem. Men of course more or less willingly visited doctors when confronted by symptoms of ill health. But there were few active efforts to encourage men to become concerned about their health. Since the early 1990s, however, activities and initiatives that seek to bring the problem of men's health to public attention, and which in particular aim to change the attitudes and behaviour of men themselves, have become a ubiquitous feature of social life.

The most obvious example of this new preoccupation is the emergence of a specialist popular literature for men about their health. Traditionally marketed for women, men's health magazines first appeared on the British market just over a decade ago.[26] It was at about the same time that campaign groups were established to 'raise awareness' of 'men's health needs'. The best-known and most influential such British group, Men's Health Forum was founded in 1994.[27] Little more than ten years later, such initiatives are numerous and very visible. Male students at the University of Kent are welcomed to their campus with posters asking them whether they have recently examined their testicles, and encouraging them to visit the doctor if they have not. Awareness campaigns of this type are now commonplace. A wide range of projects seek to promote the need for male awareness of conditions ranging from prostate, testicular and breast cancer, to anorexia and bulimia, post-natal depression and heart disease. What are the features of this new health concern? Four themes can be identified.

The bifurcation of health concerns

One of the most notable aspects of men's health concerns is the way advocates of their recognition often self-consciously challenge sex-based distinctions associated with health campaigns in the past. Men are the 'forgotten victims' of post-natal depression, argues the author of one book on the subject, since 'becoming a father can have a huge impact on a man and yet all the attention seems to be focused on the woman'.[28] Male cancers such as prostate and testicular cancer are promoted as important health problems that should be taken as seriously as breast cancer, and breast cancer itself is now defined as an under-recognised men's health problem. The menopause has also crossed the sex divide, with some claiming it affects men in middle age as well as women.

The health of young men and boys has become a particular focus for claims of this kind. Anorexia and deliberate self-harm in the past considered psychological problems associated most often with young women, are thus represented as disorders that affect more and more young men. The problem of 'poor sexual health' is also now widely considered to be a male as much as female problem with claims made that boys in particular need to be targeted in programmes that aim to improve sexual health, and combat teenage pregnancy. The process of 'medicalization' – the definition of social experience in medical terms – has, as was noted earlier, been strongly associated in sociological literature with the experiences of women. As Rosenfeld and Faircloth detail however, this sort of contemporary experience suggests there is now a strong tendency for men's lives to also be increasingly medicalized.[29]

A common diagnosis for a range of conditions

A second feature of the problem of men's health is that a wide range of different diseases and complaints, which have very little in common in a medical sense, are united by one common diagnosis. Taking as their central trope the idea of 'traditional masculinity', advocates of greater recognition for the problem of men's health blame ill health in men – in whichever form it might appear – on a particular set of attitudes and sensibilities. Regardless of which men's health problem is at issue, the ultimate cause of the problem – 'masculinity' – is always the same.

Thus argued one early advocate of the need for more to done about men's health, 'The road to improvement in men's health lies in puncturing typical myths of masculinity such as that it's good to be daring, unemotional and in control'.[30] In this framework, it is men's attitudes, their alleged 'daring' and 'unemotional' outlook that constitutes the barrier to health, regardless of which medical problem is at issue.

Social psychologists Lee and Owens also centre their analysis on 'hegemonic masculinity', defined as 'toughness, unemotionality, physical competence, competitiveness and aggression'.[31] Illness-inducing behaviours associated with 'hegemonic masculinity', they claim, include 'relative reluctance to seek help for medical and psychological problems', 'avoidance of the expression of emotion', and 'a high level of involvement in risky behaviours, which include both the socially sanctioned risks involved in dangerous sports and the more deviant masculine-type risks such as crime and violent behaviour'. Similarly, according to one health website, it is 'male stereotypes' that damage men's health, centrally the 'macho' stereotype that centres on 'an inability to admit vulnerability'.[32] In this framework, ill health of all types is thus commonly caused by a particular form of identity, that which is 'masculine', meaning it is only when men adopt a different set of attitudes, crucially those that involve a 'feminine' acceptance of vulnerability, and embrace the need to seek help, that health can be attained.

'Men's health' as a socio-cultural problem

The speed at which men's lives and experiences have been medicalised points to the conclusion that developments in science and medicine cannot be solely responsible for this development. It would be difficult for even the most energetic and enthusiastic 'medical imperialists' to generate the degree of interest in men's behaviour and attitudes that now exists, suggesting there has been a *broader socio-cultural shift*. Certain perceptions of what is positive or negative about attitudes and behaviour have come to be socially and culturally validated, and these perceptions have been imported into debates about health. The idea that 'masculinity' is a plastic set of attitudes and behaviours that can and should be modified is associated originally with the fields of sociology and social psychology.[33] Through a process of cultural transmission, it seems such theories about men and their (allegedly problematic) behaviour have come to influence much wider arenas, including the medical.

A problem definition that influences the medical world

> The way that men think about themselves can be quite unhelpful ... Most men don't like to admit that they feel fragile or vulnerable, and so are less likely to talk about their feelings with their friends, loved ones or their doctors. This may be the reason that they often don't ask for help when they become depressed.

Concerns about 'masculine', 'unhealthy' behaviour and attitudes, if non-medical in origin, have come to be strongly endorsed by the medical world. The degree to which 'masculine' values and attitudes have been stigmatised (and 'feminine' ones validated) is indicated by the extent to which the claim that men need to be encouraged to be less 'tough', 'invulnerable' and 'in control', and more 'open', 'soft', and prepared to 'seek help' informs health-related institutions, and the medical profession itself. Despite the dubious efficacy of almost all interventions for men justified on such grounds many medical bodies endorse the idea that there is need to address men's health in this way.[35]

The Royal College of Nursing, the British Medical Association and the Royal College of Psychiatrists all have initiatives that aim to encourage men to seek help and which aim to counter the allegedly detrimental effects of 'masculinity' for health. In 2005 a range of international medical societies came together in Vienna for a 'World Congress on Men's Health and Gender'. '[M]en's health is much more than just about diseases that affect men', argues the doctor who organised the conference. 'It is also about the consequences of male attitudes to health in general', he claimed.[36] Official health promotion programmes in Britain explicitly target men on just this basis[37] and key organisations also promote the need to change 'men's attitudes'.

In summary, the growing visibility of the problem of men's health implies cultural stigmatisation of particular attitudes, for example resilience, and the validation of others, for example risk aversion and help-seeking. This in turn implies a significant increase in the medicalisation of men's lives, as men are encouraged to seek help, if possible in advance of any symptom of ill health. It is for this reason that, on the one hand, the alleged reluctance on the part of men to go to the doctor is bemoaned, and on the other, regardless of their dubious efficacy, programmes that seek to encourage more men (and women) to take up preventative health measures are championed.

It is perhaps the advocacy of screening programmes for cancer that illustrates most clearly the central aspects of the changing definitions of gender and health discussed so far. It is to this case study of the 'feminization' of health that we now turn.

Cancer and cancer screening

> It is hardly possible to take up one's residence in the kingdom of the ill unprejudiced by the lurid metaphors with which it has been landscaped.[38]

In the 1970s Susan Sontag wrote, in her book *Illness as Metaphor*, about the social stigma of the cancer sufferer. She described the metaphors and mythology surrounding cancer, and the way this mystification made it harder for cancer sufferers to come to terms with their illness as an illness.

In recent years, cancer has been demystified, both in medical terms, and also in terms of public discourse. The gradual introduction of more effective treatments, in some cases cures, alongside development of a more interventionist model of palliative care have meant that in western societies, the burden of physical suffering caused by cancer is considerably reduced.

The theories Sontag describes about the psychological basis of cancer, from Galen's description of 'melancholy women' in the second century to the 1970s 'cancer personality' (depressive, repressed, with poor relationship skills) have been overturned, and now seem unscientific and indeed cruel, as we have learned more about the genetic and environmental causes of the disease. Sontag describes a French oncologist who told her that less than a tenth of his patients knew they had cancer. Only 30 years later, this level of denial seems unimaginable.

It would be wrong to draw the conclusion that mythology about cancer has disappeared, however. Some of today's beliefs about cancer are summed up in the opening paragraphs of the Haynes *Men's Cancer Manual* from 2004: 'although about one man in three will develop a cancer at some time in his life, the most common forms are almost entirely preventable or treatable through early diagnosis'. In other words, it is suggested that if we behave responsibly, by reporting suspicious symptoms to our doctors, and following the type of lifestyle advice contained in the Haynes manual, we may avoid cancer altogether or certainly drastically improve our chances of survival. The message of this campaign is that 'awareness saves lives'. As we shall see however, this simple apparently commonsensical message is unfortunately not borne out by the evidence. The real impact of 'awareness campaigns' is not less cancer, but ironically a higher incidence of cancer, along with a new consciousness of the possibility of becoming sick, and further legitimation of help-seeking behaviour.

Breast cancer

Cancer campaigns have gained enormous popularity and publicity in the UK and USA. Take the example of breast cancer. Three-quarters of a million women were expected to take part in the 'Race for Life' in 2006, a three-mile run organised by the UK charity Cancer Research. Over a million take part in the annual 'Race for the Cure', the US equivalent. Barbara Ehrenreich wrote about this popular movement after she was diagnosed with breast cancer herself:

> Culture is too weak a word to describe all this. What has grown up in just the last fifteen years more nearly represents a cult – or given that it numbers more than two million women, their families and their friends – perhaps we should say a full-fledged religion.[39]

The roots of this 'religion' arguably lie in aspects of the feminist movement of which Ehrenreich herself was a part. In the 1970s, the impact of the women's movement in relation to breast cancer was two-fold. First, women were encouraged to be more open about their bodies and diseases. Various American celebrities of the time 'went public' about their breast cancer and treatment, notably First Lady Betty Ford, newsreader Betty Rollin, tycoon's wife Happy Rockefeller and former child actor Shirley Temple Black. Black justified her decision to speak out in early 1972 as one made 'for all my sisters who have lost a breast, for all my sisters who fear they may'. Second, the women's movement was an important part of the drive towards more conservative, less disfiguring treatment for breast cancer, which formed part of its criticism of medical control of women. In the words of Black again: 'The doctor can make the incision, I'll make the decision'.[40]

This challenge to medical paternalism had a real impact. Combined with new medical advances and understanding about the way cancer spread, it brought improved treatment to sufferers. The contribution of feminism to the eventual death-knoll of the radical Halsted mastectomy (involving removal of the breast, chest muscles and axillary lymph-nodes) practised since the 1890s has been described this way:

> Transforming the prevailing mind-set would take more, much more, than data, statistics and refereed articles in scientific journals. American surgeons did not come around for years, not until the sexual revolution and modern feminism altered the cultural and political landscape, changing forever American attitudes about power, eroticism and physical beauty.[41]

What is different about today's breast cancer campaigners? The emphasis on the 'survivor' speaking out is still with us. Indeed, for breast cancer sufferers in the public eye, it now seems almost obligatory. When pop singer Kylie Minogue was diagnosed in 2005, the details of her subsequent surgery made headline news. There was never any question that Minogue had a choice in the public discussion of her medical problems, as her surgeon gave daily press briefings on the hospital steps. She was congratulated by the press as she issued statements denying that she was using alternative therapies, conscious of the influence attached to her celebrity.

But Minogue's case shows how the aim of 'speaking out' has changed. Her situation was used not to challenge medical control, but as an opportunity to educate others about 'breast cancer awareness'. Television news interviewers approached random young women in the street, asking them whether they examined their own breasts for signs of cancer and sought medical advice. Rates of young women requesting mammograms soared in Minogue's native Australia. The role of the celebrity survivor today is thus not to help women find an independent way to respond to an illness, but rather to encourage as many people as possible to be 'aware' and take the advice of cancer campaigners and charities, and seek help from doctors in the form of cancer screening.

Rather than struggling to free women from unnecessary tests and overtreatment by a conservative medical profession, today's campaigners seem relatively unquestioning about the need for as many tests and as much treatment as possible. The charity Breast Cancer Care has thus recently organised a specific campaign to raise breast awareness among black and ethnic minority (BME) women in Britain, and publicised the following comment:

> 43 per cent of BME women said they never look at or feel their breasts. 45 per cent of BME women of screening age (50 to 70 years) had never attended the NHS breast cancer screening programme. Breast Cancer Care is committed to ensuring that everyone in the UK has access to high quality breast awareness and breast cancer information. We believe this is an essential part of strategies to increase early detection.[42]

The justification for raising awareness here is increasing early detection, as women will be encouraged to examine their breasts and go for screening. Although this is not spelled out, the implicit presumption is that this will also improve women's chances of surviving breast cancer, yet problems can be identified with this idea.

Perhaps surprisingly this idea is not borne out by the medical evidence. Take breast self-examination, until recently a central facet of awareness campaigns. For many years, women were encouraged to use a technique similar to that used by medical practitioners to examine their own breasts, looking for suspicious signs of cancer. Several trials have discovered that not only is this not beneficial, it is overall a harmful exercise.[43] Groups of women who were taught how to examine their breasts were compared with those who were not, and the results showed no difference in mortality between the two groups, but an increase in potentially harmful benign breast biopsies in the group examining themselves.

The benefits of mammography, used widely to screen for breast cancer, are also contested in medical circles. A review in October 2006, by the highly respected Cochrane group, suggested that

> for every 2000 women invited for screening throughout 10 years, one will have her life prolonged. In addition, 10 healthy women, who would not have been diagnosed if there had not been screening, will be diagnosed as breast cancer patients and will be treated unnecessarily. It is thus not clear whether screening does more good than harm. Women invited to screening should be fully informed of both benefits and harms.[44]

This caution regarding efficacy is rarely expressed by breast cancer charities, and it is particularly the failure to provide clear information and advice to women which incenses critics of breast cancer screening. Informed choice, one of the buzzwords of modern medicine, is often overlooked in promotion of mammography according to the UK breast surgeon Professor Michael Baum:

> Tensions exist between the demands of the screening industry's 'pursuit of good uptake' and properly promoting informed choice of patients ... Most women who are screened have neither suffered nor been educated about the reality of the uncertainties, harms, and limitations of screening or the consequences of finding pathology of borderline importance.[45]

One Australian study reviewed 58 leaflets given to women to explain mammography.[46] The researchers found that the leaflets were much more likely to quote the statistics for lifetime risk of breast cancer (1 in 10 by the age of 85) rather than the lifetime risk of dying from breast cancer (about 3 in 100). Benefits of mammography were explained in terms of relative risk reduction, with estimates from 30–50 per cent improved survival (estimates which it would be difficult to support from medical literature). No leaflets at all cited the more prosaic 'number needed to treat' format, as used by the Cochrane review mentioned earlier.

This disregard for medical evidence seems to indicate that the goal of awareness has become an end in itself. Indeed, in the words of Breast Cancer Care's literature, 'The campaign seeks to emphasise that anyone can be affected by breast cancer, whatever their background, and everyone should be breast aware'.[47] There is a moral imperative here, in the demand that all of us should live life with an awareness of mortality and human susceptibility to disease, regardless of the relatively low risks the disease poses for a particular individual. In this regard, it has been argued that some contemporary cancer campaigns misrepresent the medical evidence. The imperative to 'be aware' also creates new difficulties.

The effects of 'awareness' are perhaps shown most clearly in the display of the pink ribbon. A tenet of breast cancer campaigning is that women are encouraged to identify their support and awareness publicly, a trend epitomised by ribbon wearing. Sarah Moore investigated this fashion in her research. She interviewed a group of women about why they wore pink ribbons, and her findings make for interesting reading.

'Because it's your worst fear, to have breast cancer', stated one woman, who Moore describes as 'often reticent ... [she] frequently spoke in a whispered tone'. She describes another interviewee whose mother had recently recovered from breast cancer. She explained wearing a pink ribbon as a means of reminding herself of the risks associated with the disease:

> Every time I put my coat on [and see the ribbon] I'm remembering that this thing's going to be in my mum's body for the rest of her life. And it could happen to me. You've got to be aware that it could

happen to you ... I obviously don't sit there everyday thinking, "Oh, I could have breast cancer. I could get breast cancer". It's just one of those subconscious things that rushes across your mind in a matter of seconds when you put your coat on and see the ribbon.[48]

Most of her interviewees described ribbon wearing in terms of worries or fears about the disease. The consciousness or awareness of illness so sought after by campaigners is thus revealed not as a positive, helpful force in their lives but as a 'constant, niggling sense of worry about this illness'. What was also interesting about Moore's interviewees is that they were mostly young women. Given that only around 2000 UK women under 40 are diagnosed with breast cancer each year, the impact of such worries seems to fall unfairly on their shoulders.

Testicular and prostate cancers

The successes of the contemporary breast cancer lobby have inspired others to follow directly in their footsteps. Charities funding research into cancers affecting men, particularly prostate cancer and testicular cancer, have followed the 'awareness-raising' model in their own campaigning. In place of pink ribbons and girly T-shirts, are beer-mats and 'Prostate cancer tool-kits^{TM}'.

Even more than is apparent in breast cancer campaigning, 'raising awareness' is promoted as a primary goal for men's cancer campaigns. The assumption underlying the men's health movement, that 'masculinity' makes men ignorant about their own bodies and health, and too reluctant to seek help, leads to the claim they need to be persuaded to do so by whatever means necessary.

Colin Osborne, who set up the Orchid Appeal, a charity raising awareness of testicular cancer, thus described himself prior to diagnosis as 'not one to go to the doctor's ... I have to be at death's door before I stop what I'm doing'.[49] It might be said that this happy-go-lucky attitude is quite reasonable for a young man in the prime of life. Testicular cancer is extremely rare, and has better cure rates than any other cancer (95%, even for those with advanced disease). There is no need for young men to worry about this disease. Yet Osborne has drawn the opposite conclusion, despite evidence to the contrary. He represents this 'masculine' disregard for ill health as dangerous and unwise and encourages other men to change their outlook on life if they are to avoid suffering from the problems he has faced.

In 2003 the Prostate Research Campaign ran a campaign called *Ignorance Isn't Bliss*. This campaign sought to encourage women to 'persuade your man to talk to his doctor about his prostate health'. Leaflets advised women to 'leave medical information leaflets lying around where he is likely to find them – i.e., the bathroom, near the remote control or on the car seat'.

'Feminine' acceptance of the need to seek help is thus envisaged as the means to change the way men behave. As one general practitioner put it, recognising the moral imperative regarding behaviour in such campaigns, 'The unfortunate conclusion I fear from reading the leaflet is that good men get PSA tests done, and good women make sure of it'.[50]

Prostate cancer is unusual in that it more often than not causes no problematic symptoms. Post-mortem studies have shown that around 40 per cent of men who die aged over 70 have prostate cancer.[51] In the past, most of them would have been blissfully unaware of this fact. The introduction of the prostate-specific antigen (PSA) blood test in the late 1980s has caused an enormous increase in the number of men diagnosed with prostate cancer (almost doubling in the USA). More than any other cancer, however, screening and early treatment for prostate cancer are highly controversial. In the UK, there is no organised screening for prostate cancer precisely because of the lack of evidence that screening is helpful, and evidence of its potential harmfulness.

Problematically, PSA testing does not differentiate between aggressive and potentially fatal cancers, and those that might have had a benign course, never troubling their host. Many more of these formerly hidden and harmless prostate cancers are now being picked up. One critic has accurately described this as 'the eradication of a disease: how we cured symptomless prostate cancer'. Formerly symptomless prostate cancer now has a new symptom, 'a disabling state of anxiety resulting from (men's) knowledge of their PSA level'.[52]

Just as we have seen in the case of breast cancer, evidence of the harms of 'awareness' and the advocacy of 'help seeking' does not, however, deter the campaigners. Medical intervention in the most personal aspects of men's lives is welcomed. For example, the Prostate Cancer Charity sells the 'Peeball™', a biodegradable ball that men can destroy by urinating on. This is marketed as a fun game to be played in pub toilets with friends, but of course it contains a serious message. The charity's website warns, 'It is not a diagnostic tool to test for prostate cancer. However difficulty passing urine whilst playing the game may indicate a prostate or urinary problem'.[53] This is reminiscent of Barbara Ehrenreich's description of the 'infantilizing trope' of merchandise such as teddy bears and crayons sold in aid of breast cancer charities.

In summary, the new discourse of health, as we described earlier, makes modifying the 'internal life' of individuals central to the pursuit of health. Campaigns for cancer awareness strongly exemplify and express this approach to 'health'. Yet such campaigns can have a highly negative effect at the level of the individual, in terms of raised anxiety levels and unnecessary medical interventions. One critic has contrasted such campaigns with the ideals of the women's movement in the 1970s, which attempted to resist the medical profession's intervention into the intimacies of everyday life:

Just as the smear test exposes women not merely to the medical gaze but to vaginal penetration, so the palpation of the prostate involves digital penetration of the male rectum. The slippery finger may be less impressive than the metal speculum, but it is no less significant an instrument of domination.[54]

On a broader social level, we have arguably moved from the state of denial described by Sontag to a position where we are all encouraged to see ourselves as 'cancer victims in-waiting'.

Conclusion

The problem of women's health came to prominence because of second-wave feminism in the 1970s. Discussion of the relationship between gender and health has a longer history however. The feminist novelist Virginia Woolf wrote in 1929:

> In a hundred years . . . women will have ceased to be the protected sex . . . All assumptions founded on the facts observed when women were the protected sex will have disappeared – as, for example, that women and clergymen and gardeners live longer than other people. Remove that protection, expose them to the same exertions and activities, make them soldiers and sailors and engine drivers and dock-labourers, and will not women die off so much younger, so much quicker.[55]

What mattered to Woolf was for women to be equal to men, and no longer the 'protected sex'. The most rewarding objective of life for women as well as men was, as far as she was concerned 'exertion and activity'. Almost 100 years later women are no longer the 'protected sex' they once were, but aspects of the new-found equality between women and men appear very different to that Woolf imagined, when she thought of the equal society of the future.

In the age of the new discourse of health a code of conduct has developed to shape the behaviour of both sexes, which is a far cry from Woolf's vision of what might lie ahead. Epitomised by advice given about men's health, it is one that upholds the 'virtues of the feminine'. Admission of vulnerability, risk awareness, and help-seeking behaviour are championed as desirable attributes for both men and women. It might be argued that, in Woolf's terms, both men women are in this way encouraged to adopt the identity of 'the protected sex'. What should we make of this outcome? Do we live in a better society because of this?

This chapter has argued that the cultural dominance of the new discourse of health, with its mantra 'prevention is better than cure', should be assessed very critically. The preventative approach now advocated so widely may appear to be 'common sense'. Yet closer examination suggests it may have the effect of encouraging *illness identities*. Our discussion has suggested that control of health 'from the inside' through 'awareness raising' involves encouraging people to adopt the identify of the help seeker, in contrast to that of the 'invulnerable' person, who assumes they are well most of the time. Could an unintended consequence of this strategy for improving the health of the nation be to make more people than ever worried about being ill? Could it even be that people come to consider themselves ill in this context?

Further reading

Lee, E. (2003) *Abortion, Motherhood and Mental Health: Medicalizing Reproduction in the United States and Great Britain.* New York: Transaction.

> This book uses the examples of Post-abortion Syndrome and Post-natal Depression to explore how women's experiences of pregnancy have been pathologised. It is also a useful read for those interested in how sociologists go about exploring the construction of social problems.

Olson, J. (2002) *Bathsheba's Breast: Women, Cancer and History.* Baltimore, MD: Johns Hopkins University Press.

> American historian James Olson explores the history of breast cancer through the ages, from the sufferings of Persian queen Atossa in 538 B.C. to Jerri Nielsen's confrontation with cancer at the South Pole in A.D. 1999. He describes how developments in medical understanding and treatment have interacted with cultural factors, in particular the rise of feminism and patient activism.

Rosenfeld, D. and Faircloth, C. A. (eds), (2006) *Medicalized Masculinities.* Philadelphia, PA: Temple University Press.

> In this edited collection, contributors discuss a range of ways in which men's lives have been medicalised; chapters discuss issues including balding, viagra, boys and ADHD and war veterans and PTSD. The Introduction provides a very useful overview of how sociology might theorise the medicalisation of masculinity.

References

1. Nettleton, S. (2006) *The Sociology of Health and Illness.* Cambridge: Polity.
2. Nettleton, S. (2006) ibid., p. 244, emphasis in the original.
3. Kimmel, M. S. (1995) Series editor's introduction. In D. Sabo and D. F. Gordon (eds), *Men's Health and Illness.* London: Sage, pp. vii–viii.
4. Rosenfeld, D. (2006) Medicalized masculinities: the missing link? In D. Rosenfeld and C. A. Faircloth (eds), *Medicalized Masculinities.* Philadelphia, PA: Temple University Press.

5 See for example, Zola, I. K. (1972/1978) Medicine as an institution of social control. In J. Ehrenreich and B. Eherenreich (eds), *The Cultural Crisis of Modern Medicine*. New York and London: Monthly Review Press, pp. 80–100; Conrad, P. (1992) Medicalization and social control. *Annual Review of Sociology*, 18: 209–32; and Gabe, J., Bury, M. and Elston, M. A. (2004) *Key Concepts in Medical Sociology* ('Medicalization'). London: Sage. Also Furedi F., this volume.
6 Conrad, P. (1992) ibid., p. 222.
7 Riessman, C. K. (1983) Women and medicalization: a new perspective. *Social Policy*, Summer: 3–17.
8 Ehrenreich, B. and English, D. (1973) *Complaints and Disorders: The Sexual Politics of Sickness*. New York: The Feminist Press.
9 Oakley, A. (1976) Wisewoman and medicine man: changes in the management of childbirth. In A. Oakley and J. Mitchell (eds), *The Rights and Wrongs of Women*. Harmondsworth: Penguin, pp. 52–3.
10 Graham, H. and Oakley, A. (1981) Competing ideologies of reproduction: medical and maternal perspectives in pregnancy. In H. Roberts (ed.), *Women, Health and Reproduction*. London: Routledge and Kegan Paul.
11 Boston Women's Health Book Collective (1995) Our bodies ourselves. In M. Schneir (ed.), *The Vintage Book of Feminism*. London: Vintage, p. 353.
12 Gordon, L. (1990) *Woman's Body, Woman's Right*. New York: Penguin.
13 Doyal, L. (1994) Changing medicine? Gender and the politics of healthcare. In J. Gabe, D. Kelleher and G. Williams (eds), *Challenging Medicine*. London: Routledge.
14 Shorter, E. (1997) *Women's Bodies*. New Brunswick, NJ: Transaction.
15 Strong, P. M. (1979) Sociological imperialism and the profession of medicine. *Social Science & Medicine*, 13A: 199–215.
16 Annandale, E. C. and Clark, J. (1996) What is gender? Feminist theory and the sociology of human reproduction. *Sociology of Health and Illness*, 18(1): 17–44.
17 White, K. (2002) *An Introduction to the Sociology of Health and Illness*. London: Sage Publications.
18 See Purdy, L. (2001) Medicalization, medical necessity, and feminist medicine. *Bioethics*, 15(3): 248–61 and Gabe, J., Bury, M. and Elston, M. A. (2004) *Key Concepts in Medical Sociology* ('Reproduction'). London: Sage.
19 Doyal, L. (1994) ibid., p. 142.
20 Miles, A. (1991) *Women, Health and Medicine*. Milton Keynes: Open University Press.
21 Figes, K. (1998) *Life After Birth*. London: Penguin, p. 40.
22 Wolf, N. (2001) *Misconceptions, Truth, Lies and the Unexpected on the Journey to Motherhood*. London: Chatto and Windus, p. 184.
23 For discussion of this subject, see Downs, D. (1996) *More Than Victims, Battered Women, the Syndrome Society and the Law*. Chicago: The University of Chicago Press; Figert, A. E. (1996) *Women and the Ownership of PMS: The Structuring of a Psychiatric Disorder*. New York: Aldine de Gruyter; Lee, E. (2003) *Abortion, motherhood and mental health: medicalizing reproduction in the United States and Great Britain*. New York: Transaction; Raitt, F. E. and Zeedyk, S. (2000) *The Implicit Relation of Psychology and Law, Women and Syndrome Evidence*. London: Routledge; and Westervelt, S. D. (1998) *Shifting the Blame: How Victimization Became a Criminal Defense*. New Brunswick, NJ: Rutgers University Press.

24 Miles, A. (1991) ibid, p. 65.
25 Fitzpatrick, M. (2001) *The Tyranny of Health*. London: Routledge.
26 Tredre, R. (1992) American magazine's target Britain's new men. The *Independent*.
27 Baker, P. (1994) Focus on men: sorry for the horrors, doctor. The Men's Health Network. The *Independent*, p. 20; Men's Health Forum. 'About Us', http//www.menshelathforum.org.uk
28 Curham, S. (2000) *Antenatal and Postnatal Depression: Practical Advice and Support for All Sufferers*. London: Vermillion, p. 72.
29 Rosenfeld, D. (2006) ibid.
30 Cited in Wainwright, D. (1996) The political transformation of the health inequalities debate. *Critical Social Policy*, 16: 67–82.
31 Lee, C. and Owens, R. G. (2002) *The Psychology of Men's Health*. Buckingham: Open University Press, p. 3.
32 Leary, C. (n.d) Men's health: worth talking about. Available at: http://www.sanitarium.com.au
33 Connell, R. W. (1995) *Masculinities*. Cambridge: Polity; Horrocks, R. (1994) *Masculinity in Crisis: Myths, Fantasies and Realities*. London: Macmillan.
34 Royal College of Psychiatrists (2004), *Men Behaving Sadly*. Available on line at www.rcpsych.ac.uk
35 Fitzpatrick, M. (2006) The men's health movement: a morbid symptom. *Journal of Men's Health and Gender*, 3(3): 258–62.
36 Meryn, S. (2005) Men's Health 2005: A small step for mankind. *Journal of Men's Health and Gender*, 2(4): 389–90.
37 Gunnell, C. (2004) Do we know how to help men? *Community Practitioner*, 77(6): 204–5; White, E. (2004) Men's health: the hard facts. *Community Practitioner*, 77(6): 206–7.
38 Sontag, S. (1978) *Illness as Metaphor*. New York: Farrar, Strauss and Giroux.
39 Ehrenreich, B. (2001) Welcome to cancerland: a mammogram leads to a cult of pink kitsch. *Harper's Magazine* (November).
40 Olson, J. (2002) *Bathsheba's Breast: Women, Cancer and History*. Baltimore, MD: Johns Hopkins University Press, p. 127.
41 Olson, J. (2002) ibid., p. 108.
42 Breast cancer care (c. 2006) *Same Difference: Breast awareness is for everyone*. Available on line at www.breastcancer care.org.uk
43 Semiglazov, V. F., Moiseyenko, V. M., Bavli, J. L., Migmanova, N. S., Seleznyov, N. K., Popova, R. T., Ivanova, O. A., Orlov, A. A., Chagunava, O. A. and Barash, N. J. (1992) The role of breast self-examination in early breast cancer detection (results of the 5-year USSR/WHO randomised study in Leningrad). *European Journal of Epidemiology*, 8: 498–502; Thomas, D. B., Gao, D. L., Ray, R. M., Wang, W. W., Allison, C. J., Chen, F. L., Porter, P., Hu, Y. W., Zhao, G. L., Pan, L. D., Li, W., Wu, C., Coriaty, Z., Evans, I., Lin, M. G., Stalsberg, H. and Self, S. G. (2002) Randomised trial of breast self-examination in Shanghai: final results. *Journal of National Cancer Institute*, 94: 1445–57.
44 Gøtzsche, P. C. and Nielsen, M. (2006) *Screening for breast cancer with mammography*. Cochrane Database of Systematic Reviews, Issue 4.
45 Thornton, H., Edwards, A. and Baum, M. (2003) Women need better information about routine mammography. *British Medical Journal*, 327: 101–3.

46 Slaytor, E. K. and Ward, J. E. (1998) How risks of breast cancer and benefits of screening are communicated to women: analysis of 58 pamphlets. *British Medical Journal*, 317: 263–4.
47 Breast cancer care, ibid, p. 1.
48 Moore, S. (2006) PhD thesis, University of Kent. 'Ribbon wearing: a sociocultural investigation'.
49 Carlowe, J. (2004) Boys don't cry. *Observer*, 10 October.
50 McCartney, M. (2004) Screening must remain a free choice. *British Medical Journal*, 328: 1023.
51 Coley, C. M., Barry, M. J., Fleming, C. and Mulley, A. J. (1997) Early detection of prostate cancer: part 1: Prior probability and effectiveness of tests. *Annals of Internal Medicine*, 126(5): 394–406.
52 Tannock, I. (2002) Eradication of a disease: how we cured symptomless prostate cancer. *The Lancet*, 359:1341–2.
53 Prostate Cancer Charity (2006) Product information. Available at: http://www.prostate-cancer.org.uk/
54 Fitzpatrick, M. (2001) ibid., p. 64.
55 Wainwright, D. (1996) ibid., p. 79.

Part 3

CAPTURING INDIVIDUAL EXPERIENCE AND GENDER CONTEXTS IN RESEARCH

12

VAGINAL POLITICS

Tensions and possibilities in *The Vagina Monologues*

Susan E. Bell and Susan M. Reverby

Source: *Women's Studies International Forum*, 28 (2005), 430–44.

Synopsis

We are feminists in our 50s who first became activists in the women's health movement when we were in our 20s. In 2002 we performed in *The Vagina Monologues* and participated in the 2002 V-Day College Campaign to end violence against women. We use our experiences "then" in the women's health movement and "now" in the College Campaign as a lens through which to introduce a "worry" about "a culture of vaginas" that the play's author, Eve Ensler does not adequately address. Our focus is the differing ways that the body, and in particular the vagina, has been politicized in these two feminist eras. Our concern relates to what we see as the unproblematized tension between a celebration of the pleasures of the body and the politics that underlie the play and the movement it has spawned. We worry whether or not our sense of disquiet and recognition signals both a recapitulation of 1970s women's health politics and their limitations and a failure to learn from critiques of this form of "globalized" feminism.

© 2005 Elsevier Ltd. All rights reserved.

... There are problems with using the female body for feminist ends.
(Wolff, 2003, p. 415)

Eve Ensler's play, *The Vagina Monologues* (TVM) opens with worries: "I bet you're worried. I was worried ... I was worried about vaginas. I was worried about what we think about vaginas, and even more worried that we didn't think about them. I was worried about my own vagina. It needed a context of other vaginas—a community, a culture of vaginas" (Ensler, 2001, p. 3). As we performed in 2002 college productions of the play, we had qualms, too. But they are of a differing sort that speak to our own feminist political histories and the productive tensions we fear are not in the play.

We are feminists in our 50s who first became activists in the women's health movement when we were in our 20s. We had very different experiences in the women's health movement: one of us worked within the self-help movement, the other on questions of political economy. Both of us are senior faculty members at US northeast liberal arts colleges where we each participated in the 2002 V-Day College Campaign and performed in the play, Susan Bell at Bowdoin and Susan Reverby at Wellesley. We have written words like Ensler's in analyzing various issues confronting the feminist women's health movements of the 1970s and 1980s. We had spoken the word "vagina" in women's living rooms, in store-front women's centers, in our classrooms, and in other college lecture halls before we said it in Ensler's play.

In this article, we use our experiences "then" in the women's health movement and "now" in our college performances as a lens through which to introduce a worry about "a culture of vaginas" that Ensler does not adequately address. Our focus will be the differing ways that the body, and in particular the vagina, has been politicized in these two differing feminist eras. Our concern relates to what we see as the unproblematized tension between a celebration of the pleasures of the body and the politics that underlie the play and the movement it has spawned.

Even though the play is less than a decade old, it has already been labeled a "feminist 'classic'" (Young, 2004, p. A17). Ensler wrote and began performing TVM in 1996, after interviewing 200 women. The play consists of a series of monologues about women's experiences with their "vaginas" (Ensler's body short hand for the vagina, cervix, clitoris, labia, and sexual experiences). Since 1998, the play has been performed annually on or near Valentine's Day to raise funds as part of a campaign to end violence against women and girls. "V-Day," as the larger movement is called, is a worldwide political movement "to end violence against women by increasing awareness through events and the media and by raising funds to support organizations working to ensure the safety of women everywhere" (Shalit, 2001, p. 173). As of December 2004, more than US$25 million had been raised for V-Day in thousands of performances by women across the globe (V-Day, 2004a, 2004b, "About V-Day"). This is a stunning achievement.

These productions—on hundreds of college campuses and in communities worldwide—have become performance vocabularies for a liberatory sexuality and anti-violence activism. Just as our own experiences teaching women to do vaginal self-exams, or to think from our bodies into the body politic did, this performance of vaginal politics seems to have opened up a new generation of women to wonderment and power and connection to women through the body. It builds upon what columnist Katha Pollitt (2001, p. 10) called the "old bones" of "sisterhood-is-powerful feminism." But at the same time, TVM is, in the words of anthropologist Sea Ling Cheng (2004), a "monologue" controlled from the center, not yet a "dialogue." It fails to acknowledge the problems of a global movement that begins with American voice-overs and interpretations of other women's lives. We worry whether or not our sense of disquiet and recognition signals both a recapitulation of some of the limitations of 1970s women's health politics and a failure to learn from critiques of "globalized" feminism.

We are very cognizant that this is a different historical moment. Feminism in the 21st century builds upon what came before and attempts to create a new politics. Neither of us thinks the 1970s feminism was our own golden moment or should or can be reproduced. We are too mindful of political, historical, and cultural change to think that the forms of political critique and agit prop from one generation can translate to another. Nevertheless, we think there are enough echoes of 1970s women's health politics in the emotional draw of TVM to give us great pause.

The vagina monologues and V-Day: a short history

Feminist performance artists and playwrights have long used interviews with other women to present as many "other women" on stage as possible and looked to "spectacle" to perform feminism (Case, 1990; Gale & Gardner, 2000; Glenn, 2000). Playwrights like Anna Deveare Smith have used methods of documentary or "verbatim theatre" to translate taped and subsequently transcribed interviews into scripts (Paget, 1987; Smith, 1993). By contrast, Ensler (2001, p. xxv) theatricalizes interview material. As she puts it, "some of the monologues are close to verbatim interviews, some are composite interviews, and with some I just began with the seed of an interview and had a good time" (Ensler, 2001, p. 7). Although she performs as if she were merely "telling very personal stories that had been generously told" to her, there is not a systematic method to her translation of the interviews into TVM (Ensler, 2001, p. xxv). In TVM, longer monologues on sexual experiences are interspersed with fantastic images of what vaginas wear, say, or smell-like and "vagina facts."

For Ensler (Braun & Ensler, 1999, p. 517), "the connection between how women regard their vaginas, and how women feel, and the state of women in the world is deeply connected." Ensler's sense of the play's power grew as she began to perform it, at first alone in the US and worldwide. In 1997, she and other activist women formed the V-Day Benefit Committee. The Committee's first project was a celebrity benefit performance of TVM on Valentine's Day 1998 to raise money to stop violence against women globally.

With its movie star cast, the benefit raised US$100,000 and launched the V-Day Movement as an organized effort beyond production of the play to end violence against women and girls (Ensler, 2001, pp. xxxii–xxxiii). A College Initiative followed to encourage college and university students to perform TVM on or near Valentine's Day to raise money to support local organizations working to stop violence against women (Obel, 2001). In addition to making violence against women visible and raising money to support local organizations, participating in the College Campaign gives students an "opportunity to learn about philanthropy, art, and activism" (Lewis, 2001, Campus Groups, para 2).

The first year, in February 1999, 65 schools in the United States and Canada participated in the College Initiative (Obel, 2001, p. 135). By February 2002, when we performed in TVM, more than 500 colleges in the US and worldwide participated in V-Day. There were more than 2000 events in V-Day (2004a, 2004b), including more than 600 performances of TVM in the College Campaign (Ensler, 2001; Lewis, 2001; Obel, 2001).

Each year, V-Day takes a different focus on violence against women and girls. Monologues are added or subtracted, and new monologues are performed, depending on V-Day's annual focus. Local performances have some flexibility, but the directors must agree to adhere to the V-Day rules in order to participate in the College Campaign. For example, students participating in the College Campaign must perform specific monologues in a particular order. But the numbers of women in the casts may vary widely: in the Wellesley 2002 production there were more than 35 women, whereas at Bowdoin there were 12. From its inception, V-Day has been "misunderstood as merely glitzy entertainment" by some, challenging its supporters to make its fundraising and consciousness-raising and social change goals explicit and clearly brought into focus for audiences worldwide (Baumgardner, 2002, para 7).

Methodology

This article is a collaborative endeavor. It is based on our experiences in the performances, as teachers of women and health courses, and as feminist activists. When TVM came to our campuses, we both decided to try out for our college's productions. We wanted to make connections with our students outside of the classroom setting where we were always the "teachers." We wanted to place ourselves in a more vulnerable position vis-à-vis our students, where our expertise (teaching and writing, not acting) would be of less use. We hoped this would give us insight into how feminist ideas and politics resonated with this generation. We also wanted to see if this new kind of performance would provide a cathartic re-engagement in our feminist work and connection to our students. We performed different monologues:

"Because He Liked to Look at It"[Reverby] and "I Was There in the Room" [Bell]. Based on an interview with "a woman who had a good experience with a man," Susan Reverby performed in the monologue that is, according to the script instructions, meant to be "ironic but male-friendly!" It is about how a woman who hated her vagina began to love it. She met a man named Bob, "the most ordinary man [she] ever met" but who loved vaginas. Bob "looked and looked" at her vagina "for almost an hour, as if he were studying a map, observing the moon, staring into [her] eyes" (Ensler, 2001 p. 57) and when she began to see herself the way he saw her, she "began to feel beautiful and delicious—like a great painting or a waterfall" (p. 57) and to love her vagina. *I chose to audition and perform this because I liked the idea that a women's studies professor would be in a "male-friendly" monologue. I didn't want to be typecast in the other monologues that were about an obviously older Jewish woman or about birthing [Reverby].*

The two directors of the Bowdoin production cast Susan Bell in "I Was There in the Room," the last monologue in the play. In her introduction to the monologue, Ensler (2001, p. 120) writes that "if I was in awe of [vaginas] before the birth of my granddaughter, Colette, I am certainly in deep worship now." The monologue is written as a poem about birthing. It compares the vagina to a "wide red pulsing heart. . . . that can ache for us and stretch for us, die for us and bleed and bleed us into this difficult, wondrous world. I was there in the room. I remember" (Ensler, 2001, pp. 124–125). *At first I thought "how boring and predictable." I was the only mother in the cast, typecast in the monologue about giving birth. Rehearsing the monologue took me back to times I had witnessed the births of others as well as the birth of my daughter. The honor of having been giving the last words, and the memories evoked by my performance, changed my feelings about this part [Bell].*

When we performed in TVM, each of us was the only faculty member in the cast, indeed the only member of the cast who was not a college student. During the time we rehearsed and then performed in the play we talked and corresponded by e-mail frequently about our experiences in the Bowdoin and Wellesley productions. Susan Bell kept a detailed journal beginning in December 2001 after the first meeting of Bowdoin's cast until after Bowdoin's last performance in February 2002. Together, we saw Ensler perform TVM in Boston. Susan Reverby, with the assistance of another member of the cast, conducted tape-recorded interviews with several cast members after Wellesley's production of the play. We asked for and received permission (informed consent) from all members of the Bowdoin and Wellesley casts to base our analysis on the two productions and to use examples from the productions. We have taken care to protect their confidentiality and privacy. Our analysis of the Wellesley and Bowdoin productions of the play and V-Day actions draws from all of these materials.

Body and body politic

On the surface, it appears that Ensler's play and the movement has inspired and helped to fund have solved what we have called elsewhere the body/body politic problem in women's health activism (Bell, 1994; Reverby, 2003). That is the play and the movement have seemingly enabled women to connect their individual body concerns with the larger structures of societal oppression. The play draws its audience in with its promise to talk openly about sexuality and personal desire, travels around the world in its monologues, and provides millions of dollars for women's anti-violence work. It has managed to transform the romanticism of Valentine's Day into fundraising and consciousness-raising about violence against women. In the United States, Valentine's Day, once owned primarily by the greeting card, flower, and chocolate industries, now competes with V-Day standing for victory, valentines, and vaginas, and (in 2004), voting.

But is V-Day simply a one-day, feel good event? We worry whether the empowerment that comes from a contemporary "speak-out" using Ensler's interpretation of other women's experiences translates into a larger political assault on the structures of oppression throughout the world. We do not wish to underestimate the power of words, especially since the play has been censored for what it says (Kahn, 2004) and shows (Bollag, 2004). But even so, is saying what is still transgressive out loud or showing it in public with hundreds of others also a political act? Does it in the end make the personal political? And whose personal life does it make political?

It is not as if these issues—of women's relationships to our bodies and the structures of power—are not dealt with anywhere else on US campuses. Many campuses (including our own) have health and sex educators, "safe space" organizations, take back the night groups, women's centers, etc. There are now hundreds of Women's Studies programs and departments with courses that focus at least some of the time on the analytic and interpretive dimensions of body politics. But in those courses, we do not show our students how to do a vaginal self-exam or explain how to masturbate. Nor do we share our personal experiences at this level, or ask them to do the same in return. When we do draw from personal experience, it is to help them make connections among their lives, cultures and social structures.

The power of TVM comes from its transgressive and carnivalesque public stance. The play, as with parts of the self-help movement and early consciousness raising groups, performs the personal publicly. It brings private experiences, hidden from others and especially from the self, literally onto a public stage (Haaken, 1998). It turns societally denigrated desire, practices, fantasies and physical body parts into public celebration. As one member of the cast told us, women "give but do not have" their own bodies.[1] No wonder that the vagina fact—the pleasure giving "8000 nerve fibers" in the clitoris that are "twice... twice... twice the number in the penis"—is the play's recurring mantra that the audience is allowed to request repeatedly and out loud and at any point (Ensler, 2001, p. 51). It is, despite disclaimers, competitive with the normative male sexual "performance." This move can be a crucial part of political action. But it runs the danger of remaining simply a transgressive moment easily reabsorbed and neutralized (Wolff, 2003, p. 418).

The play is a reclamation project, taking back the female body for women, as did the feminist health bible, *Our Bodies, Ourselves (OBOS)* (Boston Women's Health Book Collective, 1971). However, even with its sections on sexuality, OBOS's reclamation project worked through primarily the language of anatomy and physiology, providing readable information and multiple women's testimonials. In TVM, the power is in the performance itself, the process of the doing in public rather than the privacy of reading, and the focus is sexuality not anatomical parts. Anatomy does of course get into the performance, but very differently than in OBOS. V-Day actions on our campuses now also include the sale of female genitalia shaped lollipops and cookies and information about sex toys. At the Wellesley performance, a rubber dildo was incorporated as a prop. The positive affirmation of female sexuality makes the "joy of sex" apparent.

The play makes the assumption that knowledge about women's ability to have and right to know about sexual pleasure has to be at the center of our politics. Ensler herself, in a recent interview has claimed that TVM did this for her. We would never assume that the empowerment that comes from becoming a sexual subject, rather than object, was irrelevant. Yet repeating the "vaginal fact" about the mighty nerve endings of the clitoris, however titillating, has its limitations.

This knowledge does little to explain to women that there is a connection between their failure to know this "fact" and speak about their bodies. We worry whether the continual refrain is for improving individual women's sex lives or for helping women make the connection between their failure to know and speak about their bodies and the causes of the constructed ignorance about sexual pleasure and violence. The play itself risks leaving its audience and performers in the exhilaration of the transgressive moment alone.

The limit of this kind of individualized transgression is illustrated by contrasting the play's monologue, "The Vagina Workshop," with the real model of the masturbation workshops it builds upon. The workshops, started in the 1970s by feminist Betty Dodson, were set up to teach women how to masturbate and how to find their clitorises. In Ensler's hands, Dodson's focus on the clitoris becomes the more euphemistic "vagina." Betty Dodson's Bodysex workshops helped women learn about orgasm by explaining the difference between the clitoris and vagina. By contrast, Ensler (Braun & Ensler, 1999, p. 515) uses "vagina" to refer to "the 'common-sense' vagina—all the bits 'down there'." Ironically, Ensler actually dissembles its original. Using the word "vagina" (as in "The Vagina Workshop") in a monologue about sexual pleasure and orgasm perpetuates the myth of the vaginal orgasm.

Feminists in the late 1960s, recapitulating insights from Alfred Kinsey, argued against the Freudian claim that the vagina is women's primary site for "mature" sexual pleasure (Koedt, 1968). Dodson wanted women to find their clitorises, "the real source of our sexual stimulation" (Dodson, n.d.). To be more specific, the play in its discussion of pleasure is really about the clitoris and the vulva as well as the vagina. But after all, how large would the audience be for a play called "The Clitoris or Vulva Monologues?" By using the somewhat vaguer term "vagina," Ensler literally births a larger audience into sexuality and the world. But in doing so, she undoes the very hard work of second wave feminists who debunked the political, not just "pleasure," consequences of the myth of the vaginal orgasm.

In addition, in Dodson's workshops, groups of women'shared the experience of learning about orgasm collectively. One after another, "the entire class looked at one person's vulva at a time" (Dodson, n.d.). This is another key tenet of feminism, connecting women to each other. By contrast, in Ensler's monologue about this, one woman tells of her experiences, which, like all the others in the room, is individualized. In "The Vagina Workshop," each woman lies on her own blue mat, looking at and learning about her own vagina and clitoris. This individualizes and privatizes the experience, undoing a feminist process Dodson and others worked hard to create.

Not everyone, even in the most radical of second wave feminist circles, thought that Dodson's workshops made enough of a connection between our bodies and the body politic. Many of us found her workshops "over the top," even for their time. Generations of feminists have argued that we are more than our bodies, more than a vagina or "the sex." Yet, TVM re-inscribes women's politics in our bodies, indeed in our vaginas alone. In the Wellesley College production, for example, each cast member in the rehearsals was asked "how her vagina was doing that day" and to have her "vagina check-in" to the group as if one key site of women's sexual being could become "ourselves." The very use of this language led us to remember the discomfort we had in the 1980s when artist Judy Chicago, in her installation "The Dinner Party," portrayed powerful women throughout history as a series of dinner plates and tapestries with various vulva shapes (Chicago, 1979).

The endless arguments in feminism over transcendence of the body or life in it are the subtexts here, but they are never acknowledged. Only the body in the play seems to have the upper hand. The real "vagina fact"—that there are and were tensions about how to think about the body/body politic connection—is erased.

Do you need to be happy about your clitoris and/or have sexual pleasure to be politically effective? Can even those whose lives do not include a dildo, a right or left hand, or pleasure-giving partners have meaningful political lives? How much does making political change require each individual woman to love her own body? Alternatively, what does speaking of pleasures and critiquing violence do? Both speaking publicly and finding pleasure are important practices. Do Ensler's play and the V-Day movement allow multiple points of entry into the body politic?

Our monologues, our political selves

Our experiences in women's health movements "situate" our concerns with TVM. Each of us became activists to transform women's health care. Each of us entered women's health activism differently.

> Susan Bell: *I joined the women's health movement thirty years ago. I worked in women's health centers, organized a range of feminist health education projects, and wrote about women's health concerns. In my political work, I began with women's bodies, and worked out from there. At first, I worked in women's health centers (Feminist Women's Health Center, Oakland California and Women's Community Health Center [WCHC] Cambridge Massachusetts), providing abortion, birth control and "well-woman" health services. Both the women's health centers were founded on the principles of feminist self-help, to share knowledge and skills, to affirm the commonality of women, and to criticize and challenge the medical system. This part of the women's health movement "placed women's sexuality, sexual self-determination, and sexual identity at the center of women's health concerns."*
>
> (Swenson, 1998, p. 647)

In addition to providing health care, my work at the women's health centers also included developing educational self-help groups to provide a forum in which women could learn about their bodies with other women, be comfortable with their own bodies, learn about their reproductive and sexual anatomies, and break down barriers which keep women apart from each other. Another goal of self-help groups is to demystify the role of experts in providing medical services and expose the experts' role in defining and treating normal female conditions—aging, pregnancy, and childbirth—as "medical" problems. Self-help groups include showing as well as telling about women's bodies. Reciprocal sharing of cervical/vaginal and breast self-examinations was central to the ethic of feminist self-help.

At the WCHC I met and worked with women from the Boston Women's Health Book Collective, authors of Our Bodies, Ourselves. *OBOS reflects the philosophy of the women's liberation movement that the personal is the political, and draws from women's health experiences to expand, enrich, and criticize textbook views of women's health. One goal of the book is to value women's experiences as a source of knowledge. A second goal is to become an organizing tool, to help women translate their personal concerns about health into matters for social and political change. The Collective invited me to become an author and I accepted. I wrote the chapter on birth control for three editions of* OBOS.

(1984, 1992, 1998)

As with self-exam, the play is a vehicle of personal empowerment for individual women in the company of others. Whereas—to put it most simply—self-exam demystifies and demedicalizes the anatomy and physiology of women's reproductive bodies, TVM demystifies pleasure and desire. These can be exhilarating experiences for cast members and audiences. Yet at the same time, both self-exam and TVM seek to translate the joy of personal discovery into a matter of social and political change. To put it slightly differently, the goals and scope of self-help go far beyond self-exam. Self-help entails affirming the commonality of women, criticizing and challenging the medical system, and transforming science and society more broadly in addition to the ability to perform self-exam and to "know your body." V-Day, as well, has more far reaching goals than TVM. V-Day aims to expose and eradicate violence against women in the world in addition to encouraging women to talk about their vaginas. Thus, at the same time as I felt the excitement and possibilities offered in TVM, I worried about the difficulties of translating these immediate experiences into viable feminist health activism.

Susan Reverby: *I came into the women's health movement only briefly through the body. As with many feminists in New York City, I worked in a legal abortion clinic in 1970 when abortions became legal in the state two and half years before Roe v. Wade. I spent about a month at the clinic before I was hired by the Health Policy Advisory Center as a feminist activist. Health PAC, as it was called, was a left liberal think tank that critiqued the politics of the health care system and published a monthly Bulletin widely read by activists, professionals and workers in the health care industry.*

I wrote and lectured widely on women's health and nursing issues. I continued to do some work as well with two feminist consumer groups that provided access, information, teaching and testimony on women's health issues. I helped write pamphlets on everything from health services to vaginal infections. When I put my body on the line (as with the research for a pamphlet with the pithy title "How to get thru the System with your Feet in the Stirrups: A Guide to Women's Health Services Below 14th Street"), I did so to make the system's limits appear more transparent and to encourage women to critique it.

Mostly I gave talks on the health care system: the interlocks among industry, government, big hospitals and health priorities. I did this as part of women's "Know your Body" courses taught by activists in storefronts, at a range of women's health conferences and at schools and colleges. While others gave lectures on birth control, sexuality or childbirth, I talked about drug companies and the need for universal health insurance.

When the self-help movement provided women with a plastic speculum and told us to find our cervixes, I did spend one evening with a friend doing just that. But I never thought finding my cervix was a moment of empowerment. I worried alone and in print about the limits of looking inward, of how to make women see the link, as I wrote once, between our vaginas and Vietnam. At the time I never thought looking through a plastic speculum was a way to see power.

My worry came because no matter how often I talked about the bigger picture, women seemed to focus only on their own bodies. If I talked about health insurance, I was asked about cures for breast cancer. If I spoke about needing to attack physician power, I was told often about a woman's vaginal infection. I was too focused on the body politic; my audience often on their bodies. I realized that women were so hungry for information that they would ask anyone who seemed sympathetic and knew something. I had not yet figured a way to move from the larger politics to the body; and the women I spoke to couldn't hear about power when they still didn't live in their own bodies. I continued to try and understand how these differences could be resolved.

Years later when, through the Boston Women's Health Book Collective's recommendation, I became the consumer representative on the U.S. Food and Drug Administration's OB-GYN Devices Expert Panel, I worried anew about the link between personal body experiences and politics. I saw in a different format how women's focus upon their bodies could easily become a site of manipulation from drug companies (Reverby, 1997). For me, the body could be an impediment to empowerment, not a way out.

The experience of going through the process of having a vagina check-in at rehearsals, of hearing our students speak about their reasons for performing, of listening to students from a wide range of cultural, ethnic and religious backgrounds discuss the meaning of the play and whether they could invite their families and friends, reminded us again of the power of body talk to bond diverse women together. The sense of energy and excitement was palpable as guards were let down, individual stories exchanged, personal moments of joy and pain shared. It was indeed like consciousness-raising of

1970s feminism all over again. Our hopes of learning about their lives were fulfilled. We saw how performing the differing parts taught them to see themselves anew and to see from the position of others. In rehearsals, we were challenged to re-interpret individual monologues and to talk about their meanings. As performances were critiqued during rehearsals, we all learned to see the complexity of the various roles and positions of the women whose words (however filtered by Ensler) we were to speak.

We were, however, always self-conscious and self-aware that we were not just "one of the girls." One of the entries in Susan Bell's journal exemplifies what we both experienced:

> *We started [rehearsal] by doing warm-ups. I am completely at sea here, not having done any acting at all and not having ever taken an acting course, even a one-shot, one-afternoon session with a visiting what, dignitary? We stood in a circle and then [the director] hemmed and hawed and tried out different exercises that we might do, and others piped in, and I stood silent, feeling, well, older, and awkward, and worried that I couldn't do this. My boots felt heavy. I was the only person there wearing boots, not sneakers or clogs ... But really I guess the feelings I had were all about feeling like the odd person out—the professor, the mother, the menopausal woman, the non-acting woman. You name it.*
>
> *(Jan. 30, 2002)*

We are as old, if not older, than our students' mothers. We were, after all, either their professors or colleagues of their professors or professors of their friends. We were privy to backstage information that most professors, even in women's studies, don't hear. We carefully acknowledged this with cast members, promising that anything said would not leave the rehearsal space. Susan Reverby intentionally skipped a rehearsal when very personal information about sexual experiences and feelings was to be exchanged (the Bowdoin group did not have one rehearsal with this focus). At other times, our age and experiences made us the source of information and advice. We found ourselves explaining what a Grace Slick moan might sound like when they didn't know about the 1960s rock group Jefferson Airplane; we brought in a speculum to use as a prop that we had from our 1970s feminist health activism; we even were asked to help coach cast members in the performance of "authentic" orgasmic moments. We talked about college matters when they asked. In sum, we were both "one of them" and not.

The limits of transgressive performances

The nights of the performances too were emotional highs for both the audiences and the actors. The students and community members, men and women, cheered us on, got into the mantras, laughed and wept at the various moments. But what both of us wondered is: What comes next? Will this be a point of longer-term engagement in a political process or just a rite of passage in a 21st century woman's college years, a chance to think of her body differently? One of the students interviewed said she had decided not to audition for the next year's performance of TVM because she wanted "to give others a chance," that is to give them the bonding experience of being in the cast.[2] Having seen women take this kind of message from the women's health movement, we knew there was no guarantee that the momentary transformations would become political engagement. Would the women perhaps have better sex lives (just as some of us learned to), or would they learn the need to question the structures of oppression and their roles in it, just as some of us did?

We had seen some of this before and wrestled with these concerns. Although in her characteristic humor, political commentator Molly Ivins (2001) has claimed, "this is not your mother's feminism" in many ways TVM was just that. When the self-help movement swept through women's health groups in the early 1970s, thousands of women learned to look at their own cervixes, to study their cervical mucus to determine their monthly cycles, or to even consider doing menstrual extractions to rid their bodies of blood. Women like Lolly and Jeanne Hirsch, a mother–daughter team on the East Coast, and Carol Downer and Lorraine Rothman on the West Coast, "performed" in front of hundreds of women's groups (Morgen, 2002; Weisman, 1998). The plastic speculum, in contrast to the metal ones used by gynecologists, became the transparent symbol of the new power, in which this physician's tool was used by women in combination with a mirror and light to be able to see for themselves (Bell & Apfel, 1995).

[The first time we read through the script] I found myself laughing particularly uncontrollably during My Angry Vagina. The reader ... was excellent, and the monologue tickled me. I don't know why, maybe because some of the lines were so close to the jokes we used to tell at the FWHC [Feminist Women's Health Center] about vaginal (self) exams, the clowning around behind the scenes we used to do. Or perhaps in part because the criticisms were so apt, so biting, so reminiscent of the criticisms I used to make during self-help presentations ...
(Bell journal, Jan. 28, 2002)

"Cold duck lips," the descriptive lines in the play that make fun of the metal speculum seemed especially riotous to me as I recalled pretending to have vaginal infections so I could investigate the treatment women received in New York's public health clinics. I laughed, too, thinking about how ludicrous and frightening that instrument can be. I brought a metal speculum I used for talks and classes to a rehearsal

> *and it became a prop in Wellesley's production. It was hilarious for me to watch it get whipped out of a woman s back jean pocket and waved at the audience. It reminded me of the demands we made on our obgyns to take away the paper drapes in the exams, to put oven mitts on the stirrups to keep our feet warmer, and to require that we be talked to before we got undressed and were lying there in wait for the "duck lips." I remembered how putting up with all those unneeded exams had led me, along with other activist women, to a confrontation with a clinic director and eventual changes in their insensitive practices (Reverby).*

All that emphasis on mucus, on visualizing the hidden, was as transgressive and shocking in the 1970s as the play's repetition of the one word "vagina" is today. Activists who did this kind of self-exam work had to defend its political implications to others even at the time. Feminists in the 1970s worried that this form of personal transgression could become a political dead-end. In 1972, political columnist Ellen Frankfort (1972, p. 239) asked whether "women's body courses, by offering instant rewards, may be the way of triggering the less-gratifying long-range work" or not. Indeed her book on *Vaginal Politics* focused as much on the political economy that structured women's experiences as it did on those experiences themselves.

But at the same time, some of the monologues are counter-narratives of pleasure and desire (Taylor, 2002). Psychologist Jill Taylor (2002) argues that monologues like "The Flood," contest both standard narratives about women and other narratives within the play of violence and repression. "The Flood" is told by an older woman who, like other women Ensler interviewed between the ages of 65 and 75, "had very little conscious relationship to their vaginas." (Ensler, 2001, p. 23). The monologue ends with, "You know, actually, you're the first person I ever talked to about this, and I feel better" (Ensler, 2001, p. 30). Thus, even in itself, the play might accomplish something by helping to rewrite narratives of desire, pleasure, and community among those performing and attending its performances. We are reminded again of how "pride and advocacy can replace shame" (Huizenga, 2005 p. 2).

Looking at these moments through our experiences in the women's health movement, we know that the performance of TVM could move beyond the immediate sense of empowerment that comes from transgression if it is a starting point and not an end point for action. More knowledge does not always lead to more power. The women's health movement in the 1970s was often co-opted by "solutions" when providers in commercial health centers for women handed you a mirror, or told you to use yogurt for your vaginal infection, or provided a birthing room, but did not give up control over decision making or expand their services. Performances of TVM also risk this kind of cooptation and commercialization.

Whose bodies, whose cultures?

The power of TVM and the subsequent V-Day movement has been its appeal worldwide. The play portrays the experiences of many groups of women. It contains monologues from women in Bosnia and Afghanistan, from the southern US to Great Britain. It engages with a range of emotions, images and stories. It is about both sexuality and violence, the Janus-like constructions of "pleasure and danger" that haunt women's experiences (Vance, 1984). TVM's humor comes in part from its naming of various words for female genitalia from differing groups of women; its pathos from its making visible the pain and sexual violence that has been visited upon individual girls and women in times of peace and war.

Those producing the college shows are encouraged to make sure the cast reflects as wide a diversity of women as possible, seemingly to make the very words in the play embodied on the stage. The directors of the college productions attend meetings with Ensler to assure that certain rules and strategies for the play and fundraising are employed. In the time leading up to the performance of TVM, students are encouraged to provide information about violence against women, organize events and "rape free zones" on campuses and in communities and generally to make vaginal politics visible. At the performances, audiences can sign up for anti-violence work, see exhibitions of survivors of violence art, and pick up pamphlets on topics ranging from domestic violence to abortion rights.

The V-Day movement has made a strategic decision in its attempt use TVM as a catalyst for raising money and awareness. It connects women's groups around the world, names the problems in particular countries, and funds women who are working for social change (Lewis, 2001). Each year, V-Day highlights one anti-violence campaign. The 2002 V-Day events shone a "Spotlight on Afghan Women," in 2003, the campaign was titled "Afghanistan is Everywhere: A Spotlight on Native American and First Nations Women," and in 2004, the "Spotlight" was on "Missing and Murdered Women in Juarez, Mexico." Ten percent of all funds raised during V-Day events are designated for women working to reduce violence in these spotlighted communities.[3] The rest of the money goes to local nonprofit organizations working to end violence or providing services for women and girls who have survived such violence. As one of the recipients of money from the V-Day effort noted, "many people who come to see TVM would never attend a conference organized by a non-profit organization." TVM has "helped [to] breath new life into . . . efforts to end violence against women" by non-profit organizations, according to some charity officials (Lewis, 2001, 'Power of an Artist,' para 2).

In a way, TVM and V-Day embody what bell hooks has called "yearning," across racial, sexual and class lines that allows for "the recognition of common commitments and serve[s] as a base for solidarity and coalition" (hooks, 1990, p. 27). But the yearning that it invokes, after years of criticism of western white feminism, seems at best romantic. According to many critics, "this version of feminism with its belief in universal sisterhood, its celebration of individuality, and its embeddedness in modernist paradigms of social action" is too narrow to contain the multiple experiences and actions of women across the world (Davis, 2002, p. 226). Having taught these critiques in our classes, had our scholarship informed by them, and lived through the arguments in various feminist organizations to which we belonged, we could not help but bring these concerns with us when we participated in the college productions.

Yet here was the "yearning" without the critique. The monologues were not just about one group of women. But the starting point, the very core of the play, is the United States. The monologues that focus upon women outside US boundaries uniformly represent those women, as sociologist Kathy Davis has written in another context, "as oppressed victims of a despotic patriarchy in need of support and salvation by their more emancipated sisters in the West" (Davis, 2002, p. 227).

One of the short "vagina facts" that serves as the play's connective tissue between the longer monologues illustrates this problem. It starts with the lines "genital mutilation has been inflicted upon 80 (million) to 100 million girls and young women. In countries where it is practiced, mostly African . . ." (Ensler, 2001, p. 67). The use of the term mutilation is done without any acknowledgment of its problematic history and the ways in which many women's groups in different African and Middle Eastern countries have turned to the word "cutting" instead of "genital mutilation" to signify the problem. The unproblematized use of the word mutilation effaces the political struggle between western and various African women's groups over even the terminology to explain this practice (James & Robertson, 2002).

Of course, TVM is a play not a political tract or a feminist scholarly article. But its movement across the boundary of entertainment into agit prop and feminist political change requires it to at least acknowledge the implications of its dualistic and potentially disempowering terminology. It need not be the feminist equivalent of Soviet era didactic theater nor boringly reductive. Theatricality, however, does not mean that the complexity of a political question must be lost.

There are to be sure powerful monologues in the play that focus on the problems of a diverse group of American women and girls. But these problems appear both individualistic and shaped by culture. As anthropologist Uma Narayan has argued about the ways "dowry murders" are presented in the West, no one discusses domestic violence in the United States as "murder by culture" yet implies this continually for women in the third world (Narayan, 1997, pp. 81–118). In the play, the lives of women in Africa (read as one country not a continent with more language groups and diverse cultural practices than any other continent in the world), Bosnia, and Afghanistan are articulated as uniform. At the same time these women's stories are performed as personal narratives in individual life circumstances, they replicate stereotyped images. The monologues do not present what has been done to overcome the problems or provide enough clues to imagining their lives differently. This is left to the action of the V-Day funding, but is not part of the play's message itself. Thus the play separates out the political analysis and action from its other feminist messages.

In order for there to be a feminist practice that crosses international borders, there has to be a sophisticated understanding of how coalitions can be formed. While V-Day itself may allow for very culturally (politically) specific organizational structures—for example its support of work in Kenya—the play itself in the way it engaged our college audiences did not provide evidence of such variety, subtlety, or self-determination.[4] In fact, the rules given to the directors of the college productions prohibited revisions such as rewording, reorganization of the monologues, or insertion of more explanatory text into the play itself.

However, Ensler has added and subtracted monologues from the play. The year after we performed in it, a new monologue about Native American women was added, as were two site-specific monologues (one by women students and one by men students). This way of revising the play places power to establish the feminist practice of border crossing mostly (if not exclusively) in the hands of Eve Ensler. It discourages student and community involvement in the practice of translation and adaptation (Cheng, 2004; Davis, 2002).

The risk that worries us is that the play will remain the only connection that its audience and performers have with women anywhere else in the world. While the money raised may easily be exchanged across borders for local currency, American women's consciousness may remain rooted in nativist soil. When performed by women outside the United States, or by women in the United States whose "identities" are depicted in TVM, the monologues still reflect images that Ensler has created. If the play is not going to recreate this view of the world from the "core out to the periphery," more will have to happen than the addition of more monologues about more women and girls from more cultures in the world. The very universality, which makes the play so powerful for North American audiences, will have to be undermined. A new and different basis for connection will have to be created.

The V-Day movement may provide the evidence for such connections and even the language for new monologues themselves. And if it does whether this changed trope will be as wildly successful as the play has been to date is also uncertain.

Danger, pleasure, and power

Ensler is not the first feminist, of course, struggling to find a balance between celebrating sexuality's potential for pleasure and acknowledging its use as a weapon of power. As a survivor of sexual violence herself, Ensler is determined to keep her audiences ever mindful but not mired in violence's consequences for women. She writes, "*in order for the human race to continue, women must be safe and empowered*" (Ensler, 2001, p. xxxvi).

Betty Dodson, more focused on sexuality's pleasure principles, criticizes Ensler for linking pleasure and violence in TVM. In her view, the main problem is that "women end up celebrating sexual violence and not the creative or regenerative pleasures of erotic love" (Dodson, n.d.). We disagree with her. Ensler did not tilt the monologues this way (Sheiner, n.d.). In the play, no one in the audience is asked to say "no more domestic violence, no more rape as a tactic of war, no more unnecessary caesarian sections" over and over as a mantra. If the play did this, the result would not be the exhilaration that comes from remembering or learning what the clitoris can do. Instead of seeing women's bodies as the sites of pleasure, it would be the constant reminder of violence and danger.

Ensler's way out of the danger/pleasure dilemma is to include several monologues on the psychic and physical costs of the violence and to put the play's money toward ending such violence. At the end of the Bowdoin performances, audience and cast members who had experienced violence or who knew women who had were asked to stand. Seeing approximately two thirds of the people in the room standing together was a powerful reminder of the reality of violence in women's lives. However, the assumption that all violence is the same (which is implied by the action of standing together), or that state controlled rape and domestic abuse are equal, does not provide women or men with a way to consider the sources of these very different kinds of violence and can give them a false sense of connection.

Separating the body and the body politic, TVM from V-Day, is a problem. When Susan Bell wrote about birth control for OBOS, she struggled to incorporate political analysis with "the facts" (Bell, 1994). When Susan Reverby lectured about the political economy of American health care or listened to women testify at FDA hearings, she tried to find ways to connect their body talk to political power (Reverby, 1997). We want and expect TVM to do this too. Transgression and speaking out loud about what has been silenced are powerful tools, as we learned in the 1970s and as the play clearly demonstrates. Its ability to shock its audience into recognition can become merely the ability to shock.

A recent critique of the 2004 V-Day march in Juarez, Mexico also points to the problems we seen inherent in the play. According to performance artist and Columbia University professor, Coco Fusco, an organization of mothers of the murdered women in Juarez, Mexico does not see their daughters' serial killer or killers and rapists as the perpetrators of domestic violence. Rather, they have argued this is about the protection of powerful men by the authorities. They were angered by V-Day and Amnesty International's linking of the play to their own "rituals of public mourning" and what Fusco writes was the failure of the march organizers to incorporate these mothers in the planning of the demonstration. While it is beyond the scope of this paper to address in detail the politics of the V-Day movement itself, this critique from Juarez suggests the difficulties we have been raising about violence, power, and representation in TVM (Fusco, 2004).

The politics of vaginas

There is much to value in the performance of TVM, beginning with the personal experiences of cast members and audiences. Our own is illustrative. We had a great time rehearsing for and performing in the play. Each of us successfully crossed the boundary between professor and student. Our lack of acting skills demystified our power in the face of our more experienced and talented students. We managed to become cast members, not merely cast mothers, although we did nurture and support them. We learned from them and crossed the multiple barriers that have separated our generation from theirs. Interviews with some of the cast members afterwards indicate that the performance had a powerful effect at the time and continued long afterwards. Not only were they educated about pleasure and desire in their own bodies in a "culture of vaginas," but at the same time their consciousnesses were raised about violence against women and girls.

Students at Wellesley and Bowdoin have continued to participate in the College Campaign, led by some of the students who were in the casts with us. Anti-violence groups that received V-Day funds from these performances have benefited, as have their clients and communities. We have seen that individual empowerment can lead to wider political action, and that the experience of political collective movements can change one's sense of self. While Ensler, and the movement her work has spurred, clearly sees "vaginas" as metaphors, we know from our feminist practices that such metaphors do not always become apparent as political actions. A better sex life and sense of self are well worth having, but recreating a false sense of connection among women is not.

The play makes no effort to explain how women's ignorance *itself* is constructed. We worry about whether the cast members and the audience could see connections between the monologues about the lack of self-awareness and knowledge about pleasure and violence and why this lack occurs. There seems to be no way to look critically at each monologue itself, to question its accuracy and representativeness within the play. Identification on the most essential grounds, rather than complexity, along with humor and pathos became the only possible responses. Realistically, we can acknowledge the limits of any performance to do everything we would want. But we worry still about the simplicity of this approach and whether in this case "less" is *not* "more." To put it simply, we would like to see explicit recognition of the tension between the body and the body politic.

Furthermore, we are not convinced that the play enables cast members or the audience to become self-reflexive about "difference." In the joy of the seeming knowability that the play makes possible, the audience and performers can imagine they have shared the "real experiences" of women whose lives are different from their own. The problem cannot be solved just by adding more monologues, as Ensler has done. If the framework remains the same, the strategy will be just "add women from (fill in the country or the latest visible form of violence) and stir," and each addition will do nothing to address problems in the framework. The play itself needs to find ways to use its humor and connection by perhaps changing the introductions to the monologues, finding ways to show how collective action has transformed the stories, not just introducing women to better sexual lives or telling them to become part of V-Day.

The play underlines the difficulties of "crossing the border" with another person's story (Behar, 1993). Ensler tries to deal with this problem by requiring actresses to read their monologues (even if they have memorized the lines) holding index cards to indicate the presence of another. Appearing to represent the experiences of another, without any focus on how their subjectivity and location have been created, is a theoretical dilemma feminist scholars have been debating for a generation (Chandler, Davidson, & Harootunian, 1991; Stone-Mediatore, 2003). But holding the index cards as if speaking for another does not adequately acknowledge or alleviate any of these tensions.

We realize the play cannot be a classroom, nor do we want it to become one. That would be redundant. For us, as Ensler intended, the process of putting together the performance and the V-Day activities was just as critical as being on the stage in front of the audience. We and our students could not have had this kind of dialogue in the classroom. Rehearsing and then performing in the play gave us an opportunity to do feminist political work differently. We do not want this to get lost in the exhilaration of transgressive performance and simple knowability of the other. We want the tensions that are in the play, both spoken and unspoken, to be used as a framework for dialogues across generational as well as other differences. Addressing these tensions requires more than revisions in the script; it demands participation in the performance itself as well as the rehearsals and conversations surrounding the performance.

The possibilities of performance and engagement can be a link between the body and body politic in a new way. Despite our worries about the limitations we believe in an advocate engagement with TVM and V-Day actions. For three decades we have been part of complicated, and at times heated disputes, among feminists about the tensions between the body and the body politic and the need to be cognizant of the essentializing discourses that have appeared in western feminisms. There is much to be hopeful about forms of political engagement engendered by connecting TVM with V-Day. But unacknowledged tensions that the play hides and does not problematize ultimately are much to worry about.

Acknowledgements

We wish to thank the cast members of the 2002 Bowdoin and Wellesley College productions for their talent, spirit and openness to us, and the permission they granted us to use their and our experiences for this paper. We are grateful to the members of the Wellesley College cast who spoke to SR or were interviewed by Erin Judge, Wellesley College 2002. SB thanks Clare Forstie, Bowdoin College 2002 and SR thanks Erin Judge for their research assistance. We thank Roberta Apfel, Kathy Davis, Clare Forstie, and Barbara Condliffe for reading earlier drafts, and Gretchen Berg for helping us to understand feminist performance. Susan Bell's work on this project was supported by a Bowdoin Faculty Leave Fellowship. We are particularly grateful to our families who came to watch us perform.

Notes

1 Susan M. Reverby, Interview with Wellesley College student in 2002 production, April, 2002.
2 Erin Judge interview with Wellesley College cast members, May 2002.
3 V-Day website, http://www.vday.org/contents/vcampaigns/indiancountry. Retrieved February 9, 2004.
4 Agnes Pareyio provides education about "cutting" to young Maasi girls and a safe house for those girls who choose not to be cut. The safe house is a space not only of protection but of replication, where girls spend 5 days in seclusion, learning from an older woman in much the same way they would have learned from their own mothers if their genitals had been cut. Pareyio reports that "Eve and V-DAY started by donating a jeep that has enabled me to reach my people—the Maasi—who are deeply rooted by their traditional cultures and who still hold their beliefs that girls cannot be a woman without the cut. With the opening of the Safe House, girls who have escaped the cut can undergo an alternative ritual which I hope my people will grow to understand and adopt." http://www.vday.org/contents/vday/press/release/020405.

References

Baumgardner, Jennifer (2002, December 2). When in Rome... *The Nation* 275:19, pp. 22–25. Retrieved February 6, 2004 from Academic Search Premiere database.
Behar, Ruth (1993). *Translated woman: Crossing the border with Esperanza's story*. Boston: Beacon Press.
Bell, Susan E. (1994). Translating science to the people: Updating *The new our bodies, ourselves. Women's Studies International Forum*, *17*(1), 9–18.
Bell, Susan E., & Apfel, Roberta J. (1995). Looking at bodies: Insights and inquiries about DES-related cancer. *Qualitative Sociology*, *18*, 3–19.

Bollag, Burton (2004, February 18). Society steps up campaign against productions of 'The Vagina Monologues' on Catholic campuses. *The Chronicle of Higher Education's Today's News* http://chronicle.com/daily/2004/02/2004021894n.htm. Retrieved February 18, 2004.

Boston Women's Health Book Collective (Eds.). (1971). *Our bodies, ourselves*. New York: Simon & Schuster.

Braun, Virginia, & Ensler, Eve (1999). Virginia Braun in conversation with Eve Ensler, public talk about 'private parts'. *Feminism & Psychology*, 9(4), 515–522.

Case, Sue-Ellen (Ed.). (1990). *Performing feminisms: Feminist critical theory and theatre*. Baltimore: Johns Hopkins University Press.

Chandler, James, Davidson, Arnold I., & Harootunian, Harry (Eds.). (1991). *Questions of evidence: Proof, practice, and persuasion across the disciplines*. Chicago and London: University of Chicago Press.

Cheng, Sea Ling (2004). Vagina dialogues? Critical reflections from Hong Kong on The Vagina Monologues as a worldwide movement. *International Feminist Journal of Politics*, 6(2), 326–334.

Chicago, Judy (1979). *The dinner party: A symbol of our heritage*. Garden City, NY: Anchor/Doubleday.

Davis, Kathy (2002). Feminist body/politics as world traveller: Translating *Our bodies, ourselves. European Journal of Women's Studies*, 9.

Dodson, Betty (n.d.). Give sex a chance: 'V-Day' and the Vagina Monologue blues, Spectator.net, pp. 1–5. http://www.spectatotr.net/1173/pages/1173_dodson.html. Retrieved February 6, 2004.

Ensler, Eve (2001). *The vagina monologues. The V-Day edition*. New York: Villard.

Frankfort, Ellen (1972). *Vaginal politics*. New York: Quadrangle Books.

Fusco, Coco (2004). "Nettime, the mothers of Jurarez's letter to Eve Ensler." http://amsterdam.nettime.org/Lists-Archives/nettime-l-0401/msg00055.html. Retrieved February 27, 2004.

Gale, Maggie B., & Gardner, Viv (Eds.). (2000). *Women, theatre and performance*. Manchester: Manchester University Press.

Glenn, Susan A. (2000). *Female spectacle: The theatrical roots of modern feminism*. Cambridge: Harvard University Press.

Haaken, Janice (1998). *Pillar of salt: Gender, memory, and the perils of looking back*. New Brunswick, NJ: Rutgers University Press.

hooks, bell (1990). *Yearning*. Boston: South End Press.

Huizenga, Judith N. (2005, January 20). *Comments during the discussion group, Vaginas: Real and symbolic*. New York City, NY: American Psychoanalytic Association Meetings.

Ivins, Molly (2001, September 17). Body bard. *Time*, 158, 66–67.

James, Stanlie M., & Robertson, Claire C. (Eds.). (2002). *Genital cutting and transnational sisterhood: Disputing U.S. polemics* (pp. 129–171). Urbana: University of Illinois.

Kahn, Joseph (2004, February 13). Beijing journal: Offended by the v-word, China mutes monologues. *New York Times*, Section A, Column 3, p. 4.

Koedt, Anne (1968). The myth of the vaginal orgasm. *Notes from the first year*. New York: The New York Radical Women. http://scriptorium.lib.duke.edu/wlm/notes/. Retrieved December 16, 2004.

Lewis, Nicole. (2001, April 19). Staging an end to abuse. *Chronicle of Philanthropy* 13:13 (pp. 7–10). Retrieved February 6, 2004 from Academic Search Premiere database.

Morgen, Sandra (2002). *Into our own hands: The women's health movement in the United States, 1969–1990.* New Brunswick: Rutgers University Press.

Narayan, Uma (1997). *Dislocating cultures: Identities, traditions and third world feminism.* New York: Routlege.

Obel, Karen (2001). The story of V-Day and the college initiative. In E. Ensler (Ed.), *The vagina monologues. The V-Day edition* (pp. 129–171). New York: Villard.

Paget, Derek (1987). 'Verbatim theatre': Oral history and documentary techniques. *New Theatre Quarterly; NTQ, 3*(12), 317–336.

Pollitt, Katha (2001, March 5). Subject to debate: Vaginal politics. *The Nation*, 9, 10.

Reverby, Susan M. (1997). What does it mean to be an expert? A health activist at the FDA. *Advancing the Consumer Interest, 9,* 34–36.

Reverby, Susan M. (2003). Thinking through the body and the body politic: Feminism, history, and health-care policy in the United States. In Feldberg Georgina, et al., (Eds.), *Women, health, and nation: Canada and the United States since 1945* (pp. 404–420). Montreal: McGill-Queen's University Press.

Shalit, Willa (2001). V-Day until the violence stops. In E. Ensler (Ed.), *The vagina monologues. The V-Day edition* (pp. 173–177). New York: Villard.

Sheiner, Marcy (n.d.). Give V-Day a chance. Daze Reader (originally published in Spectator.net), http://www.dazereader.com/sheinervday.htm. Retrieved February 27, 2004.

Smith, Anne Deveare (1993). *Fires in the mirror.* New York: Anchor.

Stone-Mediatore, Shari (2003). *Reading across borders: Storytelling and knowledges of resistance.* New York: Palgrave/Macmillan.

Swenson, Norma (1998). Women's health movement. In Mankiller Wilma, et al., (Eds.), *The reader's companion to U.S. women's history.* New York: Houghton Mifflin.

Taylor, Jill McLean (2002). 'But what's at stake?' Older women talking about sexuality. *Narrative Inquiry, 12*(2), 423–429.

Vance, Carol (Ed.). (1984). *Pleasure and danger: Exploring female sexuality.* Boston: Routledge & K. Paul.

V-Day. (2004a). About V-Day http://www.vday.org/contents/vday/aboutvday. Retrieved December 16, 2004.

V-Day. (2004b). College campaign. Participating schools, http://www.vday.org/contents/vcampaigns/college/schools. Retrieved February 8, 2004.

Weisman, Carol S. (1998). *Women's health care activists and institutional change.* Baltimore: Johns Hopkins University Press.

Wolff, Janet (2003). Reinstating corporeality: Feminism and body politics. In Amelia Jones (Ed.), *The feminism and visual culture reader.* London: Routledge.

Young, Cathy (2004, February 23). Feminism's troubling 'classic'. *The Boston Globe*, A17.

13

TOWARDS TRANSNATIONAL FEMINISMS

Some reflections and concerns in relation to the globalization of reproductive technologies

Jyotsna Agnihotri Gupta

Source: *European Journal of Women's Studies*, 13:1 (2006), 23–38.

Abstract

This article discusses the emergence of the concept of 'transnational feminisms' as a differentiated notion from 'global sisterhood' within feminist postcolonial criticism. This is done in order to examine its usefulness for interrogating the globalization of reproductive technologies and women's right to self-determination over their own bodies by using these technologies. In particular, women's use of technologies for assisted conception, and the local and global transactions in reproductive body parts form a testing ground for transnational feminisms. Does the construction of individual reproductive rights still leave some ground for women's collective struggles? It is proposed that, if at all, transnational solidarity on this issue is possible, it will have to be built on the concept of universal ethical norms regarding human dignity.

Transnational feminisms: a new concept

In the early 1980s, I was a student pursuing the 'women and development' (sub) specialization within the masters programme in development studies, at the Institute of Social Studies in The Hague. This programme was one of the pioneers in the field of women's studies in the Netherlands, under the stewardship of Maria Mies and Kumari Jayawardena. We were a group of international students drawn from all continents. For our first International Women's Day celebration on 8 March 1982, we made a poster with the slogan 'Divided in Culture, United in Struggle' and launched a newsletter called *Insisterhood*. During the course, we had become aware of the differences in our social positioning due to our diversity not only in terms of culture, but also race, class, religion, sexual orientation, etc. And yet we felt the bond of sisterhood in terms of the shared discrimination, subordination and oppression that either we had experienced personally as women or had learnt of through our work, as well as the need for feminist scholarship and political organizing to fight against it. Were we being too naive then in discounting our differences? And were we too optimistic regarding forging solidarity, speaking from our own privileged positions within our own societies, or could we actually see the commonalities beyond the differences?

Now, we are more than 20 years further. Over the years, in our postmodern, 'posthuman', and perhaps for some, even 'postfeminism' (Braithwaite, 2002) times, the idea of 'universal truths' has been replaced by 'diversity'. The category 'woman' has been deconstructed to take cognizance of the differences among women. Also, the idea of our individual 'situatedness' within intersections has gained ground, and there is a multiplicity of world's feminisms. At the same time, the concept 'transnational feminisms' has been introduced to mark the shift from 'global sisterhood' (Morgan, 1984), which according to some bears the bias of ethnocentrism. 'Transnational feminisms' is a fairly new concept to emerge in western academia. So, what does this term encompass? What does it have to offer feminists at the beginning of the 21st century? Is it just a new buzzword, or does it have an added value over the old concept of 'global sisterhood' used during the second wave of the women's movement mainly by first world, white, middle-class feminists, a term that allegedly glossed over the differences between women? Is the concept 'transnational feminisms' adequate to describe women's organizing across the globe from their different social positioning and interests? Is transnational solidarity possible and on what grounds will it be built under the conditions of transnational capitalism in this era of globalization? In particular, women's use of technologies for assisted conception and the local and global transactions in reproductive body parts form a testing ground for transnational feminisms.

As a point of departure for reflecting on these questions, I make use of the insights of Breny Mendoza (2002) and Chandra Talpade Mohanty (2003a). According to Mendoza, the concept 'transnational feminisms' builds on feminist postcolonial criticism within western academia, and seems to imply a shared context of exploitation and domination across North and South. Used in the plural, it 'points to the multiplicity of the world's feminisms and to the increasing tendency of national feminisms to politicize women's issues beyond the borders of the nation state, for instance, in United Nations (UN) women's world conferences, or on the Internet. The term points simultaneously to the position feminists worldwide have taken against the processes of globalization of the economy, the demise of the nation state and the development of a global mass culture, as well as to the nascent global women's studies research into the ways in which globalization affects women around the globe' (Mendoza, 2002: 296). 'But foremost', Mendoza continues, 'it takes its meaning from Third and First World feminist theorizations on race, class and sexuality, and feminist postcolonial studies that make us aware of the artificiality of the idea of nation and its patriarchal nature' (Mendoza, 2002: 296). It envisages the desirability and possibility of a political solidarity of feminists across the globe transcending race, class, sexuality and national boundaries, based on the concrete experiences of transnational organizing of women.

While 'global sisterhood' starts out from the commonalities between women, 'transnational feminisms' departs from the differences between women. Mendoza (2002: 310), however, puts the finger on the problem in saying that although committed to intersectional analysis and transversal politics as well as dedicated to praxis rooted in postcolonial critiques of racism, ethnocentrism, sexism and heteronormativity and committed to the subversion of multiple oppressions, transnational feminist debates still reveal important gaps between the intentions – in terms of its theory and tactics – and outcomes of transnational feminist mobilizations. Many of these gaps derive from an undertheorization or an inadequate treatment of political economic issues within feminist postcolonial criticism and their entrapment in cultural debates. I share this concern of Mendoza and find the insights developed by Mohanty (1986, 2003a, 2003b) useful to approach these concerns.

Mohanty (1986) argued that 'cross-cultural feminist work must be attentive to the micropolitics of context, subjectivity, and struggle, as well as to the macropolitics of global economic and political systems and processes'. Inspired by Maria Mies's and Vandana Shiva's writings, she places feminist solidarity firmly within a broad framework of anti-capitalist struggles. UN conferences – such as the International Conference on Population and Development in Cairo (including its NGO counterpart) and the World Conferences on Women – as well as the campaigns around WTO negotiations, such as the popularly known 'Battle of Seattle', have acted as important catalysts for global solidarity, and not only among feminists. For instance, events such as the regional Social Forums, and the World Social Forum last held in Mumbai in January 2004, were manifestations of global solidarity of men and women, on myriad issues, and in particular against the neoliberal development model now also embraced by many developing countries. These transnational forms of politicization and social movements, invoking the idea of a global citizenship, have also been referred to as 'globalization from below'.

Global feminist solidarity and alliances for future campaigns may not be difficult on issues such as violence against women, the global trafficking in women and children, gender justice in terms of equal opportunities for education and employment, health, food and shelter, security and environmental concerns. However, other issues including translocation and outsourcing of jobs and services to the global South, or religious fundamentalist prescriptions regarding dress codes, may pitch women on different sides of the fence and could form a testing-ground for feminist solidarity. One such issue I focus on here to problematize the question of transnational feminisms is that of the right to self-determination of women over their own bodies. While most feminists would posit that this is a non-negotiable right, the development and globalization of new reproductive technologies for (1) sex-determination or genetic testing of the embryo/foetus, (2) conception through artificial reproduction technologies (without heterosexual intercourse) such as in vitro fertilization (IVF) and (3) the transactions in reproductive body parts – such as eggs, sperm, embryos and the renting of the uterus (surrogacy), pose complex and unforeseen challenges and dilemmas for feminist solidarity worldwide.

Women's right to self-determination over their own bodies – a testing-ground for transnational feminisms

In 1989, I embarked upon a study of new reproductive technologies (NRTs) in three areas – contraception, assisted conception and screening of the embryo/foetus for genetic purposes and for sex selection – looking at their effects on the health and autonomy of women within an international comparative perspective. My research focused in particular on India and the Netherlands, two societies in which I lived and followed the application of NRTs. Many a colleague and layperson in the Netherlands told me they did not see the point of 'comparing apples and pears' (a typical Dutch expression). To me, however, the point of comparison was quite clear, namely the global processes and forces and ideologies (factors and actors) that operate openly and invisibly behind the technologies to influence women's choices and lives, within their different local situatedness. This became even clearer to me in my follow-up research on transactions in reproductive body parts.

I became aware that the goals of the second wave of the feminist movement, such as access to free and safe abortion, had united many, though not all, women's rights activists in different parts of the world, as pointed out by Angela Davis (1981) among others. At the International Conference on Population and Development in Cairo in 1994, I witnessed how the women's health and rights activists formed a broad front against the unholy alliance of the Holy See and Islamic fundamentalist regimes which attempted to restrict women's right to abortion. They demanded provisions to ensure reproductive health and rights for individuals the world over. Also, they exposed and strongly condemned target-oriented, coercive population control programmes in India and Bangladesh and China's one-child population policy, which violated the principle of women's self-determination. The trend towards the use of (coercive) sterilization and provider-dependent, long-acting hormonal methods in state family planning programmes, without provision of adequate information and medical back-up services, was questioned on grounds of adverse effects on women's health and autonomy.

However, both nationally and transnationally, feminist solidarity showed cracks when it came to the question of sex-selective abortion. Faced with the contrary demands of the state for population control that forces them to have no more than one or two children on the one hand, and patriarchal ideologies of son-preference on the other, women in India started taking advantage of the liberal abortion laws of the country and resorting to sex-determination tests and abortion of female foetuses in their desire to have one or more male children. Also, with the birth of sons they wished to secure their status within the family and financial security in the present and future. This practice became so widespread that some feminists and other concerned citizens united under the Forum Against Sex-Determination and Sex-Preselection Techniques and successfully fought for national legislation banning the tests in 1994. They did so primarily on grounds of (1) discrimination against and devaluation of the female sex; (2) unnecessary medicalization of healthy women; (3) the objectification of women as son-producing machines; and (4) skewed male–female sex ratios. Also, they exposed the commercial interests of service providers who had turned it into a highly lucrative business. Feminists in India were divided on whether legislation adopted to ban the practice was an effective measure or counterproductive, as it punishes the woman who goes for these tests (Kishwar, 1993). Some used ethical arguments to justify the practice, arguing that female foeticide is better than female infanticide (Macklin, 1999), and upheld women's right to choose to abort the female foetus, as a key freedom, for to deprive them of the same would be a violation of feminist moral principles (Zilberberg, 2004).

In Europe too, women increasingly undergo prenatal diagnostic tests routinely. They do this, in contrast with India, to ensure the health of the foetus, by preventing the birth of a handicapped child, which is usually burdensome for women, who are the main carers. This, too, remains a controversial subject as, with the availability of various technologies for pre-conceptional and prenatal diagnosis, pregnancies become increasingly medicalized and more and more women fall under the (self) disciplinary regimes as theorized by Foucault. Feminists have expressed this anxiety by asking whether the 'right' to choose is not gradually turning into a 'duty' to choose and that there is a foreclosure of certain choices, for instance, to choose to continue a pregnancy even if the foetus is affected. Some fear the 'state eugenics' practised in several European countries and the US in the earlier half of the 20th century being set forth now as 'private eugenics'.

Also, women demand reproductive health services to meet the needs of infertile women/couples. Some radical feminists and lesbians in the West see in the technologies for assisted conception an opportunity to secure the right to these services not only for heterosexual couples but also for single women and lesbian couples. Some feminists, however, find these technologies as re-essentializing women by reinforcing the ideology of motherhood and exploitation of their reproductive potential, while health advocates warn of the adverse effects of fertility drugs.[1]

It is clear from the above that NRTs have brought 'new freedoms' in the form of opportunities for some women – for instance, to prevent unwanted pregnancy and births through contraception and abortion; to some extent, the prevention of birth of undesired children (the 'wrong' sex, 'unhealthy') through prenatal diagnosis technologies; and the possibility of motherhood for infertile women/couples and single and lesbian women through artificial insemination or IVF. Concomitantly, they have also brought 'new dependencies', on technologies and on service providers. Also, often these technologies come at a heavy price, not only financially, but also in terms of adverse effects on women's physical and mental health (Gupta, 2000). While for some women use of these technologies has meant a shift from being 'objects' and 'victims' to 'knowing subjects' and 'agents' of control over their own bodies, for others they have brought more outside control and expropriation.

Considering the divisions between women who profit from NRTs and those who are exploited by them, feminists are divided in their response to NRTs, making it difficult to formulate effective common feminist strategies of resistance to the medicalization of women's bodies and the adverse effects of certain technologies (such as long-acting hormonal contraceptives, prenatal diagnosis technologies and fertility drugs[2]) on the health of women and their offspring. Apparently, not all women have the same interests and moral values regarding NRTs, even as there are differences in their socio-economic and cultural circumstances. Corresponding with differences among women, the increasingly global hegemony of enterprise culture, the rise of fundamentalism, increasing disparities characterizing various forms of domestic and international inequalities, a woman's right to choose can be seen to be in crisis (Himmelweit, 1988). This crisis is perhaps nowhere sharper than in relation to the transactions in reproductive body parts and reproductive services made possible through the globalization of NRTs on the one hand and information and communication technologies (including the Internet) on the other.

Local and global transactions in reproductive body parts and reproductive services

In order to understand the global transactions in reproductive body parts and reproductive services, some distinctive features of globalization in general are highlighted here. Globalization is a process that is changing the nature of human interaction across a wide range of spheres (economic, political, sociocultural, etc.). Most prominent is the erosion of boundaries of time, space and knowledge hitherto separating individuals and societies; however, increasingly other types of boundaries that have defined human experience, temporal (e.g. instantaneous communication) and cognitive (e.g. cultural beliefs, academic disciplines) are being changed. It is marked in particular by transnational capital and trade liberalization. Neoliberal economic policies facilitate the globalization of technologies (through the import of high-tech equipment) and ideas (through the global electronic media, including satellite television), also made possible by faster modes of transport of goods, persons (through aviation) and knowledge (through the Internet).

The global development of capitalism is nothing new, but what characterizes its most recent phase is the 'cultural convergence' of cultures and lifestyles around the world in the societies it impacts. Although, the market is the primary motor of globalization, its implications are not limited to the commercial arena alone. In the field of biological reproduction, globalization – understood as the rapid growth of global capitalism – has brought in its wake an extension of consumer culture creating 'new regimes of consumption'. Not only have women's whole bodies been thrown onto the world market (Truong, 2001; Wichterich, 2000) for trafficking, the human body and its parts (organs, tissues, cells) have been turned into commodities that are exchanged and traded (Kimbrell, 1993; Scheper-Hughes, 2000; Sharp, 2000). Initially confined to solid organs such as kidneys, livers and hearts, with the development and expanded use of IVF technology, the last decade of the 20th century saw this extended to reproductive body parts, such as sperm, ova and embryos, which have become discrete entities – commodities that can be donated or traded, by individuals themselves as well as infertility specialists, IVF brokers, etc., for profit. There is an unregulated trade in body parts and fertility tourism within and across countries; in particular, increasing access to the Internet has contributed immensely to the trade's further proliferation. Several centres all over the world, mainly in the US and Europe, but also in India, are profiting from the 'fertility business', including the commercial transactions in reproductive body parts.

Globalization involves an interaction between economic and cultural factors whereby changes in production and consumption factors can be seen as producing new shared identities. High-tech reproductive technologies are available in many developing countries, too. Not only Indian infertile couples but those from neighbouring South Asian countries as well as the Middle East throng Indian infertility clinics where they can avail themselves of the latest technologies for assisted reproduction including IVF and intra cytoplasmic sperm injection. The last decade saw the number of service providers in this field increase dramatically, proliferating beyond the metropolitan cities.[3] In 1999, a popular Indian weekly carried the story of an Indian woman in a village in Gujarat who acted as a surrogate for a German couple.[4] In January 2003, an Indian grandmother in a small town in Gujarat acted as a surrogate and gave birth to twins for her own London-based daughter and son-in-law.[5] Earlier, similar cases of grandmothers acting as surrogates and giving birth to their own grandchildren were reported from South Africa and the US.

With the help of reproductive scientists and gynaecologists, women now assert their rights to their eggs and embryos and sperm of their (living or even deceased) partners. With the aid of information technology they trade in their own eggs and embryos and those of other women on the Internet. In the US, female university students use the Internet to sell their eggs and surrogacy services to pay their way through university. Karla Momberger (2000: 1–2; 32), a graduate student at Columbia law school, relates her story: 'I began my feminist/activist career trying to escape the confines of my body, and that now I take refuge in the solid reality of me-ness that my body brings.... I donated ova to pay for law school. That's what I did. I am the mythical $50,000 woman. My finishing law school and becoming a lawyer depended, quite literally, on my body and how much it is worth.'

Also, specialized agencies mediate between infertile women and potential 'egg donors' (primarily college girls recruited through advertisements on college noticeboards and the Internet) to choose from, with photos and complete profiles regarding IQ and other characteristics. However, attempts to set up commercial surrogacy bureaus have been largely unsuccessful in most Western European countries, including the UK, due to restrictive legislation, where also the sale of human gametes is banned by law.

In India, on the other hand, egg donors are usually younger sisters, cousins and sisters-in-law, although according to the guidelines issued by the Indian Council of Medical Research in December 2004, this is to be banned, which is likely to increase trade in eggs and embryos. Some clinics also run egg-sharing programmes where anonymous egg donors receive some compensation for their treatment costs from the couple they have donated to. In the Netherlands, where commercial egg donation and surrogacy are banned, IVF clinics at hospitals run egg-sharing programmes. Egg donors are generally friends and acquaintances. However, more recently it has come to light that Dutch infertile women are travelling to Spain for eggs donated by university students.[6] Since July 2003, Baby Donors, an Amsterdam-based company, claiming to be the first in Europe, has been advertising its services on its website, operationalized in September 2003. It offers to act as an intermediary for the sale of tailor-made, personalized sperm insemination and egg donor packages through the Internet.[7] It seeks entrepreneurs from around the world for franchising or joint venture partners at a licence fee of €5000. Taking advantage of loopholes in national legislation, such enterprises are able to operate in a particular country and take their business to another when their practices are outlawed in one.[8] While selling solid organs[9] is illegal in many countries, this is not always the case with egg selling, or surrogacy, whether for commercial or altruistic motives. The Internet as marketplace makes legislation even more difficult, if not impossible. Women operate on this marketplace both as buyers and sellers.

Can there be common gender interests?

While the forces of globalization have repositioned women in new systems of inequality, among themselves as well as vis-a-vis men, can there be common gender interests? Mohanty (2003b: 7) spells out the requirements for transnational feminism in our times. It must, she argues, be based on a 'politics of solidarity' – one that comprises 'mutuality, accountability, and the recognition of common interests as the basis for relationships among diverse communities'. Can the need of infertile women for donor eggs or surrogacy services and the financial need of women that drives them to offer the same, thus creating a relationship of mutual dependency, be a basis for mutual solidarity? Should we view these cases as examples of women's agency, self-determination and solidarity, of 'global sisterhood' between the fertile/infertile, first world/third world, rich/poor and support them? If only things were that simple!

Women who 'donate' their eggs to non-related recipients may profess acting out of altruistic motives, such as 'giving the gift of life' to infertile women. However, they do it for a fee – €600 are paid to Spanish students who are egg donors and US$6000–10,000 to students in the US; therefore, to call it 'donation' is a misnomer. Thanks to women willing to sell their eggs or rent their wombs as surrogates, helping infertile women has become a thriving global business. A whole range of professionals – such as infertility specialists, psychologists, lawyers, middlemen – also profit from it.

The transfer of reproductive materials is, at several levels, a market transaction. While not all individual practitioners may be motivated by profit, entities and actors operate within a market that spans many sectors of production including biomedical engineering firms, multinational pharmaceutical companies, research institutes and hospitals. IVF is a big 'money-spinner', being the basis for a wide range of research products, genetic and hormonal, that contribute to the growing multinational drug and genetic industries (Steinberg, 1997). Women undergoing IVF provide the raw material in the form of embryos for research in stem cells and human cloning; not to forget that it is they who are hyperovulated to obtain multiple eggs used for 'donation' to infertile couples as well as for research. The process of surplus production (normally only one egg matures during a woman's monthly cycle, whereas through hyperstimulation as many as 30 eggs can be matured) and its linkages to (global) capital as well as to asymmetrical gender, class and other power systems remain underexposed. This is particularly so with egg selling and surrogacy. Within global capitalism women's cheap labour is not only used to produce for the world market, but also to 'reproduce' for the world market.

Some feminists see surrogacy as valorizing women's 'labour' as otherwise it is done 'for free'. Lori Andrews (quoted in Mies, 1988) and some others argue for a liberalization of almost all laws that stand in the way of full-fledged commercialization of reproduction. They do this on the basis of women's right to self-determination over their own bodies, and as long as women do it knowingly and voluntarily. Mies, however, sees this position as an ideological legitimization for the new reproduction industry, a new 'growth industry' for the production of children, which in its greed for maximization of profit has to do away with the integrity of the individual. Within this 'supermarket of reproductive alternatives', a whole person is reduced to saleable and disposable parts. In the ensuing market relationships, women are objects of use and children are created as products. The right to choose is reduced to a right to consume. Neoliberal ideologies play a significant role in constructing choice in terms of individualism and consumerism.

It is debatable whether women are choosing freely to become surrogates, or that their will is socially and economically constructed. It is clear from the profiles of women who act as surrogates and those who are the commissioning parties that the two are not equals. Women do not have the same opportunities as men for making money. Usually women with a low education, low or no income (e.g. students), or in low-paying, low-status jobs, choose to become surrogates. From infancy women are socialized to be self-sacrificing, please others, and put others' needs above their own, and made to believe that childbearing is the most valued activity they can engage in. In surrogacy, they can combine this idea of benefit to others while at the same time fulfilling their 'natural' function in life – bearing children. Surrogate motherhood 'is a curious *ad hoc* compromise of biological and social connection which conforms to no principle whatsoever, but merely serves the interests of whoever possesses the economic and social power to turn generative capacities, technological innovations and economic advantages to their own personal use' (Dworkin, 1983, quoted in Williams, 1986: 22). Surrogacy is exploitative, alienated labour, exploiting women as 'breeder women' (Corea, 1985). Women are being encouraged to treat their bodies and body parts as commodities for consumption, thus extending the market relationships. Many women, who, like Momberger, are brought up to be subservient to others, have come to see themselves as having the right to do as they wish with their bodies. To them the possibility of selling their eggs or renting their wombs seems like an act of empowerment.

Dilemmas around choice and self-determination

From the credo 'our bodies, our selves' popularized by the Boston Health Book Collective in the 1970s there has been a shift to 'my body, my body parts' since the 1980s. 'Choice' and 'self-determination' were key concepts during the second feminist wave. Now, these terms are also used indiscriminately by service providers to justify women's right to sell their eggs and embryos or rent their uterus, just as they are used as a justification to provide sex-determination tests followed by abortion of the 'unwanted' female foetus in the name of 'family balancing'. While the contraceptive pill is said to have ushered in the first sexual revolution, assisted reproduction technologies have been responsible for the second sexual revolution. But problems with the tenet 'a woman's right to control her body' soon arise. If a woman can use the pill to postpone pregnancy, why should it be a problem if she wants her embryos frozen to be implanted in her at a time more convenient to her? So, how far does the right of self-determination regarding one's body go? May the capacity to reproduce be turned into earning money by selling or renting one's body parts?

The 'Baby M'[10] case brought out the dilemmas inherent in the language of control that made it difficult to come out with 'the' feminist response. Women's use of assisted reproduction technologies can be considered as a means of escaping the constraints of the 'given'. Some feminists see this as a part of the pro-choice extension of the right to self-determination over their own bodies; they believe women can use these technologies to their own advantage, and to break the traditional heterosexual patriarchal structure of the family, for instance by lesbian women using donor insemination to fulfil their desire for a child. They accuse feminists who oppose technological reproduction of portraying women as helpless victims incapable of making decisions in their own interest, and of undermining women's rights. The enormous stigma related to infertility compels women themselves to use the latest technologies (including donor ova or surrogacy) as part of strategies in their own interest, as ethnographies on infertility demonstrate (Becker, 2000; Inhorn and van Balen, 2002). Similarly, there are women who sell their ova or surrogacy services voluntarily. Depending on the kind of surrogacy used, some even profess non-monetary motivations, such as experiencing the pleasures of pregnancy for themselves and the fulfilled desire for a child for the commissioning couple (Ragoné, 1994). These women apparently do not see themselves as 'objects' and 'victims' or even 'cultural dopes', but as acting as 'knowing subjects' and exerting their 'agency', to borrow metaphors from Kathy Davis's (1995) work on women undergoing cosmetic surgery.

Ethical universals and transnational feminisms

Transnational feminist analyses and practices require an acknowledgement of the fact that one's privileges in the world-system are always linked to another woman's oppression or exploitation. This implies that the perpetual inequalities between women produced by their location in the world-system in themselves foreclose the possibility of solidarity (Grewal and Kaplan, 1994). Transnational feminist practices require comparative work rather than the relativistic thinking of 'differences' undertaken by proponents of 'global feminism'; that is, to compare multiple, overlapping and discrete oppressions rather than to construct a theory of hegemonic oppression under a unified category of gender. Amrita Basu (1995), too, has shown the importance of attending to 'local feminisms' instead, even if the cost of doing so means abandoning hopes for a 'master theory' of gender or a unified feminist agenda. Mohanty (2003b: 250) is more optimistic, and believes that 'global capitalism' both destroys the possibilities [for a transnational feminist practice] and also offers up new ones'. She suggests the thorough embeddedness of the local and the particular within the global and the universal, and envisions a feminism without borders to address the injustices of global capitalism.

The challenges posed by new socioeconomic and political developments in a globalized world constantly require new responses and new strategies at a practical level; at an analytical level, they require re-examining old concepts and theoretical paradigms and developing new ones. Mohanty (2003a: 518) suggests that a 'comparative feminist studies' or 'feminist solidarity' model is the most useful and productive pedagogical strategy for feminist cross-cultural work. 'It is through this model that we can put into practice the idea of "common difference" as the basis for deeper solidarity across differences and unequal power relations.'

It is apparent that there is an urgent need for a redefined feminist engagement with reproductive politics encompassing the issue of repercussions of the trade in artificial reproduction technologies for the health and integrity of individual women and men and their offspring. While multi-sited ethnographic research at the local level is absolutely necessary, it is worthwhile to analyse the data also in a cross-cultural comparative perspective. Whether as producers (of consumer goods as well as ova), or as consumers, women are co-implicated in the capitalist global economy that needs women and yet marginalizes women's labour both as producers and reproducers in search of profit. Due to globalization, the implementation of transnational ethics and legislation, so that procedures and practices banned in one country may not be available in another, becomes imperative, though it may prove difficult. Perhaps transnational solidarity on this issue could also be based on the concept of bioethics – that some things are integral to a human being and should not be for sale – whether it is solid organs taken from impoverished individuals, or ova, embryos, semen, cells and genes – and to prevent the excesses of the market.

Acknowledging local and contextual knowledges, and realities in diverse cultures as essential should not prevent us from thinking transnationally. A shared common goal of commitment to enhancing women's health and well-being across the globe requires a moral framework that values individuals as ends in themselves and not as tools. By dehumanizing their body and treating it as a machine, thereby reducing human reproduction to a mere production process, as in surrogacy, women's capacity for moral self-development is undermined (Tao, 2004). We need to call upon universal moral values, ethical universals, global ethics, terms used within (feminist) bioethics discourses (Dickenson, 2004; Donchin, 2004), which encompass individual rights claims but go beyond the narrow focus of individualism and autonomy for the protection of women's self-respect and human dignity. I see this as an ongoing challenge not only for reproductive rights activists and feminist scholars, but also for transnational feminisms.

Acknowledgements

The research on the transaction in body parts for this article was conducted within a research project, 'Body Parts, Property and Gender', funded by a grant from the Netherlands Foundation for the Advancement of Tropical Research (NWO-WOTRO), project number WB 52–871 during my affiliation as postdoctoral researcher at Leiden University Medical Centre. I am extremely grateful to Professor Dr Annemiek Richters, Leiden University Medical Centre, Department of Culture, Health and Illness, for comments and suggestions on earlier drafts of this article and to Professor Dr Indu Agnihotri, Centre for Women's Development Studies, New Delhi, for her input. I also thank the anonymous reviewers for their sharp comments and suggestions.

This article is a revised version of my presentation at the conference 'Passing on Feminism' held to commemorate the 10th anniversary of the *European Journal of Women's Studies*, Belle van Zuylen Institute, Amsterdam, 23 January 2004.

Notes

1. See Thompson (2002) for an excellent historical overview of feminist debates on infertility.
2. The adverse effects of fertility drugs include hyperstimulation of ovaries and tubes, which can even be fatal, as well as long-term risks such as cancer of the reproductive organs and multiple births. The latter can be risky for the mother and a cause of morbidity in the children born.
3. In 1990, there were just about a dozen centres; in January 2003, the Indian Society for Assisted Reproduction listed 186 members.
4. Anosh Malekar, 'Carrying for her Kids', *The Week*, 30 May 1999, Cochin, India.
5. *Nation Feature*, 18 February 2004.
6. Mariël Croon, 'Vrouw voor donor eicel naar Spanje', *NRC Handelsblad*, 25 July 2004.
7. www.babydonors.com (accessed November 2003).
8. *De Volkskrant*, 25 September 2003.
9. By 'solid organ' is meant those internal organs including the heart, liver, kidneys and lungs that have an anatomical boundary in contrast to blood, bone marrow and so on.
10. This refers to Baby Melissa, born to a surrogate mother who refused to hand over the child to the commissioning couple, but was ultimately forced to do so, on the basis of the contract she had signed earlier.

References

Basu, Amrita, ed. (1995) *Women's Movements in Global Perspective*. Boulder, CO and Oxford: Westview Press.

Becker, Gay (2000) *The Elusive Embryo: How Men and Women Approach New Reproductive Technologies*. Berkeley: University of California Press.

Braithwaite, Ann (2002) 'The Personal, the Political, Third-Wave and Postfeminisms', *Feminist Theory* 3(3): 335–44.

Corea, Gena (1985) *The Mother Machine: Reproductive Technologies from Artificial Insemination to Artificial Wombs*. New York: Harper and Row.

Davis, Angela (1981) *Women, Race and Class*. London: The Women's Press.

Davis, Kathy (1995) *Reshaping the Female Body: The Dilemma of Cosmetic Surgery*. New York and London: Routledge.

Dickenson, Donna L. (2004) 'What Feminism Can Teach Global Ethics', pp. 15–30 in R. Tong, A. Donchin and S. Dodds (eds) *Linking Visions: Feminist Bioethics, Human Rights and the Developing World*. Lanham, MD: Rowman and Littlefield.

Donchin, Anne (2004) 'Integrating Bioethics and Human Rights: Towards a Global Feminist Approach', pp. 31–56 in R. Tong, A. Donchin and S. Dodds (eds) *Linking Visions: Feminist Bioethics, Human Rights and the Developing World*. Lanham, MD: Rowman and Littlefield.

Grewal, Inderpal and Caren Kaplan, eds (1994) *Scattered Hegemonies: Postmodernity and Transnational Feminist Practices*. Minneapolis and London: University of Minnesota Press.

Gupta, Jyotsna Agnihotri (2000) *New Reproductive Technologies, Women's Health and Autonomy: Freedom or Dependency?* New Delhi: Sage.

Himmelweit, Susan (1988) 'More Than a Woman's Right to Choose?', *Feminist Review* 29: 38–57.

Inhorn, Marcia, C. and F. van Balen, eds (2002) *Infertility around the Globe: New Thinking on Childlessness, Gender and Reproductive Technologies*. Berkeley: University of California Press.

Kimbrell, Andrew (1993) *The Human Body Shop: The Engineering and Marketing of Life*. Penang: Third World Network.

Kishwar, Madhu (1993) 'Abortion of Female Fetuses: Is Legislation the Answer?', *Reproductive Health Matters* 2: 113–15.

Macklin, Ruth (1999) *Against Relativism: Cultural Diversity and the Search for Ethical Universals in Medicine*. New York: Oxford University Press.

Mendoza, Breny (2002) 'Transnational Feminisms in Question', *Feminist Theory* 3(3): 295–314.

Mies, Maria (1988) 'From the Individual to the Dividual: In the Supermarket of "Reproductive Alternatives"', *Reproductive and Genetic Engineering* 1(3): 225–37.

Mohanty, Chandra Talpade (1986) 'Under Western Eyes: Feminist Scholarship and Colonial Discourses', *Boundary 2* 12(3): 333–58.

Mohanty, Chandra Talpade (2003a) '"Under Western Eyes" Revisited: Feminist Solidarity through Anticapitalist Struggles', *Signs: Journal of Women in Culture and Society* 28(2): 499–535.

Mohanty, Chandra Talpade (2003b) *Feminism Without Borders: Decolonizing Theory, Practicing Solidarity*. Durham, NC: Duke University Press.

Momberger, Karla (2000) 'Breeder at Law', *Columbia Journal of Gender and Law* 11(2): 1–51.

Morgan, Robin (1984) *Sisterhood is Global: The International Women's Movement Anthology*. New York: Anchor Press/Doubleday.

Ragoné, Helena (1994) *Surrogate Motherhood: Conception in the Heart.* Boulder, CO: Westview Press.

Scheper-Hughes, Nancy (2000) 'The Global Traffic in Human Organs', *Current Anthropology* 41(2): 191–224.

Sharp, Lesley A. (2000) 'The Commodification of the Body and its Parts', *Annual Review of Anthropology* 29: 287–328.

Steinberg, Deborah Lynn (1997) *Bodies in Glass.* Manchester and New York: Manchester University Press.

Tao Po-Wah, Julia (2004) 'Right-Making and Wrong-Making in Surrogate Motherhood: A Confucian Feminist Perspective', pp. 157–79 in R. Tong, A. Donchin and S. Dodds (eds) *Linking Visions: Feminist Bioethics, Human Rights and the Developing World.* Lanham, MD: Rowman and Littlefield.

Thompson, Charis M. (2002) 'Fertile Ground: Feminists Theorize Infertility', pp. 52–78 in M. C. Inhorn and F. van Balen (eds) *Infertility around the Globe: New Thinking on Childlessness, Gender and Reproductive Technologies.* Berkeley: University of California Press.

Truong, Thanh-dam (2001) *Human Trafficking and Organised Crime*, Working Paper series No. 339. The Hague: Institute of Social Studies.

Wichterich, Christa (2000) *The Globalized Woman: Reports from a Future of Inequality.* Australia: Spinifex Press and London and New York: Zed Books.

Williams, Linda S. (1986) 'But What Will They Mean for Women? Feminist Concerns about the New Reproductive Technologies', *Feminist Perspectives/Perspectives Féministes*, No. 6. Ottawa: CRIAW/ICREF.

Zilberberg, Julie M. (2004) 'A Boy or a Girl: Is any Choice Moral? The Ethics of Sex-Selection and Pre-Selection in Context', pp. 147–56 in R. Tong, A. Donchin and S. Dodds (eds) *Linking Visions: Feminist Bioethics, Human Rights and the Developing World.* Lanham, MD: Rowman and Littlefield.

14

FEMINISM MEETS THE "NEW" EPIDEMIOLOGIES

Toward an appraisal of antifeminist biases in epidemiological research on women's health

Marcia C. Inhorn and K. Lisa Whittle

Source: *Social Science & Medicine*, 53 (2001), 553–67.

Abstract

This essay explores an alternative paradigm for epidemiology, one which is explicitly informed by a feminist perspective. We intend to expand upon recent critiques and debates within the emergent fields of "critical", "popular", and "alternative" epidemiology to examine how epidemiology's conceptual models — which are meant to contribute to the prevention of social inequalities in health, but may instead reinforce social hierarchies based on gender, race, and class — constrain our understanding of health and disease. Specifically, we examine persistent antifeminist biases in contemporary epidemiological research on women's health. Issues highlighted include: problem definition and knowledge production in women's health; biological essentialization of women as reproducers; and decontextualization and depoliticization of women's health risks. As part of this critique, we include suggestions for an emancipatory epidemiology that incorporates an alternative feminist framework.

© 2001 Elsevier Science Ltd. All rights reserved.

Introduction

If the biological finality of death can only be explained in wider social context then the complex realities of women's sickness and health must be explored in similar ways. In order to do this, traditional epidemiological methods have to be turned on their head. Instead of identifying diseases and then searching for the cause, we need to begin by identifying the major areas of activity that constitute women's lives. We can then go on to analyze the impact of these activities on their health and well being.

Lesley Doyal (1995, p. 1)

Epidemiology is currently engaged in a moment of critical self-reflection, debating its models, theories, methods, levels of analysis, guiding principles, ethics, and future role in protecting the public's health.[1] These debates have been precipitated by the increasing concern over the "reductionism" of mainstream, university and government-agency-funded epidemiology in the United States (Pearce, 1996; Susser & Susser, 1996a, b; Wing, 1994; Winkelstein, 1996). Namely, critics from within epidemiology have argued that epidemiology, as the "basic science" of public health, has adopted a biomedical, clinical science model (Charlton, 1997) for the study of disease "risk factors", which has taken epidemiology away from its fundamental roots in public health (Lawson & Floyd, 1996; Pearce, 1996; Susser & Susser, 1996b; Weed, 1995). In particular, the myopic focus of biomedicine on microlevel causes of diseases in individuals (e.g., human genes, infectious agents) has subsequently been translated within "modern", "analytical", "risk factor" epidemiology into a "single exposure–single disease" paradigm of illness that does little to generate effective preventive health strategies (Wing, 1994), especially for chronic illnesses (Scribner, 1997; Susser & Susser, 1996a, b).

Historically, epidemiology *has* employed various models that consider the broader social context, including political-economic conditions that impinge upon human well-being (Krieger, Rowley, Herman, Avery, & Phillips, 1993; Pearce, 1996; Trostle, 1986; Weed, 1995; Wing, 1994). There are many such examples in the history of epidemiology (Pearce, 1996; Wing, 1994), with John Snow's "pump-handle diplomacy" over *Vibrio cholera* in the streets of London being epidemiology's most popular historical story (Weed, 1995). However, as lamented by many a contemporary critic, the true "public health" dimension of epidemiology so apparent in the early days of Snow, Virchow, Goldberger, and other epidemiological pioneers has been lost — and replaced instead by the prevailing and hegemonic disease model in epidemiology, which frames health problems in terms of decontextualized exposures to risk factors, including the isolated behaviors of individuals (Wing, 1994). Thus framed, dominant, mainstream epidemiological research encourages public health policies that: (1) blame individuals for their poor health by portraying risk as a lifestyle choice (Lupton, 1993; Pearce, 1996); (2) limit our understanding and prevention of disease causation by ignoring meaning as a determinant of human behavior (Lawson & Floyd, 1996);[2] (3) leave unquestioned social hierarchies of gender, race, and nation by ignoring how these relationships mediate an individual's power, personal agency, and available choices relating to their health (Farmer, Connors, & Simmons, 1996; Krieger et al., 1993; Krieger & Zierler, 1995, 1996); and (4) overlook how local and global political economies, including policies of nation-states, affect health and disease.[3] As one critic (Brown, 1997, p. 137) notes, "Epidemiology ... has been transformed in recent decades to a largely laboratory science model, often more concerned with protecting the increasingly rigid standards of scientific procedures than with safeguarding public health."

How to "reform" epidemiology has been the focus of some discussion, with most commentators advocating the "reintegration" of epidemiology into "public health". Beyond this general calling, suggestions for change include: (1) new "socialization" efforts for epidemiologists (Susser & Susser, 1996b), in order to alter their epidemiological "mind set", which has become a "conceptual ghetto" (Weed, 1995); (2) new multidisciplinary approaches, which privilege social context and systems analysis (Koopman, 1996; Krieger et al., 1993; Pearce, 1996; Wing, 1994), so that epidemiologists can "know about disease" in its entirety (Diez-Roux & Nieto, 1997); and (3) development of explicit epidemiological theory, drawing from the humanities (Weed, 1995), ethics (Weed, 1995), human ecology (Krieger & Zierler, 1995; Wing, 1994), political-economy (Krieger & Zierler, 1995, 1996), and even postmodernism (Pearce, 1996). However, as noted by Wing (1994, p. 84), there has yet to emerge a "coherent set of theories, assumptions and techniques that could constitute a real new paradigm" in epidemiology.

"New" epidemiologies and their articulation with feminism

In this essay, we hope to contribute to an alternative paradigm for epidemiology, one which is explicitly informed by a feminist perspective. To this end, our thinking clearly has been informed by three emerging forms of "new" epidemiology, including: (1) the critical epidemiology of Krieger & colleagues (Fee & Krieger, 1994; Krieger et al., 1993; Krieger & Fee, 1994; Krieger & Zierler, 1995, 1996); (2) the popular epidemiology of Brown (Brown, 1992, 1997); and (3) the alternative epidemiology of Wing (1994) and Turshen (1984). We outline these three new approaches; then we propose a fourth approach, "feminist epidemiology", which articulates with the other three approaches but also moves beyond them in ways to be described in this essay.

Critical epidemiology

The critical epidemiology of Krieger and colleagues,[4] which includes provocative, feminist-informed insights on the nature of contemporary epidemiological practice, provides a crucial springboard for the more explicit feminist epidemiological approach to be described below.

Krieger and colleagues criticize the empirical methods and underlying constructs of US epidemiological research and describe a newly emerging approach for investigating the relationship between racism, sexism, classism, and health "that has yet to be synthesized into a well-defined paradigm"

(Krieger et al., 1993, p. 99). Although Krieger and her colleagues do not explicitly mention feminism, critical gender theory, or women's studies in their "new approach", feminist methodological strategies and research principles appear to be guiding their work, including their pathbreaking epidemiological studies of race, class and gender oppression in women's health outcomes.[5]

The critical, feminist-informed stance advocated by Krieger and her colleagues includes all of the following elements: (1) collapsing binary constructions of biological/social, body/mind, physical/spiritual to explore the dynamic interplay between exposure and susceptibility in determining "risk"; (2) continuously and reflexively asking how gender/race/class/nation function on the individual, family, societal, and global levels in shaping daily life and experiences of health and illness; (3) investigating how these combined factors affect everyone (including professionals, whites, and males) in dialectical relationships of privilege and oppression, protection and risk, rather than exclusively studying how they affect those who have historically been construed as "other" than the "norm"; (4) engaging in a "consciousness raising" of public health and epidemiological researchers which involves (a) critically questioning theoretical constructs, (b) examining the historical legacy of racism, classism and sexism in the profession, and (c) imagining alternative ways of creating epidemiological knowledge; (5) recognizing that the politics of science and our social locations within it preclude an "objective" view of the "facts", and demanding that we examine not only the biases we bring to research but also that we value experiential knowledge as scientific; (6) foregrounding concern for the ethical implications of research including the exploitation of women and members of "minority" groups as research subjects; and (7) emphasizing action-oriented research which includes liberatory goals and transformation of hierarchical institutions.

Popular epidemiology

Popular epidemiology, as forwarded by Brown (1992, 1997), shares some similarities with the aforementioned critical approach. Both of these "new" epidemiologies challenge the epidemiological status quo, and both insist on health activism to unearth and eliminate the causes of poor health. But popular epidemiology, as its name implies, diverges from the feminist-informed critical epidemiology of Krieger and colleagues in its privileging of grass-roots, participatory approaches to epidemiological knowledge production. Namely, as defined by Brown (1997, p. 137), "Popular epidemiology represents two related phenomena: (1) a form of citizen science in which people engage in lay ways of knowing about environmental and technological hazards, and (2) a type of social movement mobilization which increasingly plays a major part in modern political culture." Brown emphasizes that popular epidemiology goes beyond mere public participation in "traditional" epidemiological research, in that it (1) challenges basic assumptions of traditional epidemiology, risk assessment, and public health regulation; (2) involves lay persons' gathering of data, as well as collaborating with experts; (3) emphasizes social structural factors as part of the causal disease chain; and (4) utilizes political and judicial approaches to remedies. As such, popular epidemiology shares much in common with recent approaches to the sociology of risk.[6] For example, Beck's (1992) well-known work, *Risk Society*, discusses public challenges to science and the emergence of new political forms of protest as risk is increasingly open to the public gaze. For Beck, we live in a "risk society" where the whole world has become a place of unforeseen danger. Although the totality of this threat quiets many people, it also provokes growing opposition from both highly educated, politically active, as well as less educated people "for whom this toxic threat is a great rupture in the routinely accepted life they had expected" (Brown, 1997, p. 154). Indeed, such popular opposition among working-class people has played a significant role in identification of disease clusters resulting from toxic waste contamination, as well as political mobilization efforts to clean up toxic waste sites. These efforts have often mirrored feminist health campaigns, in that women, including working-class women, have generally played key roles in the toxic waste movement. As Brown explains (1997, p. 145):

> Women are the most frequent organizers of lay detection, partly because they are the chief health arrangers for their families, and partly because their child care role makes them more concerned than men with local environmental issues... These roles lead women to be more aware of the real and potential health effects of toxic waste, and to take a more skeptical view of traditional science. They often undergo a transformation of self, based on changes noted by Belenky, Clinchy, Glodberger and Tarule, (1986) in their concept of 'women's ways of knowing'. That perspective traces the ways that women come to know things, beginning with either silence or the acceptance of established authority, progressing to a trust in subjective knowledge, and then to a synthesis of external and subjective knowledge. This kind of knowledge framework makes it logical that women toxic activists would gravitate to a popular epidemiology approach.

Alternative epidemiology

An approach that is less concerned with feminist issues or women's health activism is the alternative epidemiology being forwarded independently by Wing (1994) and Turshen (1984). Like Krieger and Brown, these critics offer a "broad critique of the dominant practice of epidemiology" and oppose "the view that the discipline is essentially on track but needs fine tuning"

(Wing, 1994, p. 83). Instead, both Wing and Turshen propose an alternative epidemiology that fundamentally challenges the "exposure-disease" model in mainstream epidemiology by attending instead to the social, economic, and political practices and arrangements that produce such exposures and diseases. Thus, for both Wing and Turshen, fundamental questions about "why" diseases are produced among particular populations at particular historical moments take precedence, and an explicit part of any epidemiological agenda must include efforts to oppose social injustice and inhumanity. Thus, Wing outlines a seven-point manifesto for how such an alternative epidemiology would be practiced, including: (1) analyzing differential effects (what is good or bad *for whom*?); (2) looking for connections between many diseases and exposures rather than always isolating exposure-disease pairs; (3) looking for side effects of exposures and interventions; (4) developing ways to utilize historical information, including developmental narratives of particular populations and even individual people; (5) addressing the conceptual framework of the research, including analyzing assumptions about the social construction of scientific knowledge; (6) addressing the essential *context* of exposure and disease rather than controlling for context as a "nuisance factor"; and (7) displaying humility about the scientific research process and an "unrelenting commitment to playing a supportive role in larger efforts to improve society and public health" (Wing, 1994, p. 84).

Feminist epidemiology

These three forms of "new epidemiology" have inspired us to propose a fourth form, which we call "feminist epidemiology". Feminist epidemiology employs many crucial insights from the three aforementioned approaches, but diverges from them by offering: (1) an *explicit* (as opposed to Krieger's *implicit*) feminist critique of what we call "antifeminist biases"[7] in epidemiological research on women's health; and (2) a feminist-informed research agenda, which draws upon the theoretical work of third world feminists (Mohanty, Russo, & Torres, 1991) and Euro-American feminists of color (Collins, 1991; hooks, 1981, 1983, 1994). As feminist epidemiologists,[8] we argue that we must focus on women's health in particular, for this area of research has been historically marginalized by both biomedicine and public health via a narrow definition of women's health revolving around reproduction and reproductive pathology (Koblinsky, Campbell, & Harlow, 1993; Lane, 1994; Sargent & Brettell, 1996).

Our feminist critique of antifeminist biases in epidemiological research on women's health focuses explicitly on mainstream, academic and government-agency-funded US epidemiology — and thus does not consider the three "new" epidemiologies described above to be part of this dominant paradigm, nor subject to our critique.[9] In other words, we challenge the hegemonic form of epidemiology currently practiced in the US, which can also be generalized to US-based research studies of health problems (e.g., AIDS) in non-Western settings, and which is published in mainstream epidemiological journals (e.g., *American Journal of Epidemiology, Epidemiology, Epidemiological Review, International Journal of Epidemiology, Journal of Clinical Epidemiology, Journal of Epidemiology and Community Health*). We view this form of mainstream epidemiology as the methodologically rigorous discipline that mediates between biomedicine and public health. Through its modeling of disease causality within an exposure-disease paradigm, epidemiology serves to inform both the individualistic, patient-oriented framework of biomedicine and the population-based, community orientation of public health. Yet, despite its methodological rigor, epidemiology remains theoretically arid and politically unsophisticated in its models of disease causation — suffering from what one critic (Nations, 1986) has called epidemiological "rigor mortis", in which the discipline as a whole has become "a set of methods without theory" (Pearce, 1996). Furthermore, it is plagued by a number of antifeminisl biases to be explored in the following section of this essay. These include (but are not limited to) issues of: (1) problem definition and knowledge production in women's health; (2) biological essentialization of women as reproducers; and (3) decontextualization and depoliticization of women's health risks. In this essay, we examine these antifeminist biases in modern epidemiological research on women's health, and suggest ways in which a feminist analytical framework can help epidemiology to engage in the task of better understanding and responding to women's health concerns. Ultimately, we hope that this essay contributes to the ongoing debates about the future of epidemiology in the new millenium, as well as new directions for women's health research.

Antifeminist biases in epidemiological research on women's health

Problem definition and knowledge production in women's health

In the new movement toward a more self-reflexive, critical epidemiology, debates often center on what epidemiologists should study — namely, what topics are worthy of epidemiological engagement and investment. Less often questions are asked about why and how epidemiologists produce knowledge, make knowledge claims, and articulate "difference" from the conjunction of knowledge/power. These epistemological (i.e., theories about the nature and scope of knowing, including presuppositions and grounds for making knowledge claims) and ontological (i.e., theories about the nature of being and living) issues become increasingly important as epidemiology moves toward multi- and interdisciplinary research and as women and groups traditionally excluded from production of scientific knowledge bring experiential knowledge that challenges prevailing perspectives.

With few exceptions, the health problems and needs of women have been defined for them by the biomedical and public health establishments, which (1) are male dominated; (2) have focused their attention since WWII on the chronic disease "epidemics" affecting middle-aged, white men, particularly coronary heart disease, lung cancer, and peptic ulcer (Susser & Susser, 1996a); and (3) have often employed a logic of "difference" and "otherness" in their approach to women's health (Whittle & Inhorn, in press). Indeed, the very "otherness" of women is evident in the major, two-volume US Public Health Service Task Force report on women's health (1987, p. 3) that reads: "Health problems are considered women's issues if they are unique to women, are more prevalent among women, are more severe among women, or involve different risk factors or control measures." Although this proto-feminist government document can be applauded for its laudatory core recommendations (see Krieger & Zierler, 1995, for an overview), still implicit but unstated in it is the assumption that women are fundamentally different from the phantom male comparison group serving as the norm against which women's health must be judged. Indeed, men's experiences of health seem to provide the implicit norm against which public health defines and measures women's health concerns. Women, as well as men in nonwhite racial/ethnic groups, have been excluded from clinical trials and cohort studies based on the acceptability of a white male norm for explaining health and disease (Hamilton, 1996). As Krieger and Fee (1994) point out, the logic guiding this epidemiological exclusion has little to do with assumptions of similarity between white men and others. Rather, historically produced notions of difference have become so firmly embedded in epidemiological research that women and men and whites and nonwhites have rarely been studied together; for the purposes of epidemiological rigor, it does not make sense to do so.

Despite the recent attention being paid to women's health — including the creation of the Office of Research on Women's Health in the National Institutes of Health and the Office of Women's Health in the Centers for Disease Control and Prevention (Rosser, 1994) — research priorities continue to be decided by the public health funders and the epidemiologists conducting scientific investigations, most of whom are white, middle-class men interested in the risk factors that affect them (Pearce, 1996). If epidemiology is to formulate models that help us understand the varying social distributions of health and illness, including their occurrence among women, people of color, and non-elite white men, then epidemiologists — who, by the very nature of their training, constitute a highly educated, elite professional corps in white, Euro-American society — must deal seriously with issues of problem definition, knowledge production, and power relationships.

From the standpoint of feminist epidemiology, the dominant epidemiological establishment must critically address the exclusion of lay women's voices from the processes of both problem definition and knowledge production — asking how epidemiology can operate within an "open" system of knowledge (de Koning & Martin, 1996; hooks, 1994). In the current "closed" system, an elite cadre of epidemiologists, biostatisticians, biomedical professionals, and public health practitioners possesses the privileged knowledge, power, and authority to identify and name diseases; collect data pertaining to these diseases; define and measure the variables hypothesized to produce disease "risk"; create and evaluate interventions aimed at preventing disease risk; and establish public health goals and policies which determine how resources are to be allocated and health issues prioritized. The lack of a feedback loop allowing for non-elite people's experiences, meanings, subjectivities, narratives, and expertise to inform the production of knowledge maintains this closed system (de Koning & Martin, 1996; Hooks, 1994). "Opening" this closed system requires more than just eliminating the barriers faced by women and members of groups excluded from the making of epidemiological knowledge; instead, it requires a fundamental questioning of the assumptions and methodologies of epidemiology itself.

Yet, challenging this closed system of epidemiological knowledge production means challenging the history of biomedicine; for, historically, the biomedical model, upon which epidemiology is based, has cultivated its prestige and power by maintaining this closed system of knowledge. Not only are there few historical examples of biomedical/epidemiological research that have incorporated the views of women — actively seeking from them information on what ails them — but there are actually many examples from biomedical history in which women's health knowledge has been devalued and even outlawed. For example, feminist historians have provided vivid accounts of how establishment biomedicine dismantled lay midwifery in the US, discrediting local women's knowledge of pregnancy and delivery, medicalizing childbirth as a pathological event, and establishing legal and economic restrictions on women's access to non-hospital-based midwifery care (Ehrenreich & English, 1973, 1978; Litoff, 1990). The implications of such restrictions were particularly severe for poor women of color, who were the main beneficiaries of such local midwifery systems in the rural American South (Dougherty, 1982; Fraser, 1995).

Today, part of the reason why women's voices continue to be excluded from problem definition and knowledge production has less to do with consolidation of professional power and authority in biomedicine than with disciplinary boundaries and methodological approaches that are exclusionary and continue to divide the intellectual landscape in women's health research. Namely, epidemiologists involved in women's health research may fear treading outside their discipline or expanding their traditional methods of scientific inquiry in order to generate new research questions and forms of data. Yet, a truly feminist-informed epidemiology requires moving away from the lamppost of conventional epidemiology, and confronting difficult epistemological, methodological, and ethical issues surrounding the nature of epidemiological research. Frankly, the "opening" of epidemiology requires that epidemiologists join forces with anthropologists, sociologists, historians, and feminist scholars, who are not only more theoretically oriented but who also value alternate, qualitative forms of data (e.g., illness narratives, life histories, participant observations, structured observations of doctor-patient interactions, popular media accounts, historical documents) that give context and meaning to epidemiologists' more quantitative analyses (Inhorn, 1995; Inhorn & Buss, 1993, 1994; Trostle, 1986). As will be described in the final section of this essay, black feminist scholars (e.g., Collins, 1991) in particular have called for an "Afrocentric feminist epistemology" that draws upon "dialogue" and "call-and-response" as methodological strategies that would privilege black women's "experiential knowledge and wisdom" and thus lead to new forms of knowledge creation. Ultimately, we believe that epidemiology as a discipline would greatly benefit from much greater methodological triangulation and theoretical engagement with women's studies, the social sciences, and the humanities. Through such engagement, the field of epidemiology as a whole could begin to be "decentered" from its masculinist, white, Euro-American axis of privilege to allow for more democratic, egalitarian and participatory ways of knowing and using knowledge.

Indeed, we anticipate that epidemiology, perhaps more than many other disciplines, has the potential to evolve toward a feminist-informed science which pursues emancipatory goals and creates open systems of knowledge and knowledge sharing. Such potential resides in: (1) epidemiology's "shoe-leather" origins, in which highly anecdotal public information — for example, lay people's observations about connections between water and cholera (Goldstein & Goldstein, 1986) — was included in early epidemiological investigations (Brown, 1997); (2) its capacity to create and enhance channels for flows of knowledge and dialogue with general and specific populations in historical moments of public health crisis; (3) its mechanisms of accountability to both the scientific community and the public; and (4) its increasing recognition of the need for self-reflection and auto-critique, as outlined in the introduction of this essay. These potentials seem to resonate most clearly in the movement toward the new form of popular epidemiology described by Brown (1992, 1997). Popular epidemiology draws upon a "science in action" approach, first outlined by Latour (1987), in which epidemiology becomes "open to the public", a form of "citizen science" (Brown, 1997). In this new feedback model of scientific knowledge production, lay persons gather data and direct and marshal the knowledge and resources of experts in order to understand the epidemiology of disease. In turn, epidemiologists "experience the citizenry" and the problem being studied before laying claims to the "real meaning of epidemiological 'fact'" (Brown, 1992, p. 275). Brown speculates that as the number of popular epidemiologists, or what he calls "maverick scientists", grows, we may see a greater number of such well-designed "public studies", in which lay people, particularly women, play a central role.

In conclusion, theorists and practitioners of liberatory education, including health educators practicing participatory research (Stein, 1997), embrace the principle that knowledge and learning can only be emancipatory when everyone claims — and is allowed to claim — knowledge as a field in which we all labor (de Koning & Martin, 1996; hooks, 1994). An emancipatory epidemiology would require the elite cadre of specialists trained in viewing illness and health from a traditional public health perspective to listen to and engage with people articulating their lived experiences of health and illness within the social, political, economic, as well as biological context of their lives.

Biological essentialization of women as reproducers

This brings us to a second antifeminist bias in contemporary epidemiological research on women's health: namely, lingering biological reductionism, or the severing of biological processes from the social, political, and economic determinants of health and illness. Because of the hegemony of a rather narrowly focused biomedical research model — aimed at "unravel[ing] the specific mechanisms of disease processes by tracing the biochemical pathways and pathological mechanisms of the body" (Fee & Krieger, 1994, p. 7) — little attention has been paid to how social conditions, including gender and racial discrimination and economic deprivation, adversely affect health (Krieger & Zierler, 1995).

Most salient from the perspective of women's health is the continuing biological essentialization of women as reproducers, with their health thought of primarily in terms of reproductive capacity and function. In other words, in current biomedical and public health models, women are seen first and foremost as reproducers, whose "health" (and that of their children) is determined by their ability to become pregnant, give birth, and adequately mother their offspring. Because women continue to be characterized as a single, universal "risk group", defined by their reproductive biology, epidemiology ignores the ways in which the social realities of gender — as opposed to simple biological sex — manifest themselves in women's bodies (Krieger & Zierler, 1995), through the creation of what one medical anthropologist has called, poetically, "life's lesions" (Finkler, 1994).

Such "life lesions" take *many* forms in women's lives, a list that would be too long to enumerate. But some clear examples of the ways in which gender relations "get into the bodies" of women (Krieger et al., 1993) — *and not only their reproductive bodies* — might include: (1) African–American women's experiences with low-birthweight babies and the accompanying grief of high infant mortality (Krieger et al., 1993); (2) US societal preoccupations with ideals of thinness which have led to epidemics of dieting, eating disorders, and even smoking as a weight-reduction strategy among adolescent girls (Berman & Gritz, 1991; Bordo, 1993; Casper & Offer, 1990; Nichter, 2000);

(3) women's day-to-day experiences of racism and sexism at work and at home that, when unnamed and socially submerged, lead to raised blood pressure readings and the risk of hypertension and stroke, particularly among black women (Krieger, 1990); and (4) women's experiences of sexual harassment, sexual abuse, rape, domestic violence, and other forms of "gender violence" (e.g., dowry deaths, honor killings, amniocentesis-aided female feticide, female circumcision), which have increasingly been recognized and prioritized in global conferences on women, health, and development, including in Cairo (1994) and Beijing (1995) (United Nations, 1995).

Indeed, explicit theory about the three major categories, "gender", "race", and "class", and the multiple, interlocking forms of oppression that accompany these three categories to produce ill health in women's lives, is lacking in contemporary epidemiology. These categories are often formulated inadequately as uncomplicated variables in epidemiological studies. Of particular concern here is that "sex" and "gender" have been historically conflated. As currently employed in feminist and social science analysis, the term "sex" often refers to a biological category, defined by biological characteristics pertaining to the ability to reproduce (Krieger et al., 1993). Thus, in the US and many other societies, sex is typically dichotomized as "male" and "female". However, "gender" is a different construct, for it is a socially (human) constructed category, regarding culturally produced conventions, roles, behaviors, and identities involving notions of "masculine" and "feminine", and "heterosexual", "homosexual", and "bisexual", which are constructed and performed in relation to each other (Butler, 1990). Consequently, it is not enough for epidemiologists to simply replace the term "sex" with "gender" in their analyses, as has been occurring in some studies since the early 1990s. Although the move to "gender" marks an important shift in epidemiological awareness, understanding the implications of "gender" on health — and especially the health-demoting consequences of gender oppression — involves more than replacing "sex" with "gender" in the text of an epidemiological manuscript. It involves understanding how sex and gender are different and gathering data that not only link women's experiences of health to their reproductive organs and physiology, but also provide answers to questions such as: (1) how do gender norms regarding reproduction per se (e.g., pronatalist cultural norms mandating women to become mothers) affect women's daily lives and well-being?; (2) what are the ills affecting women that are unrelated to their reproductive biology?; (3) how are women's daily lives and well-being influenced by gender norms and expectations concerning femininity, masculinity, hetero-sexuality, and homosexuality?; (4) how are the health effects associated with sexism complicated by other aspects of women's social identities, including race, ethnicity, class, nation, religion, and age?; and (5) how does gender inequality perpetuated by institutional structures (including those of biomedicine) affect women's lives and health care?

However, such questions are rarely asked in contemporary epidemiological research on women's health. As noted by Krieger et al. (1993, pp. 88–89):

> Studies on the contribution of sexism — and not simply sex — to women's and men's patterns of health and disease, however, are a new phenomena. [sic] Until fairly recently, the predominant assumption has been that women and men have different health profiles because they are distinct biological sexes who differ essentially in their basic natures. According to this view, women and men have different disease risks not only because of differences in reproductive organs and physiology but also because of biologically determined differences in their social roles, which result in men's and women's exposures to different situations that can benefit or harm their health.

The narrowing of the epidemiological lens to this simple view of women as the "reproductive sex" is pervasive, and its negative consequences are manifold. First, women today continue to be seen as "controlled" by their reproductive physiology, although the discourse has changed from 19th-century Victorian notions of the frail and irrational woman with diseased ovaries and hysteria-producing wombs to views of the 20th-century woman controlled by her sex chromosomes and female hormones. As Krieger and Fee (1994, p. 15) point out, this combination of sex chromosomes and hormones has been imbued with almost magical powers to shape human behavior in gendered terms; thus, "women [are] now at the mercy of their genetic limitations and a changing brew of hormonal imperatives". The medicalization — indeed, psychopathologization — of such normal reproductive events as menstruation and menopause, including the creation of disease categories such as "premenstrual syndrome" and "estrogen-deficiency disease" (Martin, 1987; Lock, 1993), bespeaks the continuing tendency to see women as irrational, untrustworthy, and unfit for public duties by virtue of their unpredictable, even dangerous reproductive processes.

Second, the continuing focus on women's reproductive biology means that "women's health" is equivalent to "reproductive health", while women's non-reproductive health concerns (e.g., lupus, multiple sclerosis, hypertension, heart disease, strokes, occupational exposures, and violence) remain hidden from public view. The most glaring example of the neglect of a non-reproductive women's health problem is cardiovascular disease, which kills half a million women in the US every year (more than twice the number who succumb to all forms of cancer combined) (Freedman & Maine, 1993) and which tops the list of disease burden (at more than 20%) for women aged 15 and above around the world (Stein, 1997). Yet, virtually all the major studies of cardiovascular disease — including the renowned US-based Multiple Risk Factor Intervention Trials (Mr. FIT study) — involved thousands of men and no women (Freedman & Maine, 1993). This glaring gender bias in research on cardiovascular health has certainly been partly responsible for the resulting gender biases in clinical decision-making, whereby men receive more diagnostic procedures and more aggressive treatment for heart disease (Freedman & Maine, 1993).

Indeed, many of the "hot" issues in women's health in recent years — including adolescent pregnancy, low birth weight, diethylstilbesterol (DES) and vaginal carcinoma, toxic shock syndrome, unnecessary hysterectomies and cesarean deliveries, sterilization abuse, unsafe abortion and maternal mortality, and breast cancer morbidity and mortality — are all related in one way or another to women's reproductive organs and reproductive potentials. Furthermore, women's reproductive problems that are not directly fertility-related — such as cervical cancer, reproductive and urinary tract infections, and uterine and vaginal prolapses — have been relatively underprivileged in biomedical and public health discourse, despite the fact that these conditions may be a significant source of suffering for many women. Interestingly and by means of comparison, there is no equivalent public health or biomedical category of "men's health",[10] and the growth of a popular men's health movement has clearly not developed around issues of men's role in reproduction. In comparison, the two major global public health initiatives aimed at women — Safe Motherhood in the 1980s and Reproductive Health in the 1990s (Lane, 1994) — both remain quite narrowly focused on women as reproducers, whose obstetrical emergencies, unsafe abortions, fertility, infertility, sexually transmitted diseases, and other reproductive complaints, impede them in various ways not as *women* but as *mothers* or potential mothers. In other words, these well-meaning, but narrowly focused initiatives have ignored the social, cultural and political issues that determine, for example, whether a woman will be able to feed herself and her children, manage the constraints and stresses of multiple roles, and live without fear of violence and premature death (Koblinsky et al., 1993).

Third, the narrow focus on reproduction means that women on either end of the reproductive life span — i.e., girls and adolescents and postmenopausal women — have received little attention in terms of their health concerns and needs. The two "key issues" of adolescent and older women's health in the US — namely, teenage pregnancy and menopause — can be shown to have been problematized not by women themselves, but by the public health and biomedical establishments in this country, for reasons that are both moral and material in nature. For example, anthropologists have recently criticized the Western biomedical model for its assumptions of universal, hormone-driven, negative physical and psychological conditions of menopause (Davis, 1996; Lock, 1993). Comparative studies of menopause cross-culturally reveal that menopause is a biological event which is also culturally constructed and shaped by power relations in the family, the labor market, and the global economy (Lock, 1993). Furthermore, although a "life-cycle" approach to studying women's health has recently become popular (highlighting women's reproductive health experiences as determined by age and biological timing), its predominant focus on biological events often ignores how the biological timing of these events and women's experiences of them are shaped by social aspects such as race/ethnicity, nationality, and class (Krieger et al., 1993).

Finally, because women are seen as reproducers and not producers of valued goods and services themselves, little attention has been paid to the health needs of women as workers, nor has consideration been given to the multiple roles women fulfill. Thus, housework, childcare, and family health caregiving — forms of unpaid labor that are inordinately shouldered by women around the world, even in the most egalitarian settings (Browner & Leslie, 1996; Colen, 1995; Mullings, 1995) — are not considered as forms of "work" with potentially deleterious consequences for women's psychological and physical well-being (Jacobson, 1993). Furthermore, with far-reaching changes in the global economy, more and more women worldwide are entering the wage labor force (Freeman, 1999). Yet, the public health and biomedical establishments have only begun to assess the health-demoting consequences of women's wage labor — including, *inter alia*, occupational exposures (Bale, 1990; Bertin, 1989; Dew, Branet, Parkinson, Dunn, & Ryan, 1989; Jacobson, 1993), stress-producing workplace "discipline" (Freeman, 1999; Ong, 1987), repetitive strain injuries (Reid & Reynolds, 1990; Reid, Ewan, & Lowy, 1991), and various forms of sexual discrimination and harassment on the job (Krieger et al., 1993) — or how these insidious "side effects" of women's work affect both worker productivity and absenteeism.

In summary, the biological essentialization of women rampant in epidemiology, public health, and biomedicine in general has generated not only untoward views of women and their bodies, but also many "blind spots" in our knowledge of women's health. Addressing these problems begins with an "opening" not only of knowledge systems but also of the epidemiological worldview and research priorities. Analytical epidemiology has a long history of moving "beyond biology" in its interest in the disease risks associated with all sorts of nonendogenous exposures (e.g., to environmental toxins, infectious agents), as well as human behavior (Inhorn, 1995). Indeed, epidemiology has proven that the context in which people work, live, eat, recreate, and procreate has profound implications for their health status. Obviously, this basic insight should apply equally to women as half of the population "at risk" from phenomena that have little, if anything, to do with their reproductive biology per se. In other words, if epidemiology can move beyond the narrow and limiting view of women as reproducers — controlled by their sex chromosomes, female hormones, and reproductive organs — then a whole world of discovery awaits epidemiology as it considers women's lives in their totality and complexity.

Decontextualization and depoliticization of women's health risks

Finally, a problem that seriously compromises epidemiology as a theoretically generative discipline is its overarching disinterest in asking the tough "why" questions concerning the *context* in which relationships occur between discrete risk factors and disease outcomes. In fact, mainstream epidemiology literally "leaves off" at the point at which a relationship between a risk factor and a disease outcome is discovered; it poses none of the important conceptual and contextual questions about why risk factors occur in the first place, how they are socially distributed among individuals and groups, and how social, political, and economic factors generate and maintain risk in certain environments (Inhorn, 1995; Turshen, 1984; Wing, 1994). Without this sociocultural and political-economic contextualization, explanations of why particular diseases affect particular individuals and groups at particular historical moments will remain obscure (Krieger et al., 1993; Trostle, 1986; Turshen, 1984). Furthermore, while epidemiologists often fear the "ecological fallacy" — in which erroneous estimates of individuals' behavior or risks are made on the basis of population-based data — a less recognized problem is the "individual fallacy", in which the larger social context is ignored by virtue of only examining individual cases (Brown, 1997). The net result is an individualizing of disease risk, often accompanied by victim-blaming. Yet, individuals are often seriously challenged in their abilities to reduce disease risk, for they face external forces, including, *inter alia*, poverty, unhealthy living environments, inflexible gender norms and hierarchies, poor health care, governmental neglect, or political involvement in their lives (e.g., state policies, military conscription, the presence of police states, civil unrest and warfare) that may make risk reduction and prevention impossible. As noted by Krieger and colleagues (1993, p. 109):

> To understand and ultimately prevent inequalities in health associated with social inequalities, we must be guided by the 'why' questions of explaining population patterns of disease, not simply the 'how' questions regarding the mechanisms of disease causation. For research to set the basis for effective disease prevention policies, it must address the structural determinants of health, not simply factors labeled as individual 'lifestyle choices.' Continuing merely to catalog individual risk factors from an amorphous 'web of causation' no longer can suffice. If our goal is to alter the web rather than merely break its strands, it is time to look for the spider.

Similarly, alternative epidemiologist Wing (1994, p. 84) has cautioned that current global public health crises demand more than a "piecemeal approach", and that "an epidemiology oriented towards massive and equitable public health improvement requires reconstructing the connections between disease agents and their contexts".

The need for understanding disease agents in social, economic, and political context — or, to use Krieger's metaphor, understanding that a spider lives in the middle of a web — has perhaps never been clearer than in the case of the global AIDS pandemic. Yet, AIDS — a disease inordinately affecting women worldwide and thus worthy of an extended discussion in this essay — provides *the* quintessential example of a case of epidemiological decontextualization and depoliticization.

For the first decade of the epidemic, AIDS was not considered to affect women, because of a narrow epidemiological definition of the disease, which restricted it to gay men, hemophiliacs, Haitians, and IV drug users (Farmer et al., 1996). When the epidemiological community eventually recognized that women were susceptible to HIV infection, their self-inflicted "behavior" — e.g., as prostitutes, IV drug users or partners of drug users — was emphasized as the key to disease risk. Only now, after more than two decades of experience with this epidemic, have researchers begun to capture the social context in which the AIDS epidemic has unfolded among women around the world. These researchers — coming not from the epidemiology/public health community, but rather from the social sciences (e.g., anthropologists Paul Farmer, Brooke Grundfest Schoepf, Elisa Sobo, Priscilla Ulim, and many others listed in the bibliography of Farmer et al., 1996) — have emphasized the ways in which poverty and gender discrimination serve as major risk factors for AIDS among women and their children, who constitute the fastest growing core of new cases. More specifically, women who are economically dependent upon men for support of themselves and their families, and/or who live in pronatalist societies characterized by marked gender asymmetries, are unlikely to be able to protect themselves from HIV infection through the "negotiation" of condom use with unwilling partners. Thus, the "risk" of HIV infection in women involves much more than individual women having unprotected sex for no apparent reason — as the epidemiological model of AIDS risk would suggest.

In order to understand *why* so many women around the world engage in this "risky" behavior, we need to understand how systems synergistically generate inequality and how inequality structures AIDS risks and burdens. For example, in Haiti, historical and transnational political and economic forces set the stage for rapid transmission of AIDS there (Farmer, 1992). The violent penetration of early European capital and neocolonial links to the US contributed to "underdevelopment", rural poverty, migration to urban centers of industry and wage labor, unemployment rates of up to 70%, international tourism and prostitution, and social disintegration (e.g., the instability of marital unions) (Farmer, 1992). These are factors which increased women's burdens of caregiving for youngsters and elders and affected women's survival strategies concerning multiple partners and commercial sex work. Ultimately, it affected Haitian women's risk and susceptibility to HIV infection (Farmer, 1992). As this example demonstrates, context is all important, and the Haitian context bespeaks multiple forms of oppression, based on gender, race, class, and global location, which women confront and deal with often at great costs to their health and well-being.

Indeed, creating a truly feminist-informed epidemiology would involve a political commitment to identify and end the multiple forms of oppression confronting women in Haiti and elsewhere around the globe. Such an emancipatory approach arises from the understanding that women everywhere, as gendered beings, face some form of oppression and exploitation, which may be deleterious to their health. As in the AIDS example, gender oppression is typically not an isolated axis of domination, but is part of interlocking structures of oppression formed by destructive social divisions and hierarchies, which include race/ethnicity, class, religion, sexual preference, age, physical abilities, and national location in the global order (Mohanty et al., 1991). These hierarchies construct and maintain each other, supported by similar institutional structures and shared notions of difference, superiority, and the right to dominate (Lorde, 1984). Thus, a truly feminist epidemiology would involve a commitment to identifying and ending the deleterious health consequences for women brought on by multiple forms of oppression, including those interwoven with gender. The ultimate goal would be a feminist-informed epidemiology committed to the radical goal of transforming society for the improvement of every woman's health and well-being.

Creating a feminist epidemiology

Having spelled out a number of antifeminist biases in epidemiological studies of women's health, we conclude this essay with a hopeful exhortation to all epidemiologists: Namely, a call for the development of an emancipatory, feminist epidemiology that is perceptive of and responsive to the great diversity of women, their multiple forms of oppression, and the breadth of their health needs *as they themselves define them*. The theorizing of Euro-American women of color (a.k.a. black feminists) (Collins, 1991; hooks, 1981, 1983, 1994) and that of third world feminists living in "developing" countries shaped by colonial legacies (Mohanty et al., 1991) informs our feminist approach in this proposed reconfiguration. Euro-American black feminists and third world feminists, perhaps more than other types of feminists (e.g., liberal, radical, Marxist, and postmodern), have been concerned with overcoming the multiple, interlocking, and simultaneous forms of oppression based on gender, race, class, and nation which many women face worldwide. Third world feminists in particular have emerged at the center of women's health politics and debates as they have struggled against the effects of late-20th-century globalization, including recessions, structural adjustment policies, new divisions of labor, environmental degradation, and the multinational exportation of hazardous industries and technologies (Doyal, 1995).

Euro-American black feminists have directed their efforts in a slightly different direction, challenging, in part, the Eurocentric, masculinist knowledge creation process, in which "elite white men and their representatives control structures of knowledge validation" (Collins, 1991, p. 201), including scholarship in biomedicine, public health, and epidemiology, where "white male interests" prevail, as shown above. Black feminists argue instead for an Afrocentric epistemological approach that may lead to a significantly enriched understanding of "how subordinate groups create knowledge that fosters resistance" (Collins, 1991, p. 207). Epistemologically similar in some respects to the popular epidemiological approach forwarded by Brown (1992, 1997),[11] black feminists call for new forms of knowledge production capitalizing on four important elements: (1) valuing of women's experiential knowledge and wisdom, including how race, gender, and class oppression are "lived" and "survived"; (2) using dialogue in assessing knowledge claims, including traditional call-and-response discourse modes common in African-American community gatherings; (3) implementing an ethic of caring, in which personal expressiveness, emotions, and empathy are central to the knowledge validation process; and (4) implementing an ethic of personal accountability, in which a researcher's personal biography and politics are considered highly relevant to the knowledge validation process.

Drawing from these third world and black feminist approaches to theory, methodology, and epistemology, a feminist epidemiology would proceed from three important assumptions. First, feminist epidemiologists would recognize that women occupy simultaneously diverse locations and identities, which shape their experiences, their struggles, their resistance strategies, and their power and strengths (Collins, 1991; Mohanty et al., 1991). From this perspective there can be no universal category of "women" who are oppressed by the same patriarchal institutions and who share identical experiences, interests, desires, life courses, and health concerns and outcomes (Mohanty, 1991). Although most women share similar biological events (e.g., menstruation, birth, lactation, menopause) which affect their health and well-being, women will often differ dramatically in how they experience and create meaning from these events, which is highly dependent on their social locations in space and time (Martin, 1987).

Second, as a truly feminist project, a feminist epidemiology would draw upon both popular epidemiological and Afrocentric epistemological approaches in order to develop new methodological and theoretical strategies that privilege four important elements:

(1) the active engagement of women themselves in the epidemiological knowledge production process; this will involve women "talking about their health",[12] defining their own health problems, and being actively *listened to* by feminist epidemiological researchers committed to empathic engagement in the lives of those they study;[13]

(2) the documentation of women's diverse experiences of illness and health, based on the multiplicity of women's global locations, social and cultural identities, interests, and experiences as both reproductive and *non-reproductive human beings*;
(3) the evaluation of how gender oppression, as well as other interlocking forms of oppression that shape women's daily lives, is itself detrimental to women's health; this will require forging new methodological approaches to show how *gender oppression* — as opposed to an uncomplicated epidemiological variable of *gender* — shapes women's health outcomes and well-being (Krieger et al., 1993); and
(4) the connection of women's local lived experiences of health and illness and the various forms of oppression they encounter to larger *social, economic and political forces*.

Finally, a feminist epidemiology would require a personal commitment from those of us engaged in the production of epidemiological knowledge and policy to unmask relationships of domination in our professional and private lives as part of our life's work (Maguire, 1996). This means examining how we and our research institutions are implicated in relations of domination and accepting responsibility for the ways gender/race/class/nation shape our own social locations. It also requires us to create new structures and relationships to replace the hierarchical ones in which we may wittingly and unwittingly participate.

If we are to take the aforementioned set of assumptions seriously, then a feminist epidemiology is about creating (1) alternative research structures that critically challenge the dominant, hegemonic production of epidemiological knowledge; (2) new theoretical frameworks that analyze historically and globally important gender, race, and class relations and the political and economic structures in which these relations are embedded; (3) grass-roots, activist agendas for examining and solving women's self-defined health problems, as well as liberating women (and all human beings) from unequal and unjust social hierarchies that promote and maintain ill health; and (4) professional and personal accountability for academic and health institutions that leave unchallenged and intact oppressive structures, including those interwoven with gender (Barroso, 1994).

Thus, the goal of the emancipatory feminist epidemiology that we are describing involves much more than just adding women or other marginalized groups into already existing paradigms for clinical trials, cohort studies, epidemiological surveillance systems, and other ways of studying patterns of health and disease among populations. And it goes well beyond convincing practitioners of conventional, mainstream epidemiology to recognize the value of interdisciplinary linkages and qualitative data in adding dimensions of context and meaning to their quantitative studies. Although these are important goals in and of themselves, they are not sufficient for the development of a new feminist epidemiological paradigm. Instead, an emancipatory feminist epidemiology demands a critical rethinking of the very ways in which "women", "gender", "oppression", and "health" are ultimately conceptualized, studied, and linked to social policy. Only through such a radical rethinking can we begin to envision a feminist epidemiology that means research *for* women rather than *on* women, and that is responsive and ultimately beneficial to women's lives, as well as the lives of *all* members of society.

Acknowledgements

We are grateful to Robert A. Hahn, of the Division of Prevention Research and Analytic Methods, Epidemiology Program Office, Centers for Disease Control and Prevention, Atlanta, Georgia. He planted the seeds of this essay and provided rich critical insights on the nature of current epidemiological practice.

Notes

1 Examples of these critiques can he found in the following recent works: Diez-Roux and Nieto (1997), Krieger et al. (1993), Krieger and Zierler (1995, 1996); Lawson and Floyd (1996), Ozonoff and Boden (1987), Pearce (1996), Savitz (1997), Susser and Susser (1996a, b). Weed (1995), and Wing (1994). In addition, medical anthropologists Trostle and Sommerfeld (1996) have written a recent review article that summarizes many of the salient issues and critiques, as well as forwarding a proposal for the development of "cultural epidemiology".
2 Lawson and Floyd (1996) point out that epidemiological studies routinely evaluate the percentage of people in a population who responded to a specific public health intervention while ignoring why people respond as they do, how people interpret the intervention, its sources, or the behaviors themselves. The nature of epidemiology's "closed" system of knowledge precludes asking or interpreting answers to these questions and ignores meaning as a determinant of human behavior.
3 Examples of this include public health actions to reduce tobacco consumption and banning of hazardous materials in the US that result in stimulating manufacturers to aggressively promote their products in countries economically poorer than the US. Pearce (1996) notes that when public health problems such as tobacco smoking are studied in individual terms rather than in population terms (which would examine tobacco production, advertising, distribution and the social and economic influences on consumption), the solution is usually defined in individual terms and public health actions result in moving the problem from rich to poor countries and from rich to poor populations in industrialized countries.
4 Krieger and colleagues do not specifically call their new epidemiological approach "critical epidemiology". However, others (e.g., Brown, 1997) have used this term to apply to Krieger's approach.
5 For numerous references to this work, see the bibliography in Krieger et al. (1993).
6 Recent examples of this literature include: Beck (1992, 1995, 1996), Clarke and Short (1993), Krimsky and Golding (1992), Luhmann (1993), and Marske (1991).

7 We prefer the term "antifeminist" to "sexist" or "chauvinist", as "antifeminist" implies opposition to the feminist principles we are advocating.
8 With respect to our authorial positionality, we are anthropologists and epidemiologists who are generally sympathetic to epidemiological approaches and who have urged greater synthesis of epidemiological and medical anthropological research perspectives (Inhorn, 1995; Inhorn & Buss, 1993, 1994). However, we are also feminist researchers concerned with issues of gender/race/class and local and global women's health; thus, we adopt a critical feminist stance for the purposes of this essay. We suggest learning from feminist researchers in other disciplines who have been grappling with difficult issues, such as the dilemmas of an activist stance, problems encountered doing collaborative work, harsh reactions of other scholars to feminist research, and difficulties in funding feminist research activities. See Fine (1993), Fonow and Cook (1991), Nielsen (1990), and Stanley (1990).
9 Some work in mainstream social epidemiology — especially work which seriously examines health inequalities among women that are linked to social class(ism) (see Krieger et al., 1993, for examples) — would also be excluded from this critique.
10 Moscucci (1990) points to the unsuccessful attempts to establish "andrology", or the study of masculinity, in the 19th and early 20th centuries. However, the "physiology and pathology of the male sexual system simply were not seen to define men's nature" (Moscucci, 1990, p. 32) in the way that women's sexual systems were seen as defining women's nature — at least those of white, socially and economically privileged women. Today, the study of men's masculine sexual characteristics is designated to the specialized area of endocrinology.
11 See also Stein's (1997) interesting discussion of "feminist participatory-action research (PAR)", which derives from the empowerment theories of Paulo Freire and feminist methodological critiques.
12 Medical anthropologist/epidemiologist Robert Hahn (personal communication) has suggested the need for a large-scale, US-based study in which women are given an open-ended opportunity to simply "talk about their health". From the standpoint of US public health and epidemiology, such a study has never been conducted. Instead, women's health problems are typically defined in a "top-down" fashion by those in the biomedical/public health communities.
13 Anthropologists have historically advocated long-term, empathic engagement in the lives of those they study.

References

Bale, A. (1990). Women's toxic experience. In R. Apple (Ed.), *Women, health, and medicine in America: A historical handbook* (pp. 411–439). New York: Garland.

Barroso, C. (1994). Building a new specialization on women's health: An international perspective. In A. Dan (Ed.), *Reframing women's health: Multidisciplinary research and practice* (pp. 93–101). Thousand Oaks, CA: Sage.

Beck, U. (1992). *Risk society: Towards a new modernity.* London: Sage.

Beck, U. (1995). *Ecological enlightenment: Essays on the politics of the risk society.* New Jersey: Humanities Press.

Beck, U. (1996). World risk society as cosmopolitan society: ecological questions in a framework of manufactured uncertainties. *Theory, Culture and Society, 13,* 1–32.

Belenky, M., Clinchy, N. R., Glodberger, N. R., & Tarule, J. M. (1986). *Women's ways of knowing: The development of self, voice, and mind.* New York: Basic Books.

Berman, B., & Gritz, E. (1991). Women and smoking: Current trends and issues of the 1990s. *Journal of Substance Abuse, 3,* 221–338.

Bertin, J. (1989). Women's health and women's rights: Reproductive health hazards in the workplace. In K. Ratcliff (Ed.), *Healing technology: Feminist perspectives* (pp. 289–303). Ann Arbor, MI: University of Michigan Press.

Bordo, S. (1993). *Unbearable weight: Feminism, western culture, and the body.* Berkeley, CA: University of California Press.

Brown, P. (1992). Popular epidemiology and toxic waste contamination: Lay and professional ways of knowing. *Journal of Health and Social Behavior, 33,* 267–281.

Brown, P. (1997). Popular epidemiology revisited. *Current Sociology, 45,* 137–156.

Browner, C., & Leslie, J. (1996). Women, work, and household health in the context of development. In C. Sargent, & C. Brettell (Eds.), *Gender and health: An international perspective* (pp. 260–277). Upper Saddle River, NJ: Prentice-Hall.

Butler, J. (1990). *Gender trouble: Feminism and the subversion of identity.* New York: Routledge.

Casper, R., & Offer, D. (1990). Weight and dieting concerns in adolescents. Fashion or symptom? *Pediatrics, 86,* 384–390.

Charlton, B. (1997). Epidemiology as a toolkit for clinical scientists. *Epidemiology, 8,* 461–463.

Clarke, L., & Short Jr., J. (1993). Social organization and risk: Some current controversies. *Annual Review of Sociology, 19,* 375–399.

Colen, S. (1995). "Like a mother to them": Stratified reproduction and West Indian childcare workers and employers in New York. In F. Ginsburg, & R. Rapp (Eds.), *Conceiving the new world order: The global politics of reproduction* (pp. 78–102). Berkeley, CA: University of California Press.

Collins, P. (1991). *Black feminist thought: Knowledge, consciousness, and the politics of empowerment.* New York: Routledge.

Davis, D. (1996). The cultural construction of the premenstrual and menopausal symptoms. In C. C. Sargent, & C. Brettell (Eds.), *Gender and health: An international perspective* (pp. 57–86). Upper Saddle River, NJ: Prentice-Hall.

de Koning, K., & Martin M. (Eds.) (1996). *Participatory research in health: Issues and experiences.* New Jersey: Zed Books.

Dew, M., Bromet, E., Parkinson, D., Dunn, L., & Ryan, C. (1989). Effects of solvent exposure and occupational stress on the health of blue-collar women. In K. Ratcliff (Ed.), *Healing technology: Feminist perspectives* (pp. 327–345). Ann Arbor, MI: University of Michigan Press.

Diez-Roux, A., & Nieto, J. (1997). Epidemiology, clinical science and beyond. *Epidemiology, 8,* 459–461.

Dougherty, M. (1982). Southern midwifery and organized health care: Systems in conflict. *Medical Anthropology, 6,* 113–126.

Doyal, L. (1995). *What makes women sick: Gender and the political economy of health.* New Brunswick, NJ: Rutgers University Press.

Ehrenreich, B., & English, D. (1973). *Witches, midwives and nurses: A history of women healers.* New York: The Feminist Press.

Ehrenreich, B., & English, D. (1978). *For her own good: 150 years of experts' advice to women.* New York: Bantam.

Farmer, P. (1992). *AIDS and accusation: Haiti and the geography of blame.* Berkeley, CA: University of California Press.

Farmer, P., Connors, M., & Simmons, J. (Eds.) (1996). *Women, poverty and aids: Sex, drugs and structural violence*. Monroe, ME: Common Courage Press.

Fee, E., & Krieger, N., (Eds.) (1994). *Women's health, power and politics: Essays on sex/gender, medicine and public health*. Amityville, NY: Baywood Publishing.

Fine, M. (1993). The politics of research and activism. In P. Bart, & E. Moran (Eds.), *Violence against women: The bloody footprints* (pp. 278–287). Newbury Park, CA: Sage.

Finkler, K. (1994). *Women in pain: Gender and morbidity in Mexico*. Philadelphia: University of Pennsylvania Press.

Fonow, M., & Cook, J. (Eds.) (1991). *Beyond methodology: Feminist scholarship as lived research*. Bloomington: Indiana University Press.

Fraser, G. (1995). Modern bodies, modern minds: Midwifery and reproductive change in an African American community. In F. Ginsberg, & R. Rapp (Eds.), *Conceiving the new world order: The global politics of reproduction* (pp. 42–58). Berkeley, CA: University of California Press.

Freeman, C. (1999). *High tech and high heels in the global economy: Women, work, and pink-collar identities in the Caribbean*. Durham, NC: Duke University Press.

Freedman, L., & Maine, D. (1993). Women's mortality: A legacy of neglect. In M. Koblinsky, J. Timyan, & J. Gay (Eds.), *The health of women: A global perspective* (pp. 147–170). Boulder, CO: Westview Press.

Goldstein, I., & Goldstein, M. (1986). The broad street pump. In J. Goldsmith (Ed.), *Environmental epidemiology* (pp. 37–48). Boca Raton, FL: CRC Press.

Hamilton, J. (1996). Women and health policy: On the inclusion of females in clinical trials. In C. Sargent, & C. Brettell (Eds.), *Gender and health: An international perspective* (pp. 292–325). Upper Saddle River, NJ: Prentice Hall.

hooks, b. (1981). *Ain't I a woman: Black women and feminism*. Boston: South End Press.

hooks, b. (1983). *Feminist theory from margin to center*. Boston: South End Press.

hooks, b. (1994). *Teaching to transgress: Education as the practice of freedom*. New York: Routledge.

Inhorn, M. C. (1995). Medical anthropology and epidemiology: Divergences or convergences? *Social Science & Medicine, 40*, 285–290.

Inhorn, M. C., & Buss, K. A. (1993). Infertility, infections, and iatrogenesis in Egypt: The anthropological epidemiology of blocked tubes. *Medical Anthropology, 15*, 217–244.

Inhorn, M. C., & Buss, K. A. (1994). Ethnography, epidemiology and infertility in Egypt. *Social Science & Medicine, 39*, 671–686.

Jacobson, J. (1993). Women's health: The price of poverty. In M. Koblinsky, J. Timyan, & J. Gay (Eds.), *The health of women: A global perspective* (pp. 3–31). Boulder, CO: Westview Press.

Krimsky, S., & Golding, D. (Eds.) (1992). *Social theories of risk*. Westport, CT: Praeger.

Koblinsky, M., Campbell, O., & Harlow, S. (Eds.) (1993). *The Health of women: A global perspective*. Boulder, CO: Westview Press.

Koopman, J. (1996). Comment: Emerging objectives and methods in epidemiology. *American Journal of Public Health, 86*, 630–632.

Krieger, N. (1990). Racial and gender discrimination: Risk factors for high blood pressure? *Social Science & Medicine, 30*, 1273–1281.

Krieger, N., & Fee, E. (1994). Man made medicine and women's health: The biopolitics of sex/gender and race/ethnicity. *International Journal of Health Services*, 24, 265–283.

Krieger, N., Rowley, D., Herman, A. A., Avery, B., & Phillips, M. T. (1993). Racism, sexism, and social class: implications for studies of health, disease and well being. In D. Rowler, & H. Tosteson (Eds.), Racial differences in preterm delivery: Developing a new research paradigm. *American Journal of Preventive Medicine*, 6(Supplement to 9), 82–122.

Krieger, N., & Zierler, S. (1995). Accounting for the health of women. *Current Issues in Public Health*, 1, 251–256.

Krieger, N., & Zierler, S. (1996). What explains the public's health — a call for epidemiologic theory. *Epidemiology*, 7, 107–109.

Lane, S. (1994). From population control to reproductive health: An emerging policy agenda. *Social Science & Medicine*, 39, 1303–1314.

Latour, B. (1987). *Science in action: How to follow scientists and engineers through society*. Cambridge, MA: Harvard University Press.

Lawson, J., & Floyd, J. (1996). The future of epidemiology: A humanist response. *American Journal of Public Health*, 86, 1029.

Litoff, J. B. (1990). Midwives and history. In R. D. Apple (Ed.), *Women, health, and medicine in America: A historical handbook* (pp. 443–458). New York: Garland.

Lock, M. (1993). *Encounters with aging; Mythologies of menopause in Japan and North America*. Berkeley, CA: University of California Press.

Lorde, A. (1984). *Sister outsider*. Freedom, CA: The Crossing Press.

Luhmann, N. (1993). *Risk: A sociological theory*. New York: Aldine de Gruyter.

Lupton, D. (1993). Risk as moral danger: The social and political functions of risk discourse in public health. *International Journal of Health Services*, 23, 425–435.

Maguire, P. (1996). Proposing a more feminist participatory research: Knowing and being embraced openly. In K. de Koning, & M. Martin (Eds.), *Participatory research in health: Issues and experiences* (pp. 27–39). New Jersey: Zed Books.

Marske, C. (Ed.) (1991). *Communities of fate: Readings in the social organization of risk*. New York: Lanham.

Martin, E. (1987). *The woman in the body: A cultural analysis of reproduction*. Boston, MA: Beacon Press.

Mohanty, C. T. (1991). Introduction: Cartographies of struggle: Third world women and the politics of feminism. In C. T. Mohanty, A. Russo, & L. Torres (Eds.), *Third world women and the politics of feminism* (pp. 1–47). Bloomington: Indiana University Press.

Mohanty, C. T., Russo, A., & Torres, L. (1991). Preface. In C. T. Mohanty, A. Russo, & L. Torres (Eds.), *Third world women and the politics of feminism* (pp. ix–xi). Bloomington: Indiana University Press.

Moscucci, O. (1990). *The science of woman: Gynaecology and gender in England, 1800–1929*. Cambridge, MA: Harvard University Press.

Mullings, L. (1995). Households headed by women: The politics of race, class and gender. In F. Ginsburg, & R. Rapp (Eds.), *Conceiving the new world order: The global politics of reproduction* (pp. 122–139). Berkeley, CA: University of California Press.

Nations, M. K. (1986). Epidemiological research on infectious diseaes: quantitative rigor or rigormortis? Insights from ethnomedicine. In C. R. Janes, R. Stall, &

S. M. Gifford (Eds.), *Anthropology and epidemiology: Interdisciplinary approaches to the study of health and disease* (pp. 97–123). Dordrecht: D. Reidel.

Nichter, M. (2000). *Fat talk: What girls and their parents say about dieting.* Cambridge, MA: Harvard University Press.

Nielsen, J. (Ed.) (1990). *Feminist research methods: Exemplary readings in the social sciences.* Boulder, CO: Westview Press.

Ong, A. (1987). *Spirits of resistance and capitalist discipline: Factory women in Malaysia.* Albany, NY: SUNY Press.

Ozonoff, D., & Boden, L. (1987). Truth and consequences: Health agency responses to environmental health problems. *Science, Technology, and Human Values, 12,* 70–77.

Pearce, N. (1996). Traditional epidemiology, modern epidemiology and public health. *American Journal of Public Health, 86,* 678–683.

Reid, J., Ewan, C., & Lowy, E. (1991). Pilgrimage of pain: The illness experiences of women with repetition strain injury and the search for credibility. *Social Science & Medicine, 32,* 601–612.

Reid, J., & Reynolds, L. (1990). Requiem for RSI: The explanation and control of an occupational epidemic. *Medical Anthropology Quarterly, 4,* 162–190.

Rosser, S. (1994). Gender bias in clinical research: The difference it makes. In A. Dan (Ed.), *Reframing women's health: Multidisciplinary research and practice* (pp. 253–265). Thousand Oaks, CA: Sage.

Sargent, C., & Brettell, C. (Eds.) (1996). *Gender and health: An international perspective.* Upper Saddle River, NJ: Prentice-Hall.

Savitz, D. (1997). The alternative to epidemiologic theory: Whatever works. *Epidemiology, 8,* 210–212.

Scribner, R. (1997). The end of the chronic disease era. *American Journal of Public Health, 87,* 872–873.

Stanley, L. (Ed.) (1990) *Feminist praxis: Research, theory and epistemology in feminist sociology.* New York: Routledge.

Stein, J. (1997). *Empowerment & women's health: Theory, methods, and practice.* London: Zed Books.

Susser, M., & Susser, E. (1996a). Choosing a future for epidemiology I: Eras and paradigms. *American Journal of Public Health, 86,* 668–673.

Susser, M., & Susser, E. (1996b). Choosing a future for epidemiology II: From black box to Chinese boxes and eco-epidemiology. *American Journal of Public Health, 86,* 674–677.

Trostle, J. (1986). Early work in anthropology and epidemiology: From social medicine to the germ theory, 1840–1920. In C. R. Janes, R. Stall, & S. M. Gifford (Eds.), *Anthropology and epidemiology: Interdisciplinary approaches to the study of health and disease* (pp. 35–57). Dordrecht: D. Reidel.

Trostle, J. A., & Sommerfeld, J. (1996). Medical anthropology and epidemiology. *Annual Review of Anthropology, 25,* 253–274.

Turshen, M. (1984). *The political ecology of disease in tanzania.* New Brunswick, NJ: Rutgers University Press.

United Nations. (1995). *The world's women 1995: Trends and statistics.* New York: United Nations.

United States Public Health Service. (1987). *Women's health: Report of the public health service task force on women's health issues,* vol. 2. Department of Health and Human Services, Public Health Service, Washington, DC.

Weed, D. L. (1995). Epidemiology, the humanities, and public health. *American Journal of Public Health, 85*, 914–918.

Whittle, L., & Inhorn, M. Rethinking difference: A feminist reframing of gender/race/class for the improvement of women's health research. *International Journal of Health Services*, in press.

Wing, S. (1994). Limits of epidemiology. *Medicine and Global Survival, 1*, 74–86.

Winkelstein Jr., W. (1996). Editorial: Eras, paradigms, and the future of epidemiology. *American Journal of Public Health, 86*, 621–622.

15
WOMEN'S STATUS AND THE HEALTH OF WOMEN AND MEN
A view from the States

Ichiro Kawachi, Bruce P. Kennedy, Vanita Gupta and Deborah Prothrow-Stith

Source: *Social Science & Medicine*, 48 (1999), 21–32.

Abstract

We examined the status of women in the 50 American states in relation to women's and men's levels of health. The status of women in each state was assessed by four composite indices measuring women's political participation, economic autonomy, employment and earnings, and reproductive rights. The study design was cross-sectional and ecologic. Our main outcome measures were total female and male mortality rates, female cause-specific death rates and mean days of activity limitations reported by women during the previous month. Measures of women's status were strikingly correlated with each of these health outcomes at the state level. Higher political participation by women was correlated with lower female mortality rates ($r = -0.51$), as well as lower activity limitations (-0.47). A smaller wage gap between women and men was associated with lower female mortality rates (-0.30) and lower activity limitations (-0.31) (all correlations, $P < 0.05$). Indices of women's status were also strongly correlated with male mortality rates, suggesting that women's status may reflect more general underlying structural processes associated with material deprivation and income inequality. However, the indices of women's status persisted in predicting female mortality and morbidity rates after adjusting for income inequality, poverty rates and median household income. Associations were observed for specific causes of death, including stroke, cervical cancer and homicide. We conclude that women experience higher mortality and morbidity in states where they have lower levels of political participation and economic autonomy. Living in such states has detrimental consequences for the health of men as well.

Gender inequality and truncated opportunities for women may be one of the pathways by which the maldistribution of income adversely affects the health of women.
© 1998 Elsevier Science Ltd. All rights reserved.

1. Introduction

Researchers have employed a variety of theoretical 'lenses' through which to view and analyze gender differences in health (Walsh et al., 1995). At the most micro level, the biomedical 'lens' seeks to explain gender differences in health in terms of genetic, hormonal, anatomic or physiological differences between men and women. The biomedical model may be contrasted with the psychosocial 'lens' which focuses on variables at the intrapsychic and interpersonal levels, including sex differences in personality, coping behaviors, self-efficacy and the experience and reporting of signs and symptoms. Further up the levels of conceptual organization, the epidemiologic 'lens' seeks to identify population patterns of 'risk factors' — behaviors and exposures — that might help to explain gender differences in health. Finally, at the most macro level of analysis, Walsh et al. (1995) have proposed the so-called 'society-and-health lens', which attempts to analyze the large-scale cultural, social, economic and political processes in society that produce differential health risks in women and men. What is distinctive about this perspective is its emphasis on how health outcomes 'are ordained and constrained by crucial mechanisms of social control and distribution of resources and power. Current epidemiological research on gender and health takes for granted a social-stratification system that allocates resources and power on the basis of gender-determined social roles and leaves the underlying social processes unidentified, unquestioned and unexplored' (Walsh Chapman et al., 1995, p.149).

According to Connell (1987), two fundamental social processes that explain and constrain the relationships between women and men are the division of labour and structures of power. The division of labour includes, among other facts, the segregation of labour markets and the associated inequalities in wages, discrimination in hiring and promotion and the distinction between paid and unpaid work. Power structures refer to the machinery of authority, control and coercion. They include government and business hierarchies, the regulation and surveillance of sexuality and reproduction and the dynamics of authority within domestic relationships.

With the exception of some innovative work on the predictors of domestic violence (Yllo, 1983), relatively few attempts have been made to incorporate the 'society and health' lens into investigations of women's health. In 1983, Yllo reported an ecological analysis (based at the U.S. state level) of the relationship between gender inequality and violence against wives. Starting with the observation that battered women are often tied to violent men by economic dependency, Yllo reasoned that in states where women were more dependent, marital violence would be more frequent. To test this hypothesis, the researcher constructed four composite indices of women's status, covering their level of economic autonomy (e.g., the size of the female/male earnings gap, the percentage of women in managerial occupations); women's educational attainment; women's political participation (e.g., percent female members in Congress and state legislatures); and an index of women's legal status (e.g., equal pay laws, property rights, rape laws). According to all four indices of women's status, rates of severe marital violence against women were highest in the states where gender inequality was the greatest (Yllo, 1983). Of interest, violence by women against their husbands tended to be higher in states which accorded greater equality to women.

Despite growing interest in the characteristics of *places* as determinants of population health status (Macintyre, 1997), researchers have not attempted to examine women's status, modelled as an ecological characteristic, in relation to female (and male) mortality and morbidity rates. In 1996, the Institute for Women's Policy Research in Washington DC released a set of social indicators that benchmarked the status of women in the fifty American states (Institute for Women's Policy Research, 1996). These indicators — which measure the economic and political autonomy of women as well as their reproductive rights — provided an opportunity to test the relationship between the status of women in society and women's health through the 'society-and-health lens'.

2. Methods

2.1. Indices of women's status

The indices of women's status used in the present analysis were developed and published by the Institute for Women's Policy Research (Washington DC, 1996). Women's status was examined in four separate domains: political participation, employment and earnings, economic autonomy and reproductive rights. The *political participation composite index* combined 4 aspects of women's political status: voter registration, voter turnout, representation in elected office and women's institutional resources. Women's representation in elected office was calculated for several levels: state representatives, state senators, state-wide elected executive officials, as well as US representatives, senators and governors. The number of women officeholders in each state was weighted according to the degree of political influence of the position, e.g., state representatives were given a weight of 1.0, compared to 1.75 for US senators. Examples of women's institutional resources include the presence of state commissions on the status of women or legislative caucuses for women. To construct the composite index, each of the 4 component indicators was standardized by subtracting the mean value for all 50 states from the observed value and dividing by the standard deviation. The standardized scores were then weighted: 1.0 each for voter registration and turnout; 3.0 for women in elected office and 1.0 for women's institutional resources. The overall index score was then calculated by summing the weighted, standardized values for the 4 component indicators. The higher the index score, the higher the level of women's political participation.

The *employment and earnings composite index* combined 4 indicators of women's economic status: their earnings, the male/female wage gap, women's representation in managerial and professional jobs and women's participation in the labor force. Each of the 4 indicators was standardized by dividing the observed value (in 50 states) by the mean value for the entire USA. The resulting ratios were summed for each state to create the composite index, with each composite indicator given equal weight.

The *economic autonomy composite index* combined 4 aspects of women's economic well-being: access to health insurance, educational attainment, business ownership and percent of women above the poverty level. Educational attainment was obtained from the 1990 Census as the percent of women aged 25 yr or older with 4 or more years of college education. Again, each component was standardized and given equal weight, before summing to give the overall Index.

Finally, the *reproductive rights composite index* incorporated each state's scores on eight legislative and political indicators reflecting women's reproductive well-being and autonomy. These included access to abortion services without mandatory parental consent laws for minors, access to abortion services without a waiting period, public funding for abortions under any circumstances if a woman is eligible, percent of counties that have at least one abortion provider, whether the governor or state legislature is pro-choice, public funding of infertility treatments, existence of a maternity stay law and whether gay/lesbian couples can adopt. To construct this composite index, each component was assigned a weight ranging from 0 to 1.0 (depending on the existence of legal provisions and services), prior to summing. Further information on the data sources for each indicator, as well as the method of weighting, are reported in detail by the Institute for Women's Policy Research (1996).

2.2. Total and cause-specific mortality

State-specific, age-standardized mortality rates for women were obtained from the 1990 compressed mortality files compiled by the National Center for Health Statistics, Centers for Disease Control and Prevention (CDC). Data were obtained using the CDC WONDER/PC software (Friede et al., 1993). Age-standardized male all-cause mortality rates were obtained at the same time.

2.3. Self-reported days of activity limitations

State-specific estimates of self-reported morbidity were obtained from the behavioral risk factor surveillance system (BRFSS) conducted by the National Center for Chronic Disease Prevention and Health Promotion. The BRFSS is a state-based, random telephone survey of community-dwelling US adults aged 18 yr and over. Between 1993 and 1996, 350 000 respondents answered the quality-of-life module of the survey, which included an item on the number of days during the previous month in which poor physical or mental health kept the respondent from performing their usual activities, such as self-care, work or recreation (Centers for Disease Control and Prevention, 1994; Hennessy et al., 1994). From this survey, we calculated for each state (with the exception of Wyoming where data were unavailable), the mean number of days in the previous month during which women reported activity limitations.

2.4. Other ecologic covariates related to health status

It has been previously reported that income distribution and poverty rates are ecologic predictors of mortality rates at the US state level (Kennedy et al., 1996; Kawachi and Kennedy, 1997). Therefore, where appropriate, we adjusted for these state-specific economic characteristics when examining the relationships between indicators of women's status and health outcomes. State-specific data on income distribution were obtained from unpublished statistics courtesy of the Luxembourg Income Study (Timothy Smeeding, Project Director: personal communication). Gini coefficients in each state were calculated from disposable income, adjusted for Federal and state income and payroll taxes, as well as for cash or near-cash benefits including food stamps, the earned income tax credit (EITC) and school lunches. Adjustment for household size was accomplished using a household equivalence scale, with equivalence elasticity set at 0.5 (Atkinson et al., 1995; Kawachi and Kennedy, 1997). Data for adjusted Gini coefficients were calculated from the pooled 1991, 1992 and 1993 Current Population Surveys (Luxembourg Income Study: unpublished data).

Data on median household income and poverty rates were obtained from the 1990 US census population and housing summary tape file 3A (US Bureau of the Census, 1993). Households were classified as being above or below the poverty level based on the federal poverty index originally developed by the social security administration in 1964. The current poverty index is based purely on income from wages and does not reflect other sources of income such as non-cash benefits from food stamps, Medicaid and public housing. Poverty thresholds are updated annually to reflect changes in the consumer price index. The poverty variable we used represents the percentage of households in a given state that were below the federal poverty threshold. In 1990, this represented an income of less than $13 359 for households with 4 family members (US Bureau of the Census, 1993).

2.5. Data analysis

Ordinary least squares regression was used to examine the relationships between indicators of women's status and health outcomes. When examining the health impact of women's political participation and reproductive rights, we simultaneously adjusted for income distribution (using the adjusted Gini coefficients), median income and poverty rates. In our analyses of women's employment and earnings, we adjusted for income distribution and poverty rates, but not median income, since women's earnings was already incorporated in the composite index. In the case of women's economic autonomy, we adjusted only for income distribution, since poverty rates were already incorporated in the composite index and median income was highly collinear with educational attainment.

3. Results

3.1. Distribution of the composite indices of women's status

The political participation index ranged from a high of 8.78 (Kansas) to a low of −7.29 (Tennessee). The employment and earnings index ranged from a high of 4.63 (Alaska) to a low of 3.34 (West Virginia). The economic autonomy index ranged from a high of 4.50 (Maryland) to a low of 3.45 (Mississippi). The reproductive rights index ranged from a high of 5.25 (Hawaii) to a low of 0.03 (Nebraska). A consistent pattern was observed whereby states in the South-East (Kentucky, Virginia, West Virginia, Tennessee, Georgia, North and South Carolina, Arkansas, Georgia, Mississippi and Louisiana) showed up in the worst third of at least two out of the four composite indices. By contrast, Midwestern states (Minnesota, Wisconsin, Iowa, Kansas, Missouri) were more likely to be represented among the best third on two or more indices. The correlation among the 4 indices were high, ranging from 0.50 to 0.89, with the sole exception of the correlation between women's political participation and reproductive rights ($r = 0.24$) (Table 1).

3.2. Relationships of women's status to women's and men's health

3.2.1. Total and cause-specific mortality

The political participation composite index was strikingly correlated with female mortality rates ($r = -0.51$): the higher the level of women's political participation, the lower their mortality rates (Table 1; Fig. 1). In regression

Table 1 Correlations among composite indicators of women's status and total mortality, major causes of death and self-reported mean days of activity limitations.

	POL	EMPL	ECON	REPRO	Mortality	Disease	Stroke	Neoplasm	DAYS
POL	1.00								
EMPL	0.50*	1.00							
ECON	0.62*	0.89*	1.00						
REPRO	0.24	0.62*	0.61*	1.00					
Total Mortality	−0.51*	−0.25	−0.42*	−0.14	1.00				
Heart Disease	−0.43*	−0.24	−0.33*	−0.08	0.53*	1.00			
Stroke	−0.38*	−0.39*	−0.50*	−0.33*	0.49*	0.12	1.00		
Malignant Neoplasm	−0.07	0.18	0.03	0.11	0.65*	0.46*	−0.06	1.00	
DAYS	−0.47*	−0.43*	−0.52*	−0.27	0.39*	0.31*	0.28	0.15	1.00

* $P < 0.05$. POL: political participation composite index; EMPL: employment and earnings composite index; ECON: economic autonomy composite index; REPRO: reproductive rights composite index; DAYS: mean days of self-reported activity limitations (from the behavioral risk factor surveillance system, based on data from 49 states).

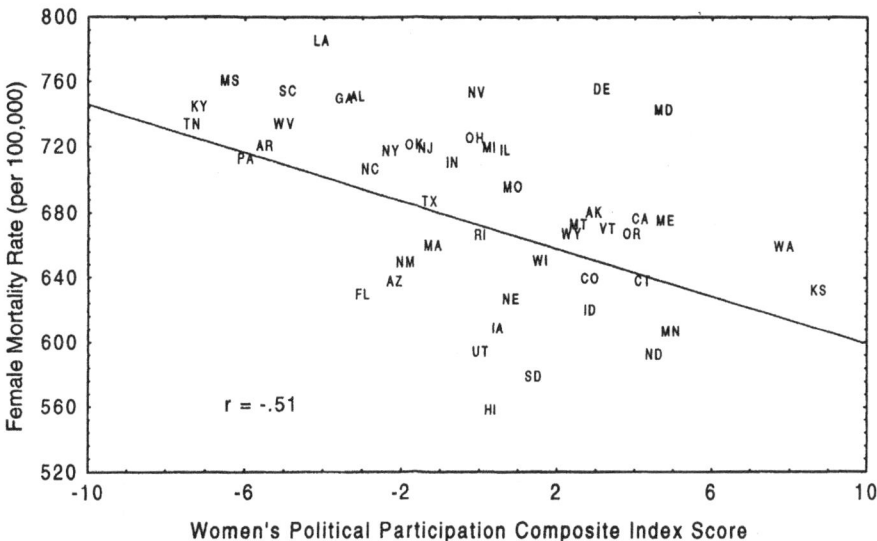

Figure 1 Women's political participation and female mortality rates.

analysis, a one unit improvement in the political participation index was associated with 7.3 fewer deaths per 100 000 women (95% confidence interval, CI: 3.8 to 10.9), equivalent to about a 11% lower age-adjusted female mortalitsy rate with each unit increase in female political participation (Table 2). In models adjusting for median income, Gini index and poverty, the political participation index remained significantly associated with overall female mortality rates ($\beta = -5.1$, s.e. = 2.1, $p = 0.02$). Interestingly, higher female political participation was also associated with lower overall mortality in men and the relationship was in fact slightly stronger than in women. A one unit increment in the political participation index was associated with 17.0 fewer age-adjusted deaths per 100 000 men (95% confidence interval, CI: 11.2 to 22.7), equivalent to about a 15% lower male mortality rate per unit increase in the index (Table 2, row 2).

Higher political participation was associated not only with lower overall female mortality, but also with certain specific causes of death (Table 2). In univariate models, higher female political participation was associated with lower rates of death from ischaemic heart disease, stroke, cervical cancer, homicide and infant mortality (where male and female infant deaths were combined). However, only the associations with ischaemic heart disease and cervical cancer mortality remained statistically significant after adjustment for median income, income inequality and poverty rates. Malignant neoplasms, breast cancer and suicide showed no association with higher political participation either before or after adjustment for income distribution and poverty rates (Table 2).

Table 2 Relationship of political participation composite index to total and cause specific mortality rates and mean days of activity limitation.

Cause of death	ICD code (9th revision)	Univariate model					Multivariate model adjusted for median income, income inequality and poverty					
		β	s.e.	adjusted R^2	$F_{1,48}$	$p <$	β	s.e.	$t, p <$	adjusted R^2	$F_{4,45}$	$p <$
Total female mortality		−7.33	1.80	0.24	16.68	0.0002	−5.09	2.15	2.36, 0.0227	0.29	6.08	0.0005
Total male mortality		−16.96	2.95	0.39	32.97	0.0000	−11.98	3.55	3.35, 0.0016	0.44	10.44	0.000
Female cause-specific mortality												
Ischaemic heart disease	410–414	−2.73	0.83	0.17	10.85	0.0019	−2.12	1.02	2.08, 0.0432	0.19	3.83	0.0092
Cerebrovascular disease	430–438	−0.75	0.27	0.12	7.87	0.0072	−0.37	0.32	1.16, 0.2535	0.18	3.69	0.0111
Malignant neoplasms	140–239	−0.27	0.53	0.00	0.26	0.6154	−0.41	0.62	0.66, 0.5119	0.1	2.38	0.0655
Breast cancer	174	−0.01	0.08	0.00	0.00	0.9572	−0.10	0.09	1.13, 0.2661	0.14	2.99	0.0285
Cervical cancer	180	−0.07	0.01	0.34	26.12	0.0001	−0.06	0.02	3.58, 0.0008	0.34	7.20	0.0001
Suicide	950–959	0.03	0.05	0.00	0.36	0.5488	−0.10	0.06	1.68, 0.1006	0.04	1.47	0.2275
Homicide	960–969	−0.20	0.05	0.24	16.31	0.0002	−0.07	0.05	1.35, 0.1848	0.49	12.97	0.0000
Infant mortality (male and female)		−0.18	0.05	0.18	11.48	0.0014	−0.11	0.06	1.70, 0.0961	0.18	3.65	0.0117
Mean days limited activity (females)		−0.05	0.01	0.21	13.62	0.0006	−0.03	0.02	1.75, 0.0871	0.25	5.05	0.002

In contrast to the political participation index, the employment and earnings composite index was statistically significantly associated with overall male mortality rates in both univariate and multivariate models, but not to female mortality rates (Table 3). Despite the lack of an association with overall female mortality, higher levels of women's employment and earnings were nonetheless significantly associated with lower mortality from specific causes after adjusting for median income, income inequality and poverty rates, including cerebrovascular disease ($p = 0.03$), cervical cancer ($p = 0.04$) and marginally to ischaemic heart disease ($p = 0.07$).

The economic autonomy composite index was strongly associated with both male and female total mortality rates, in univariate as well as multivariate models (Table 4). Once again, the association was stronger for males than for females. In multivariate models, women's economic autonomy was related to female death rates from cerebrovascular disease, cervical cancer, homicide and to infant mortality.

The reproductive rights composite index was the only index that was not associated with female total mortality, nor any specific cause of death except infant mortality (Table 5). Higher reproductive rights for women was marginally significantly ($p = 0.06$) associated with male mortality rates (Table 5, row 2), but this association did not hold up in analyses adjusting for income inequality, poverty and median income.

In sum, indices of women's political participation and economic autonomy were strikingly related to overall female and male mortality rates. For various reasons that we will discuss below, male mortality rates appeared to be even more strongly linked to indices of women's status than female mortality rates. Turning to cause-specific mortality among women, deaths from cerebrovascular disease and cervical cancer (and less consistently, heart disease, homicide and infant mortality) were associated with the status of women in both univariate and multivariate models, even in instances where the composite indices were not related to overall female mortality. Among the major causes of death, breast cancer was unrelated to any of the indices of women's status, even indicating a weak positive relationship to the index of women's economic autonomy ($p = 0.09$, Table 4).

3.2.2. Self-reported mean days of activity limitations among women

Three of the 4 indices of women's status were significantly and inversely correlated with the mean number of days of activity limitations reported by women residing in the fifty states: political participation ($r = -0.47$); employment and earnings ($r = -0.43$) and economic autonomy ($r = -0.52$) (Table 1). In regression models, women's political participation was only marginally related to activity limitation ($p = 0.09$) after adjusting for median income, inequality and poverty (Table 2, bottom row). On the other hand, two of the composite indices — employment and earnings (Table 3) and

Table 3 Relationship of employment and earnings composite index to total and cause specific mortality rates and mean days of activity limitation.

Cause of death	ICD code (9th revision)	Univariate model					Multivariate model adjusted for income inequality and poverty					
		β	s.e.	adjusted R^2	$F_{1,48}$	$p <$	β	s.e.	$t, p <$	adjusted R^2	$F_{3,46}$	$p <$
Total female mortality		−46.98	26.12	0.04	3.23	0.0783	−36.87	31.69	1.16, 0.2507	0.24	6.16	0.0013
Total male mortality		−143.16	45.04	0.16	10.53	0.002	−119.99	53.17	2.26, 0.0288	0.37	10.61	0.0000
Female cause ± specific mortality												
Ischaemic heart disease	410–414	−19.55	11.57	0.04	2.85	0.0976	−27.13	14.53	1.87, 0.0682	0.18	4.60	0.0067
Cerebrovascular disease	430–438	−10.03	3.45	0.13	8.44	0.0055	−10.16	4.53	2.25, 0.0295	0.19	4.95	0.0046
Malignant neoplasms	140–239	8.79	6.75	0.01	1.70	0.1988	1.12	8.84	0.13, 0.8997	0.09	2.57	0.0654
Breast cancer	174	1.28	1.02	0.01	1.58	0.2144	−1.32	1.28	1.03, 0.3067	0.15	3.93	0.014
Cervical cancer	180	−0.50	0.21	0.09	5.59	0.0222	−0.56	0.26	2.14, 0.0379	0.24	6.14	0.0013
Suicide	950–959	−0.31	0.67	0.00	0.21	0.6450	0.66	0.90	0.73, 0.4693	0.00	0.91	0.4451
Homicide	960–969	−1.07	0.72	0.02	2.17	0.1473	0.51	0.73	0.70, 0.4905	0.47	15.2	0.0000
Infant mortality (male and female)		−1.75	0.70	0.10	6.26	0.0158	−1.36	0.90	1.50, 0.1397	0.18	4.66	0.0063
Mean days limited activity		−0.54	0.17	0.17	10.56	0.0021	−0.49	0.22	2.24, 0.0299	0.26	6.70	0.0008

Table 4 Relationship of economic autonomy composite index to total and cause specific mortality rates and mean days of activity limitation.

Cause of death	ICD code (9th revision)	Univariate model					Multivariate model adjusted for income inequality					
		β	s.e.	adjusted R^2	$F_{1,48}$	$p <$	β	s.e.	$t, p <$	adjusted R^2	$F_{2,47}$	$p <$
Total female mortality		−82.58	25.55	0.16	10.45	0.0022	−54.55	25.11	2.17, 0.0349	0.29	11.11	0.0001
Total male mortality		−217.39	41.40	0.35	27.57	0.0000	−170.87	40.49	4.22, 0.0001	0.46	21.72	0.0000
Female cause-specific mortality												
Ischaemic heart disease	410–414	−28.19	11.76	0.09	5.75	0.0204	−17.69	11.96	1.47, 0.1458	0.18	6.22	0.0040
Cerebrovascular disease	430–438	−13.56	3.38	0.24	16.06	0.0002	−11.63	3.57	3.25, 0.0021	0.26	9.41	0.0003
Malignant neoplasms	140–239	1.42	7.17	0.00	0.03	0.8432	−6.22	9.29	0.67, 0.5067	0.06	2.66	0.0801
Breast cancer	174	1.57	1.05	0.02	2.22	0.1427	1.93	1.13	1.71, 0.0938	0.02	1.51	0.2311
Cervical cancer	180	−0.71	0.21	0.18	11.52	0.0014	−0.51	0.21	2.43, 0.0187	0.26	9.80	0.0003
Suicide	950–959	−0.35	0.69	0.00	0.25	0.6187	−0.29	0.75	0.38, 0.7002	0.00	0.14	0.8647
Homicide	960–969	−2.44	0.69	0.19	12.56	0.0009	−1.37	0.60	2.28, 0.0272	0.46	21.98	0.0000
Infant mortality (male and female)		−2.63	0.68	0.22	15.03	0.0003	−2.17	0.17	3.06, 0.0037	0.26	9.59	0.0003
Mean days limited activity		−0.68	0.16	0.26	17.84	0.0001	−0.56	0.17	3.35, 0.0016	0.31	11.56	0.0000

Table 5 Relationship of reproductive rights composite index to total and cause specific mortality rates, and mean days of activity limitation.

Cause of death	ICD code (9th revision)	Univariate model					Multivariate model adjusted for income inequality, poverty, median income					
		β	s.e.	adjusted R^2	$F_{1,48}$	$p <$	β	s.e.	$t, p <$	adjusted R^2	$F_{4,45}$	$p <$
Total female mortality		5.97	5.92	0.00	1.01	0.3188	−6.53	6.59	0.99, 0.3278	0.22	4.51	0.0038
Total male mortality		−20.61	10.63	0.05	3.75	0.0585	−11.84	11.44	1.03, 0.3065	0.31	6.52	0.0003
Female cause-specific mortality												
Ischaemic heart disease	410–414	−1.38	2.64	0.00	0.27	0.6033	0.21	3.11	0.07, 0.9452	0.11	2.51	0.0552
Cerebrovascular disease	430–438	−1.89	0.78	0.09	5.79	0.0199	−1.00	0.94	1.06, 0.2926	0.18	3.62	0.0121
Malignant neoplasms	140–239	1.16	1.52	0.00	0.59	0.4461	−0.89	1.81	0.49, 0.6235	0.10	2.32	0.0709
Breast cancer	174	0.08	0.23	0.00	0.11	0.7374	−0.18	0.27	0.69, 0.4952	0.12	2.74	0.0398
Cervical cancer	180	−0.07	0.05	0.03	2.39	0.1282	−0.07	0.06	1.23, 0.2235	0.18	3.60	0.0124
Suicide	950–959	−0.16	0.15	0.00	1.23	0.2728	−0.04	0.19	0.19, 0.8502	0.00	0.73	0.5757
Homicide	960–969	−0.18	0.16	0.00	1.23	0.2733	−0.17	0.15	1.17, 0.2462	0.49	12.75	0.0000
Infant mortality (male and female)		−0.37	0.16	0.10	5.84	0.0195	−0.39	0.18	2.08, 0.0431	0.20	4.10	0.0064
Means days limited activity		−0.07	0.04	0.05	3.55	0.0657	−0.03	0.05	0.71, 0.4817	0.12	3.19	0.0325

economic autonomy (Table 4; Fig. 2) — remained strongly associated with fewer days of activity limitations among women, even in multivariate models. No relationship was observed between reproductive rights and activity limitations (Table 5).

3.2.3. Relationships of individual component indicators of women's status to women's health

Given the strength of the associations found between composite indices of women's status and the health of both men and women, we proceeded to examine the relationships with the individual, component indicators that made up each index of women's status (Table 6). Of the 4 indicators that make up the political participation composite index, the percentage of women who voted in each state had the strongest inverse relationship to female mortality rates ($r = -0.54$), followed by women's representation in elected office ($r = -0.38$) and the percent women registered to vote ($r = -0.35$). Among the 4 indicators that make up the employment and earnings composite index, the percent of women in the labor force ($r = -0.55$) and the female/male earnings ratio ($r = -0.30$) showed the strongest relationships to mortality. All 4 indicators that make up the economic autonomy composite index were about equally correlated with female mortality rates (Table 6). In all, 8 of the 12 component indicators of women's status were statistically significantly correlated ($p < 0.05$) with women's reported mean days of activity limitation (Table 6).

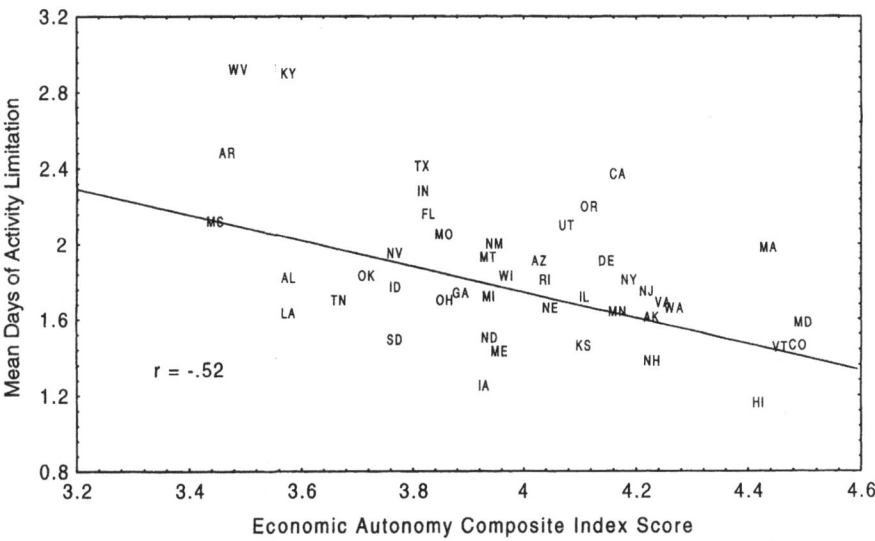

Figure 2 Women's economic autonomy and mean number of days of self-reported activity limitation.

Table 6 Correlations between component indicators of women's status and mortality rates and activity limitations.

Component indicators	Female mortality rates	Male mortality rates	White female mortality	Black female mortality	Mean days of activity limitations (females)	Mean days of activity limitations (males)
Political participation composite index						
Women in elected office	−0.38*	−0.55*	−0.26	−0.33*	−0.34*	−0.35*
Percent women registered to vote in 1992/94	−0.35*	−0.26	−0.42*	−0.18	−0.39*	−0.29*
Percent women who voted in 1992/94	−0.54*	−0.56*	−0.53*	−0.20	−0.49*	−0.47*
Number of institutional resources available to women	0.16	0.10	0.18	0.13	0.13	−0.01
Employment and earnings composite index						
Median annual earnings for full-time women	0.02	−0.19	0.10	−0.01	−0.23	−0.21
Earnings ratio between women and men	−0.30*	−0.29*	−0.28*	−0.25	−0.31*	−0.14
Percent women in labor force	−0.55*	−0.54*	−0.55*	−0.09	−0.55*	−0.44*
Percent women in managerial or professional occupations	−0.12	−0.31*	−0.05	−0.16	−0.27	−0.22
Economic autonomy composite index						
Percent women with 4 or more years of college	−0.33*	−0.49*	−0.29*	−0.20	−0.50*	−0.38*
Percent women without health insurance	0.36*	0.39*	0.30*	0.13	0.37*	0.37*
Percent women in poverty	0.39*	0.55*	0.26	0.14	0.45*	0.48*
Percent of businesses owned by women	−0.31*	−0.50*	−0.19	−0.26	−0.21	−0.27

* $P < 0.05$.

3.2.4. Relationships of women's status indicators to men's health

At the state level, female mortality rates were extremely tightly correlated with male mortality rates ($r = 0.93$). As a result, predictors of female mortality rates could be expected to correlate with male mortality rates. As described above, 3 of the 4 composite indicators of women's status also predicted male mortality rates. The correlations were -0.64 for political participation, -0.60 for women's economic autonomy, -0.42 for employment and earnings and -0.27 for reproductive rights. These correlations may partly reflect the fact that gender inequalities are manifestations of *general* inequalities. For example, the indices for female political participation and economic autonomy were both correlated ($r = -0.49$ and -0.36, respectively) with the Gini coefficient of income inequality (although neither the index of women's employment and earnings ($r = -0.14$) nor reproductive rights ($r = -0.08$) were correlated with the Gini index).

In turn, income inequality has been previously demonstrated to be strongly correlated with both male and female mortality rates at the cross-country (Wilkinson, 1992; Wilkinson, 1996) and cross-regional level (Kaplan et al., 1996; Kennedy et al., 1996). Thus, measures of gender inequality may be confounded by more general processes (such as income inequality) or alternatively, truncated opportunities for women may be a potential pathway through which income inequality produces adverse health effects for both sexes. Both types of effects are plausible and given the tight correlation between male and female mortality rates at the state level, our analyses could not distinguish between the two.

In multivariate regression models adjusting for income inequality, indices of women's political participation, employment and earnings and economic autonomy continued to predict overall male mortality rates. The strength of these associations were undiminished when we examined the *difference* in male/female mortality rates across states: where women's status was low, women's mortality rates were higher, but male mortality rates tended to be even higher, so that the difference in male/female mortality rates were, if anything, even greater.

In contrast to mortality rates (where males have higher rates), morbidity rates are almost always higher in women. The zero-order correlations between indices of women's status and reported days of activity limitations among men were -0.49 for political participation, -0.34 for employment and earnings, -0.46 for economic autonomy and -0.20 for reproductive rights. However, in contrast to mortality, none of the indices of women's status predicted male activity limitations in multivariate regression models after adjusting for income inequality, poverty rates and median income, whereas they continued to predict women's activity limitations. Close examination of the individual component indicators of women's status (Table 6) similarly indicates that the associations are generally stronger for activity limitations among women than among men.

3.3. Women's status and mortality among white women versus black women

As can be seen on Figs. 1 and 2, the Southern states in the USA tend to score poorly in terms of indices of women's status. These also tend to be the states where more African-Americans live and hence our findings could reflect confounding by other processes such as the effects of racial discrimination on health (Kennedy et al., 1997). However, when we separately examined the relationships of women's status to mortality rates among white women and African-American women, we found that whereas the component indicators were consistently related to mortality rates among the former, none of them (with the exception of % women elected to political office) were related to mortality rates among black women (Table 6). Such a pattern suggests that confounding by racism is unlikely to explain our principal findings. The lack of association with black women's mortality may reflect the aggregated nature of our composite indices, i.e., the results may have been different if indicators had been developed specifically to reflect African-American women's status.

There were too few African-American women in the behavioral risk factor surveillance system to derive stable state-specific estimates of the mean days of activity limitations in this group.

4. Discussion

Public health has increasingly recognized that women's unequal status in society jeopardizes their health and well-being (Cook, 1994; Fee and Krieger, 1994; Doyal, 1995). The 1994 Cairo Conference on Population and Development expanded the conceptual framework of women's health to encompass previously unacknowledged components of health, including socioeconomic inequality, women's empowerment, unequal burdens of domestic labour, constraints on women to determine their own sexuality and reproduction, political participation, literacy and the epidemic of male violence against women (United Nations, 1994). In seeking to uncover the societal level determinants of women's health, the present study examined four composite indices of women's status: women's political participation, employment and earnings, economic autonomy and reproductive rights. Indicators of women's status in society turned out to be closely linked to female total and cause-specific mortality (with breast cancer, all malignant neoplasms and suicide being notable exceptions), as well as to morbidity.

4.1. Women's status predicts men's health

A noteworthy finding of our study was that indices of women's status also strongly predicted male mortality rates (though not male activity limitations).

A possible interpretation of these results is that states with greater gender inequality are also more unequal in general, thereby raising both male and female mortality rates. For example, high poverty rates among women may be correlated with (and hence act as a proxy for) high prevalence of poverty among men, so that female poverty rates end up predicting both male and female mortality rates. Alternatively, it is possible that indices of women's status are confounded by other ecologic variables that are detrimental to the health of both sexes — such as the degree of inequality in household incomes — which have been shown previously to explain variations in health status across states (Kaplan et al., 1996; Kennedy et al., 1996), as well as between countries (Wilkinson, 1992, 1996). We attempted to overcome this potential confounding by adjusting for known ecologic predictors of mortality, including the Gini index of household income, percent of households under the poverty threshold and median household income. Nevertheless, indices of women's status continued to predict both male and female mortality rates in multivariate regression models. The processes by which patriarchy and unequal status for women might spill over into worse health status for men therefore need to be further explored.

One mechanism for the association between women's status and male mortality is the fact that factors which adversely affect women's economic security also affect the material wellbeing of male members of the households to which women belong: including spouses, partners, sons and fathers. Some of the indicators of women's status examined in the present analysis — for example, women's labor force participation and median earnings — could potentially affect the wellbeing of both men and women. Since dual earners characterized 70 percent of married-couple families in 1994 (Institute for Women's Policy Research, 1996), women's labor force participation and earnings could directly influence the economic well-being (and thereby the health status) of such families, including any male members.

In contrast to total mortality, our analyses of activity limitations yielded more unambiguous associations with between women's status and women's health. Greater economic autonomy, as well as employment and earnings among women were strongly associated with less activity limitations in women but not in men.

4.2. The societal costs of gender inequality

Discussions of patriarchy have tended to focus on the subordination of women by men, where the latter are assumed to benefit from such arrangements. Thus: "the material base of patriarchy is men's control over women's labor power. That control is maintained by excluding women from access to necessary economically productive resources and by restricting women's sexuality. Men exercise their control in receiving personal service work from women, in not having to do housework or rear children, in having access to women's bodies for sex and in feeling powerful and being powerful" (Hartmann, 1994, p. 572). While none could deny that men benefit from patriarchal arrangements in all the manners described, an overlooked feature of patriarchy is the costs of such a system for society as a whole. Hartmann (1994) has argued that it is crucial to examine hierarchy *among* men and their differential access to patriarchal benefits. Thus, certain types of gender inequality, such as reduced female earnings, are themselves patterned by class, race and other socioeconomic characteristics. In other words, the ill health burden of gender inequality is disproportionately borne by women — and men — with preexisting socioeconomic disadvantage. As well, women of different class, race, martial status or sexual orientation are subjected to different degrees of patriarchal power. Women may themselves exercise class, race or national power, or even patriarchal power (through their family connections) over men lower in the patriarchal hierarchy than their own male kin (Hartmann, 1994). Men's exploitation of women may be most evident when patriarchal systems are observed at the level of individual relationships, e.g., within domestic settings. But when society itself becomes the focus of analysis, the costs of patriarchy are no longer borne solely by women. Considered as a whole, a society that tolerates gender inequalities is also likely to be a more unhealthy place to live for both men and women, compared to a more egalitarian one. To paraphrase the Beijing Declaration and Platform for Action, the well-being of a society depends upon women's economic and political status within that society (United Nations, 1995).

4.3. Limitations

A number of important limitations should be noted about our analyses. The cross-sectional and ecologic nature of the data limits our ability to make causal inferences and to draw inferences about individuals. For instance, we were unable to exclude the possibility of reverse causation, i.e., that higher geographic concentrations of unhealthy women result in diminished economic autonomy and political participation in those areas. Ecologic analyses similarly do not permit us to say whether *individual* women with diminished economic autonomy suffer from increased mortality or disability risks. Statements of this type involve the risk of committing the ecologic fallacy. Our findings would have been strengthened if data were available on the health of individual women residing in different states. Such data would help to identify which subgroups of women (and perhaps men) — defined by class, age or race/ethnicity — are most vulnerable to the risks of ill health imposed by gender inequality. Ecologic analyses of the type presented here only permit us to observe that more unequal states are unhealthier in general compared to more egalitarian places. A further caveat regarding the interpretation of our data is the possibility that some as yet unidentified, omitted variables could have confounded the observed relationship between indicators of women's status and women's health. Although we attempted to adjust for some of the major predictors of population health status, we lacked data on some variables (e.g., household division of labour and economic resources), while still other variables (e.g., patriarchal culture) remain poorly conceptualized.

Most of the economic indicators of women's status (e.g., median earnings, female:male earnings ratio, poverty level and educational attainment) were obtained from the 1990 Census of Population (Institute for Women's Policy Research, 1996). However, other indicators, such as those related to women's political participation, were based on data collected from 1993 onwards, so that strictly speaking, they post-dated our mortality data (which were from 1990), though not our morbidity data (which were obtained between 1993 and 1996). Given the varying timing of the data assembled in our analyses, we have had to assume that there was sufficient stability in the rankings of states vis à vis women's political circumstances reaching back in time. This assumption may not be warranted, since certain indicators such as legislation affecting women's reproductive rights, may change over a relatively short span of time. Additionally, we have not taken account of induction times between the start of exposure to a particular social environment and specific health outcomes. For instance, mortality from cardiovascular diseases (heart attack and stroke), homicide and infant mortality may respond more quickly to changes in the social milieu than other causes of death such as neoplasms. The finding in the present study of a relationship between women's status and mortality from cervical cancer was notable in that the disease possibly reflects the extent of women's control over sexual relationships (e.g., negotiating around use of barrier contraceptive methods). If the finding on cervical cancer is real, then this would suggest to us that the indices of women's status reflect stable, long-term processes.

Finally, analyses of the type presented here need to be repeated and tested for a much fuller set of health outcomes, including domestic violence, mental health, functional status, health behaviors and other measures that capture women's health experience across the life course.

5. Conclusion

Despite the limitations mentioned, the present study has demonstrated the potential utility of extending studies of gender inequality and women's health to the societal (ecologic) domain. Geographic and political units even within a single country vary in the level of status accorded to women, in ways that have measurable consequences for the health of women (and men). Women's health and the formulation of effective strategies for improving women's status must thus be a central concern not only in feminist politics, but in broader campaigns for public health and social justice.

Acknowledgements

Kawachi and Kennedy are recipients of the Robert Wood Johnson Investigator Awards in Health Policy Research.

References

Atkinson, A. B., Rainwater, L., Smeeding, T. M., 1995. Income Distribution in OECD Countries. Evidence from the Luxembourg Income Study. Organization for Economic Co-operation and Development, Paris.

Centers for Disease Control and Prevention, 1994. Quality of life as a new public health measure — Behavioral risk factor surveillance system, 1993. MMWR 43 (20), 375–380.

Connell, R. W., 1987. Gender and Power. Stanford University Press, Stanford, CA.

Cook, R. J., 1994. Women's Health and Human Rights. World Health Organization, Geneva.

Doyal, L., 1995. What Makes Women Sick: Gender and the Political Economy of Health. Rutgers University Press, New Jersey.

Fee, E., Krieger, N. (Eds.). 1994. Women's Health, Politics, and Power. Baywood Publishing Co., New York.

Friede, A., Reid, J. A., Ory, H. W., 1993. CDC WONDER: a comprehensive on-line public health information system of the centers for disease control and prevention. Am. J. Public Health 83, 1289–1294.

Hartmann, H., 1994. The unhappy marriage of Marxism and feminism: towards a more progressive union. In: Grusky, D. B. (Ed.), Social Stratification in Sociological Perspective, westview Press, Boulder, CO, pp. 570–576.

Hennessy, C. H., Moriarty, D. G., Zack, M. M., Scherr, P. A., Brackbill, R., 1994. Measuring health-related quality of life for public health surveillance. Public Health Rep. 109, 665–672.

Institute for Women's Policy Research, 1996. The Status of Women in the States. Institute for Women's Policy Research (Library of Congress Card Catalogue Number 96-79874), Washington, DC.

Kaplan, G., Pamuk, E., Lynch, J. W., Cohen, R. D., Balfour, J. L., 1996. Inequality in income and mortality in the United States: analysis of mortality and potential pathways. BMJ 312, 999–1003.

Kawachi, I., Kennedy, B. P., 1997. The relationship of income inequality to mortality — Does the choice of indicator matter? Soc. Sci. Med. 45, 1121–1127.

Kennedy, B. P., Kawachi, I., Prothrow-Stith, D., 1996. Income distribution and mortality: cross sectional ecological study of the Robin Hood Index in the United States. BMJ 312, 1004–1007.

Kennedy, B. P., Kawachi, I., Lochner, K., Jones, C. P., Prothrow-Stith, D., 1997. (Dis)respect and black mortality. Ethnic. Disease 7, 207–214.

Macintyre, S., 1997. The black report and beyond: what are the issues? Soc. Sci. Med. 44 (6), 723–745.

United Nations, 1994. Programme of Action of the International Conference on Population and Development, Cairo. United Nations, New York, NY.

United Nations, 1995. Report of the Fourth World Conference on Women, Beijing Declaration and Platform for Action. United Nations, New York, NY.

US Bureau of the Census (1993). CD-ROM, income and poverty. US Bureau of the Census, Washington, DC.
Walsh, D., Sorensen, G., Leonard, L., 1995. Gender, health, and cigarette smoking. In: Amick III, B. C., Levine, S., Tarlov, A. R., Chapman Walsh, D. (Eds.), Society and Health. Oxford University Press, Oxford.
Wilkinson, R. G., 1992. Income distribution and life expectancy. Br. Med. J. 304, 165–168.
Wilkinson, R. G., 1996. Unhealthy Societies. The Afflictions of Inequality. Routledge, London.
Yllo, K. (1983). Sexual equality and violence against wives in American states. J. Comp. Fam. Stud. XIV, No. 1 (Spring), 67–68.

16

GENDER EQUITY AND SOCIOECONOMIC INEQUALITY
A framework for the patterning of women's health

Nancy E. Moss

Source: *Social Science & Medicine*, 54 (2002), 649–61.

Abstract

This paper explores the interrelationship of gender equity and socioeconomic inequality and how they affect women's health at the macro- (country) and micro- (household and individual) levels. An integrated framework draws theoretical perspectives from both approaches and from public health. Determinants of women's health in the geopolitical environment include country-specific history and geography, policies and services, legal rights, organizations and institutions, and structures that shape gender and economic inequality. Culture, norms and sanctions at the country and community level, and sociodemographic characteristics at the individual level, influence women's productive and reproductive roles in the household and workplace. Social capital, roles, psychosocial stresses and resources, health services, and behaviors mediate social, economic and cultural effects on health outcomes. Inequality between and within households contributes to the patterning of women's health. Within the framework, relationships may vary depending upon women's lifestage and cohort experience. Examples of other relevant theoretical frameworks are discussed. The conclusion suggests strategies to improve data, influence policy, and extend research to better understand the effect of gender and socioeconomic inequality on women's health.
© 2002 Elsevier Science Ltd. All rights reserved.

Introduction

Gender equity and socioeconomic inequality represent two different paradigms for understanding women's health and well-being. They often draw their sources from different disciplines: gender equity from the law, political sciences, development economics and the humanities; and socioeconomic inequality from economics; sociology, epidemiology and public health.

This paper develops a unified model that brings gender equity and socioeconomic inequality together in a common framework. A comprehensive framework should improve our understanding of the social and economic patterning of women's health outcomes and offer new directions for research, interventions, and policy. A criterion for a unified approach is that it should be relevant to women across cultures and nations, while allowing for country-to-country and culturally specific fine-tuning. The advantage is that researchers can learn something from the gender equity approaches developed particularly for women in less industrialized southern countries, while northern researchers can contribute insights from research on socioeconomic inequalities in health among higher income nations.

Socioeconomic inequality

Despite unprecedented prosperity in the US, the tentative extension of democratization to many countries worldwide, and rapid economic development of some countries, the gaps in income between the poorest and the richest individuals and countries continue to widen (Smeeding & Gottschalk, 1995). In 1960, 20% of the world's people had 30 times the income of the poorest 20%. In 1997, the figure was 74 times as much (United Nations Development Program (UNDP), 1999). Countries such as Russia, China, Indonesia, and Thailand that had achieved more equitable income distribution prior to the early 1980s have seen a marked growth in income inequality along with their emerging market economies (UNDP, 1999). The UK, US, and Sweden also experienced rapid growth in income inequality in the 1980s and 1990s. Among industrialized nations, Sweden moved from having one of the most equal income distributions to being one of the most unequal. During the 1980s and early 1990s there continued to be large earnings inequalities between men and women in the Western industrialized nations (Gottschalk & Smeeding, 1997).

The growth of income inequality has been accompanied, in European countries and the US, by an increase in the number of families living in poverty, which grew during the 1980s by 60% in the UK, and by nearly 40% in the Netherlands. In Australia, the UK, the US, and Canada, more than half of single-parent households with children have incomes below the poverty level; in the vast majority of cases, these single parents are women (UNDP, 1999).

Worldwide, the number of people living on less than $1 a day is increasing and was projected to reach 1.5 billion by the end of 1999 as a result of the economic crisis in Asia and its aftermath. It is now acknowledged that the international lenders' structural adjustment policies of the 1980s contributed to worsening hardship and inequality among debtor nations (Lewis, 1999;

Science and technology, 1995; Dahlgren, 1990). Because structural adjustment usually imposed user fees on health services, schools, and transportation, among other services, the burden often fell disproportionately on women. As the World Bank's policies have been forced to change, gender equity has become a cornerstone of the Bank's recent anti-poverty strategy (World Bank, 2000).

Impoverishment in southern nations and unequal development in industrialized countries contrasts, according to the UNDP, with "the staggering concentration of wealth among the ultra-rich" (UNDP, 1999, p. 37) and with an increasing fascination with celebrity culture, money and greed among the high income nations (Rich, 1999; Frank, 1999). It is against this background that we turn to a discussion of gender equity and its intersection with socioeconomic inequality as they affect women's health.

Gender equity

In contrast to the dismal picture of international trends in income inequality in the 1990s, the adoption of a gender perspective in health and development research and programs and new legal frameworks for protecting women's rights were major advances of the past decade. The Platform for Action of the Fourth World Conference on Women in Beijing (1995) emphasized a wholistic and life-cycle approach to women's health. In addition to tackling the problems caused by harmful social and economic policies, the Platform targets the discrimination and gender inequalities that underlie women's health. The foundations for the Beijing Platform were laid at the International Conference on Population and Development that took place in Cairo in September, 1994, addressing women's right to control all aspects of their health and affirming the equality of the relationship between women and men in sexual relations and reproduction (UNFPA, 1999). The Convention for the Elimination of All Forms of Discrimination Against Women (CEDAW) provides a legal framework for the promotion of gender equity in health and reproduction, as well as in social and economic life (Sullivan, 1995). As of 1999, virtually all nations had ratified CEDAW, the major exceptions being Afghanistan and the United States (UNDP, 1999).

Gender equity and economic structures are closely linked. Gender equity has been promoted by the international development organizations (e.g., the World Bank) because it is positively associated with lower fertility and better health for women and children as well as with economic development (Barrett, 1995; Razavi, 1997; World Bank, 1998). A literature with theoretical origins in neo-classical economics has focused especially on male–female equity in intrahousehold decision-making and allocation of resources, and on the economic and social benefits of education for girls and women as a form of human capital investment (World Bank, 1994).

In this approach, intra-household processes involving the exchange of resources among men and women are assumed to affect nutrition, reproductive decision-making and health (Dollar & Gatti, 1999). It singles out the balance of power, fairness and justice of gender relationships, as an analytic criterion on a par with social and economic equity. But gender equity and socioeconomic equality are not synonymous. UN data suggest that gender equity is somewhat independent of economic inequality, at least at the country level (UNDP, 1999).[1]

Socioeconomic inequalities and health

One reason for the recent interest in socioeconomic determinants of women's health is the recognition that the two decades between 1973 and 1993 were a period of striking growth in income and wealth inequality in the US and other developed nations (Karoly, 1996; Wolff, 1995), paralleled by increasing socioeconomic disparities in health. The increases in income inequality are attributable to a number of causes, including increases in differential wage rates for more and less skilled workers, devolution of publicly funded social services or "structural adjustment", tax policies favoring the rich, and the decline of labor unions. The increased proportion of female-headed households and the concentration of females' earnings gains in higher-income households also contributed to overall inequality (Karoly & Burtless, 1995). A number of recent studies in the US and in Europe have shown that growing income and wealth inequality is associated with widening differentials in mortality (although estimates of the impact on women have varied) (Wilkinson, 1996). A widely cited study found that from 1960 to 1986 the death rates in the US for blacks and whites and for men and women showed an overall decline, but the difference in mortality rates between those in higher and lower income and education categories actually increased. By 1986 there was actually a greater disparity between mortality rates of women in the higher and lower educational categories than there had been in 1960 (Pappas, Queen, Hadden, & Fisher, 1993).

At the aggregate level, there is a relationship between how income is distributed in the population (percent of income going to a particular segment of the population) and life expectancy, such that countries or regions where a larger share of income goes to the less well-off have higher life expectancy than countries or regions where income distribution is skewed to the better-off. Countries with a more equitable income distribution (such as Japan) enjoy higher life expectancy. The fact that it may be relative rather than absolute aspects of income that affect people suggests a strong psychosocial component (Wilkinson, 1992; Haan, Kaplan, & Syme, 1989). In other words, it may not be occupation and its rewards, per se, that determine health, but job characteristics (e.g., job strain—low control, high demands), limited psychological and social resources, perceived hostility and discrimination, lifestyle "incongruity", and related frustration. The literature is well-summarized in Krieger, Rowley, Herman, Avery, and Phillips (1993) and Wilkinson (1996). In formerly Communist states such as Russia, Czechoslovakia, and Hungary, social disintegration and dramatic income polarity have led to decreased life expectancy, more so for men than for women (UNDP, 1999, pp. 79, 85).

Significantly, the association of societal and state level income inequality with mortality appears to be independent of the proportion of the population engaged in risk behaviors such as smoking, and of access to health services. In other words, something in the nature of inequality itself appears responsible for socioeconomic differences in mortality patterns (Wilkinson, 1996; Kennedy, Kawachi, & Prothrow-Stith, 1996; Kaplan, Pamuk, Lynch, Cohen, & Balfour, 1996). Despite the burgeoning literature examining how gender roles interact with socioeconomic position, the extent to which societal patterns of gender equity condition the impact of economic inequality on women's (or men's) health is unknown.

Social capital as a bridge among inequity, inequality, and health

Recognizing how inequality and disparities among gender and income (as well as ethnic) groups create a burden of psychosocial, functional, and health risks, brings us to the threads of human life that create and support well-being. These threads, woven into a cloth that we call social capital, include kin and community ties and social networks (Wilkinson, 1996; Coleman, 1988). As defined by Coleman (1988), social capital is a resource inherent in the relationship among people or among organizations. Mark Granovetter, an American sociologist, wrote

> ... the analysis of processes in interpersonal networks provides the most fruitful micro–macro bridge. In one way or another, it is through these networks that small-scale interaction becomes translated into large-scale patterns, and that these, in turn, feed back into small groups.
> (Granovetter, 1973, p. 1360)

It is through interpersonal and inter-group behaviors, and the extent to which they augment or diminish personal resources and well-being, that macro-level events may have their effects at the individual level (Kawachi, 1999; Kawachi, Kennedy, & Glass, 1999). Social capital refers to the resources people experience in their everyday interactions, and thus helps to connect the quality and experience of everyday life with the more abstract experience of aggregate events. Women's interpretation, judgment and experience of events differ from men's (Gilligan, 1982); their experience of the "micro–macro bridge" may differ also.

A comprehensive model of socioeconomic inequalities and gender equity

Epidemiologists and demographers have only recently begun to consider the processes within households and in women's daily lives that may actually shape their health, or the health of men. Conversely, development economists, researchers and advocates concerned with gender equity are often focused on intra-household processes or women's status in the community, but may pay less attention to socioeconomic inequality as one of the driving engines that ends in women's disadvantage (Schultz, 1997). The World Bank's prioritization of global poverty reduction has been motivated partly by the drastic effects of the structural adjustment policies of the 1980s (World Bank, 2000). While attention to household and community may provide effective guidance for planning programs and services for women, it is by stepping back to the geopolitical context that we can most effectively create and target policies that diminish gender inequality and promote health (Östlin, Sen, & George, 2001). Ideologies of power, economic reward and exchange, and gender roles and relations are expressed through macro- and micro-level institutions and behaviors. Recent research has demonstrated how variations in economic and social policy contribute to household decisions, role patterns, and health (Khlat, Sermet, & Le Pape, 2000; Lahelma, Arber, Kivelä, & Roos, 2001).

Explicating how socioeconomic and gender inequality affect women's health demands a comprehensive model that encompasses the multiple ways in which women's health is shaped. Fig. 1 presents a framework for this integrated, comprehensive approach. It takes into account the historical, geographical, legal, and political frameworks that provide the overarching context in which men and women live. It includes the cultural and normative dimension that has a profound effect on individual behaviors, and demographic characteristics such as race, place of birth, education, marital status and age. At a level more proximate to health, the focus is the household, the locale for the exchange of the resources that are basic to life, sex, food, warmth, and emotional sustenance. Women's roles in reproduction and production are simultaneously determined by what occurs within the household and community, and also help to shape them. Related, but not identical, are the psychosocial aspects of life: stress, coping strategies, including spirituality, and, more biologically rooted, mood, and other psychological characteristics. Women's roles in family and social networks determine the extent to which they have access to "social capital". Life stage and cohort experience, while difficult to show on this two dimensional framework, provide the dynamics shaping women's health. Finally, and most proximate to health outcomes are

Geopolitical Environment	Culture, Norms, Sanctions	Women's Roles In Reproduction & Production	Health-Related Mediators	Health Outcomes
Geography	Discrimination: Ethnic	Household: Structure	Social capital/ Social networks/	Chronic Disease Infectious Disease
Policy & Services: Transportation Welfare Employment Health care Child care	Gender Age Sociodemographic Characteristics: Age Gender	Div of labor Ownership/property Support/caretaking Equality of access to Household resources, e.g:	Support: Friendship Family Work mates Other ties	Disability Functioning Mortality Mental health/ illness
Legal rights: Women's Health Human Employment	Ethnicity Birthplace Education Marital status Language	Wages Other income Land Other assets Community roles Labor market role	Psychosocial: Stress Mood Coping Spirituality	
Organizations: Banks Credit coops Political parties Advocacy Unions		Workplace: Sector: Formal Home/market-based Hierarchies, control, Authority, discretion, Sex segregation/ discrimination	Health services: Availability/use Behaviors: Sexual Substance use Physical activity Diet Contraception Breastfeeding Smoking, drinking Violence	
Economic: Policy Extent of Inequality				

Figure 1 A comprehensive framework of factors influencing women's health.

the biological endowments of individual women. While part of this biological endowment is genetically determined, a large part is not, and is shaped through a process of foetal experience and exposures in infancy and early childhood, as well as in adult and later years. A woman's biological characteristics and inheritance, together with institutional, social, and psychological processes, affect her subsequent health and well-being. Like others (Link & Phelan, 1995; Williams, 1997; Williams & Collins, 1995), I argue that there are fundamental causes of health differences among women, and that they are rooted in the economic, political, historical, and social arrangements that structure how women live.

Geopolitical environment

The geopolitical environment includes the economic, political and social structures, as well as characteristics of the actual physical environment in which people live. It is here that ideologies find their expression in institutional structures including laws and policies. Welfare, health, child care, and labor policies and laws have a particular impact on women (Östlin et al.,

2001). Environmental quality and regulation are also important, because they determine the degree of cleanliness or pollution to which people are exposed, and the protections to which they are entitled. The legal framework may include laws that protect women's rights in different spheres and that do or do not give women equal protection under the law. The ratification of CEDAW provides a fundamental marker for the support of women's legal rights among nations. However, legislation concerning rights may offer necessary but not sufficient institutional protection for women and may even be inimical to it by encouraging complacency or siphoning programmatic resources into legal, but less interventionist directions (Sharma, 1995; Plata & Calderon, 1995; Scheper-Hughes, 1996). Women's reproductive and health rights are a special kind of rights that have immediate and direct impact upon health. In the geopolitical environment are formal organizations that provide vehicles for women's empowerment or women's oppression. These might include labor and trades unions, or women's welfare unions, microcredit organizations and grameen banks, or other vehicles for collectivized resources, but they might also include organizations opposed to women's reproductive and household rights.

The geopolitical environment includes the degree of economic equality or inequality measured at an aggregate level, such as a city, state, province or nation. Included are social and economic policies such as retrenchment and structural adjustment. These affect health services, transportation, and other publicly funded services through the imposition of user fees, in ways that may pose differential burdens for women, depending upon their resources. Finally, in this area, we should include such expressions of ideology as sexism, racism and ageism, all of which both contribute to laws and policies and result from them (Krieger et al., 1993).

Culture, religion, norms, and sanctions

Culture, religion, norms and sanctions are closely related to but not identical with the legal and institutional structures that regulate peoples' lives. Hammel (1990, p. 457) proposed a "theory of culture for demography" that moves far beyond the "culture as identifier" approach used by most epidemiologists and demographers. His key idea is that

> Explanations of individual-level demographic (or any other) social behavior must be situated at a micro-level that not only reflects immediately relevant economic and ecological considerations and overarching social institutions, but also includes especially the identity of significant co-actors in a social network.
>
> (p. 45)

He continues

> Culture is an evaluative conversation constructed by actors out of the raw materials afforded by tradition and ongoing experience. It is continually modified by them in processes of social interaction, and their behavior is guided by anticipation of such cultural evaluation.
>
> (p. 45)

Culture provides the explanations and guidelines for individual behavior (including reproductive and health-related behaviors) but it is collectively and socially constituted within a framework of economic and social institutions. A thoughtful consideration of culture moves us beyond the language of the dominant institutions into the understandings that women themselves have about their health-related behaviors, and into a more rounded consideration of the ways in which equity and power are expressed in every day life (Bledsoe, Hill, Langerock, & D'Alessandro, 1994; Watkins, Goldstein, & Spector, 1992). The interplay of culture, institutional hegemony, and deprivation often forces women to make choices that appear self-defeating (Scheper-Hughes, 1992). Cultural preferences, including religious norms, help to explain variations in gender inequality (Dollar & Gatti, 1999).

Women's roles in reproduction and production

Women's roles in reproduction and production are framed at the household level. It is in the household that intimate relations are structured and issues of the allocation of resources between sexual partners and between generations are organized and expressed. Important issues to consider are women's role in the formal labor market or the informal sector such as market and home-based work, and how work roles are integrated with household labor (Nathanson, 1980; Arber, 1991); the division of labor within the household; and other family and household members for whom the woman may be responsible (Matthews & Power, 2001). Closely related, but conceptually distinct, is the intra-household allocation of material, informational and psychosocial resources, in other words, the pattern of exchange in the household. Here, too, relationships of power, control, authority and equity may be played out with varying consequences for women's health (Nanda, 2000). Another dimension, for many women, of their responsibilities, is care, nurturance, and support of household members (in many cases, this caring and nurturing is extended beyond the physical confines of the household, within the kin or social network, and should be taken into account). Support and caretaking are a double-edged sword. The provision of support and care may be emotionally satisfying and may also provide some future social credit or capital for the woman's own needs that she can draw upon from children, siblings, or friends. At the same time, supporting and caretaking can be tremendously draining. Many women experience the "double" or even the "triple" day (Hochschild, 1997b).

Simply providing more schooling for women is not sufficient to reduce the gender inequality in control of resources within the household. Schultz (1997) estimated income inequality in the world from 1960 to 1994 at three levels of aggregation: countries, households within countries, and between women and men within households. He found that despite women's gains in education there is persistent unequal control of resources in the household.

Also, within the household, women are producers of human capital. In rearing their young they produce human capital through the promotion of their own and their children's health, nutrition, child care, and the teaching of language and other skills that have labor market value, and gender preferences are expressed through these activities, also (Sen, 1984, Chap. 15; Thomas, 1990). They also contribute to human capital by the feeding and caretaking of partners and other working members of the household. Depending on other resources and constraints on women, these activities may have positive or negative effects on health.

The way in which women share in community activities is often interwoven with their household tasks (Barrett, 1995). In western industrialized countries this may include volunteer activities in children's schools, involvement in local political campaigns, or involvement in children's recreational sports. In non-industrialized nations it may include household maintenance chores performed in public or communal settings such as washing clothes, drawing water, or shopping for food, as well as the participation in local market organizations. Increasingly, women are playing roles in non-governmental organizations in their communities and integrating these roles with household labour. Women's credit co-operatives alter the relationship between market and reproductive roles and diminish the impact of socioeconomic inequality on the organization of women's lives (Brill & Kobre, 1999). These bridging roles are crucial to the formation of social capital (Kawachi, 1999; Kawachi et al., 1999).

The household is the most intimate setting for the playing out of dramas of power, authority and control, all of which may affect women in a number of ways. Male partners, and sometimes in-laws, may control women's access to children, food, money, health services, and even life itself. The expression of violence, a product of cultural, socioeconomic and power relations, towards women is a direct and indirect risk to women's health. Violence towards women is associated with higher rates of sexually transmitted disease, including HIV/AIDS, and adverse birth outcomes (Jaspard & Saurel-Cubizolles, 2000; Gielen, Ocampo, Faden, Kass, & Xue, 1994). Violence towards women takes a large toll on women's psychological health, as well as on the health and well being of children in the household. There is evidence, too, that intra-household and community violence against women is an expression of socioeconomic inequality at the interpersonal level (Ocampo, Gielen, & Faden, 1995).

The workplace, too, provides a setting for dramas of control, authority, and relative power, much of which is gender-based (Wolf & Fligstein, 1979; McGuire & Reskin, 1993). The decline of the power of labour and trades unions, combined with the increase in contract and temporary labour, have diminished the status and rights of individual workers, many of whom are now isolated in space (as home workers) or in time, as employment tenure shortens. In California, until the 1960s, thousands of Mexican-origin women found employment in fruit and vegetable canneries. Despite the often poor working conditions, cannery culture promoted close ties among women workers that often spilled into the organization and maintenance of the household, and the work had seasonal predictability that allowed women to integrate home chores with wage labour (Zavella, 1987; Ruiz, 1987). More recently, immigrant women have found employment as domestic servants, janitors, or low-wage workers in electronics and garment industries, work that is often isolating and demeaning, and offers no opportunity for advancement (Segura, 1989). Globalization and the proliferation of free trade zones have led to the proliferation of workplaces where "discretion" and "job control" are non-existent. Women's occupational as well as household roles, separately and together, relate to their physical and mental health and to their mortality risks (Smith & Waitzman, 1994).

Health-related mediators

The way in which resources such as money, food, and emotional warmth are exchanged in the household influences psychosocial health, nutritional well-being, access to health services, and the expression of violence. Resource exchange mediates the effects of geopolitical, cultural, and household patterns of equity and inequality on health status and outcomes. Health-related mediators of inequality and equity include health behaviours; access to and use of health services; stressors; and psychosocial resources and strategies including social ties, coping and spirituality.

Health behaviours include eating patterns, use of tobacco, alcohol and other mood-altering substances, and exercise and physical activity, by others in the household as well as by women themselves. Other behaviors that affect women's health include contraception, breast-feeding and the use of different forms of prescription and over-the-counter medications, and the growing use of therapies such as homeopathy and meditation in Western industrialized nations. Although these are often viewed and "treated" as individually determined, they are almost always the result of a complex pattern of causes including marketing, pricing, and social and cultural meaning (Graham, 1994). One of the most fascinating phenomena in epidemiology is how behaviors become more or less accepted by women. For example, smoking rates among women vary with social class in ways that are culturally and nationally quite specific. As better educated women (and men) in the US have rejected smoking as unhealthful (e.g., National Center for Health Statistics, 1998), cigarette companies have aggressively turned their marketing efforts towards adolescents, especially females, and to populations in newly emergent market nations such as China, which had, until recently, quite low rates of cigarette smoking.

Access to health services is differentially available to women depending upon their geographic location, insurance status or ability to pay, their ease in handling the bureaucratic and authoritarian structure of health care delivery, the presence of traditional or non-bureaucratic providers of care, and the extent to which families support women's access to and use of services (Weisman, 1998, Chap. 3). Once within the health care system, women may experience differential diagnosis or treatment depending upon their status, social power, and socioeconomic standing, as well as upon racial, ethnic, linguistic or cultural background (Clancy, 2000, Chap. 5).

Stress, and stressful life events, are related to a number of disorders, both psychological and physical, among women (Hogue, 2000, Chap. 2; Williams & Umberson, 2000, Chap. 44). Effective coping strategies such as support from social networks, and spirituality, can reduce stress, promote physical and mental well-being, and improve health. A woman's role in formal and informal labor markets, her position in a kin network and household, and her marital and parental status, shape the number and extent of her social ties. The "family" may come to be workmates with whom a woman spends much of her day (Hochschild, 1997a). The effect of social ties and support networks on women's health depends on a variety of demographic and environmental factors such as age, occupational position and role including discretion and control on the job, whether she lives in an urban or rural setting, and genetic resilience.

One coping strategy, spirituality, is helpful to women in two ways. By promoting internal resources (coping) women are able to come to terms with personal and social hardship, and obtain a feeling of well-being and calm. Spirituality as expressed through church, mosque, or synagogue attendance or participation in prayer or meditation groups, provides a form of social capital, extending an individual's caring networks, that may be protective and assist in difficult times (Jarvis & Northcott 1987; Levin & Vanderpool, 1989; Miller 1995).[2]

In virtually all societies, powerful market forces, often globalized, shape women's behaviours and expectations through the manipulation of cultural symbols and their commodification. Market forces reinforce existing socioeconomic patterns of women's psychosocial response by playing on the importance of children and partners. Qualitative research conducted by Hilary Graham in the UK suggests that women's choice among commodified coping mechanisms (e.g., smoking and certain foods) is socioeconomically determined (Graham, 1994). Class-based strategies sell products that demonstrate rank (designer handbags); reduce stress (food, tobacco); or assist in coping (cosmetics, "labour-saving" devices).

Mood, personality disorders, depression and anxiety are mediators of other health outcomes and mental health endpoints in themselves; their incidence varies by age, class and ethnicity. Depression and other adverse psychological states place women at risk of violence, including sexual assault, and, via the immune system, may lead to increased incidence of chronic and infectious disease (McDonough, Walters, & Strohschein, 2001). We are only beginning to understand how the natural hormonal fluctuation over the life course affects women's mood, health and well being, independently, and jointly with other mediators, such as diet and physical activity (Seeman, 2000, Chap. 78). Complicating the picture is evidence that perceptions of hormonal variations, such as the symptoms of menopause, may be culturally determined (Sowers, 2000, Chap. 92).

Health outcomes

Many health outcomes, including disability, perceived health status, and the presence or absence of disease and mortality risk, are shaped by a complex process of environmental, social, behavioral, psychosocial, and genetic events. Socioeconomic factors, including education, poverty, income, income inequality, and occupation, are some of the strongest and most consistent predictors of health and mortality. Gender (in)equity, combined with socioeconomic inequality, together form a powerful explanatory framework for variations in women's health. We have seen how the geopolitical environment, with its legal, political, and economic institutions, in turn contributes to patterns of inequality in the household, where the more proximal actions that affect health often take place. Psychosocial resources, whether positive, such as social networks and systems of support, or negative, such as stress and its physiological expression, also mediate expressions of inequality. Recent research is examining the extent to which repeated hardship, or "allostatic load", carried by some individuals may depress the immune system and contribute to disease (e.g., Seeman, Singer, Rowe, Horwitz, & McEwen, 1997).

A life course perspective

Health is the result of a complex interplay of biological, including genetic, demographic, socioeconomic, psychosocial and behavioral factors. Much of the research on women's health is based upon a snapshot of a small part of this complexity. A dynamic perspective that takes account of intergenerational, foetal, childhood, and adolescent precursors to adult health, as well as of cohort experiences, will deepen our understanding of the social and economic patterning of women's health. This is often constrained by the absence of longitudinal data sets that include socioeconomic and health variables, with some exceptions (e.g., Power, Matthews, & Manor, 1998; Matthews & Power, 2001). In the US, the Health and Retirement Survey and the AHEAD Survey are filling in our picture of socioeconomic-health relationship for older men and women of different ethnic groups. In the UK, the British birth cohort studies (e.g., Wadsworth & Kuh, 1997; Matthews & Power, 2001) allow researchers to test causal hypotheses about health trajectories of men and women over time.

Examples of integrated social and economic frameworks of women's health

Several researchers in the English-speaking world have attempted to develop theoretical approaches to women's health that integrate inequality in social and economic position with women's roles in production and reproduction. I present examples from the US–UK literature, but their theoretical implications are applicable cross-culturally and cross-nationally.

The "weathering" hypothesis, or analytic framework, proposes that women age in different ways depending upon how varying life circumstances undermine or promote health, and that women's health and mortality experience reflects a cumulation or cascade of advantages and disadvantages (Geronimus, 1992). The strength of this approach is that it unites lifespan and environmental factors and is applicable to many aspects of women's health The theory helps to explain ethnic as well as socioeconomic differences in the development of chronic conditions since women of different ethnic backgrounds "weather" or age at different rates, and it encompasses age-based trajectories of behaviors such as smoking, as well as environmental exposures and access to health services. The weathering framework also helps to explain the intergenerational transmission of the link between SES and health, by connecting physical manifestations of accelerated aging such as hypertension to infant's and children's health (Geronimus, Anderson, & Bound, 1991; Geronimus & Hillemeier, 1992). The weathering hypothesis emphasizes how the chronic burdens of everyday deprivation and environmental exposures affect health and how age-related patterns of childbearing and caretaking are responses to perceived vulnerability.

The analytic framework that integrates women's roles in the household (and the consumption patterns that follow from these roles) with structural measures such as occupational class and other socioeconomic indicators, inherently captures aspects of equity and equality (Arber, 1991; Khlat et al., 2000; Walters, McDonough, & Strohschein, 2001). This approach is particularly useful for capturing socioeconomic factors in women's lives, since paid employment is both a potential stressor (when added to child care and marital roles) and also an indicator of potential material and social resources. It takes account of the differing day-to-day realities of men's and women's lives within a socioeconomic framework. Consumption measures, such as housing tenure and car ownership, have been shown to be equally or more revealing of a woman's class position than occupation, perhaps because they are resources that make a difference in women's everyday lives. The interaction effects of work and home roles differ depending on gender and household configuration and several studies have found that lone mothers are particularly disadvantaged with regard to physical and mental health (Arber & Cooper, 2000; Lahelma el al., 2001). The socioeconomic factors as well as the family and occupational roles that influence health in women may be different from the factors that influence health in men. Women are more likely to experience role strain and overload that occur when familial responsibilities are combined with occupation-related stress. These are compounded (or alleviated) by material circumstances. For men, occupational class and employment status explain more of the variation in health than do familial roles and responsibilities (Arber, 1991). In southern countries, similarly complex relationships occur among gender, family, and labor market role variables, although effects may be in different directions. For example, working does not always enhance women's control over resources. The roles played by consumption variables, culture and level of development differ. In one Indian study, possession of a pressure cooker freed women's time, but the presence of a sewing machine increased servitude within the household (Nanda, 2000).

In the UK, Hilary Graham uses a combination of qualitative and quantitative methods and data drawn from a variety of sources to examine how women, especially women with children, make different kinds of decisions about health-related behaviors (Graham, 1984; Graham, 1994). She looks at how the interplay of economic circumstances and household structure influence individual family members. Both social class and gender structure the organization of family life and it is in family life (for the most part) where health is produced. Graham writes

> Assumptions about the needs and obligations of men and women play a primary role in shaping the distribution of resources *within* families . . . However, their effects are not restricted to the domestic domain. In the labour market, too, there are sex differences in employment and earnings. With the increasing numbers of female-headed families, these differences have become an important factors in fueling inequalities *between* families.
>
> The patterns of resource allocation within and between families are seen to reflect a structure of sexual divisions as deep-rooted and pervasive as the class divisions traditionally associated with Western societies. This structure is linked to family health in obvious and important ways . . .

... [T]he theme of justice, power, and fairness, in how social environments and life chances are structured and how roles are allocated within social institutions, including the workplace, the household, and the family, lies just below the surface ... [S]ocioeconomic circumstances, in combination with culturally appropriated women's roles, produce differing patterns of health, disability, and mortality.
(Graham, 1984, pp. 58–59)

Graham's work explores how the arrangement of space, the preparation and distribution of food, and the provision of heating relates to gender relations within the household, given the impact of socioeconomic relations or social class on household resources. Because of the symbolic significance of food, when resources are short women often accommodate first to children's and men's needs, putting their own nutrition last, a pattern that is found in a number of cultures.

HIV/AIDS provides, perhaps, the most vivid example of how women's lack of power within and outside of the household, and the forces of social and economic inequality and marginalization, lead to disease, social disintegration, and death. The burden is especially great on the most vulnerable women in the most vulnerable economics (often, but not exclusively, southern). It is in HIV/AIDS that the geopolitical and historical vivdly transect socio-economic and gender relations. A paper by Bassett and Mhloyi (1991) provides a dramatic illustration of how these processes occur in Zimbabwe. The paper's underlying theoretical premise, that a historical, geographically specific legacy of economic and gender relations poses epidemiologic vulnerability for women, is universally true. Other examples include son preference (for example, in India and China) resulting in female infanticide (Östlin et al., 2001), and female genital mutilation.

Operationalizing a multi-level framework

Introducing historical, policy- and institutional-level constructs into empirical studies of health mediators and outcomes is not an easy task, theoretically or statistically (Diez-Roux 1998; Von Korff et al., 1992). Much, if not most, of the research in women's health has been focused on the right-hand end of the framework shown in Fig. 1, with demographic characteristics used as "control" variables. On the other hand, there is a very long tradition in public health and in the social sciences that recognizes the importance of the environment to individual behavior and health, as well as the difficulty in estimating it (Mason, Wong, & Entwisle, 1983; Wong & Mason, 1991). Our task as researchers on women's health is to move towards the left-hand side of Fig. 1, carefully defining what we mean by "environment", making certain that it is appropriately measured, and choosing the correct statistical techniques for our models (Wiggins, Joshi, Bartley, Gleave, & Lynch, 2001).

In Fig. 1, geopolitical environment, culture and norms refer to aspects of the environment that cannot be measured by aggregating individual-level data. Aggregate data *are* important in characterizing group-level phenomena such as the portion of women in a community engaged in employment out of the household, or the role of social networks and social capital (e.g., Kawachi et al., 1999). While many environmental characteristics are measurable, others are not and may be unobserved or unmeasured (e.g., norms or perceived social and economic opportunities) but are an important part of causal thinking (Brewster, 1994). But we also need to include the more "macro" or geopolitical factors in our models. Particular care is needed when taking a cross-national or comparative approach because some constructs, such as "ethnicity", "household" or even marriage, are not really comparable across societies (Wong & Mason, 1991). An example of a cross-national multi-level analysis of an issue integral to women's health is provided by Mason and Smith (2000). They use data from communities in Pakistan, India, Malaysia, Thailand and the Philippines that have different gender traditions to explore how gender context in different types of communities in each country influences the joint goals of husbands and wives in desire for children, and their use of contraceptives.

What can be done to improve understanding of the social and economic patterning of women's health?

Elite research institutions and international governmental and non-governmental organizations have rushed during the past 15 years to make gender a focus of research, policy and program activity. Gender equity is viewed as a cornerstone of economic development. Policy initiatives have made primary school for girls nearly universal during the past decade, an investment that results in lower fertility, lower infant mortality, and better nutrition and health practices in the household. Reproductive health services for women have proliferated, and there is increased interest in the health and well being of the growing elderly segment of the population which is predominantly women. I propose a variety of ways that we can continue to make progress in research and policymaking as they promote gender and socioeconomic equity and women's health.

(a) *Put pressure on the leading research and development organizations to develop integrated approaches to women's health*, using frameworks, like the one developed for this paper, that consider jointly gender equity and socioeconomic inequality, and that situate health in specific historical, political, legal and social contexts. Research and programs that do this are in the minority. More typically, researchers use sex and socioeconomic status as control variables, and clinicians persist in developing programs or treatment regimens that focus on one limited aspect of women's health or behaviors. Disciplinary boundaries reinforce the difficulties of integrating social, economic, and epidemiological approaches to women's health. Strategies such as conferences and research initiatives that challenge the boundaries will provide a substantial contribution to our understanding of the patterning of women's health.

(b) *Domestic and international funders should continue to support research initiatives* that encourage detailed and sophisticated tests of a variety of hypotheses about the social and economic patterning of women's health. The framework presented in this paper can guide studies that examine how gender equity and socioeconomic inequality jointly shape women's and men's health across the lifecourse. It demands a multi-level perspective, taking account of contextual and individual level variables. Comparative research will lead to a better understanding of how policies and culture shape socioeconomic and household structures and roles. Attention to the methodological issues posed by a multi-level approach to women's health, and the sharing of problems, techniques, and solutions across disciplinary and national boundaries, will deepen our understanding and improve policy and programmatic strategies.

(c) *Use ethnographic techniques to provide new insights.* Survey research and vital and disease registries are necessary but not sufficient. The insights that generate theory and advance testable, quantifiable hypotheses often come from detailed qualitative field work (e.g., Graham, 1984). The recent integration of ethnographic methods by demography and epidemiology has produced exciting insights, often about marginalized populations. Applying some of this research creativity to women in the mainstream may open new lines of inquiry.

(d) *Create and maintain appropriate data systems for monitoring and reporting on socioeconomic inequalities and gender equity*, both in themselves and as they affect women's health. Even in the affluent developed countries, such systems are far from perfect and they are often weak in poorer nations (Braveman, 1996). Vital and disease registries and periodic surveys such as the Demographic and Health Surveys (DHS) can inform communities and policy makers about problems and prospects in improving women's health. Through the MEASURE project, the DHS now includes questions on gender relations and empowerment and questionnaires are administered to men as well as to women.[3] In order for the data to be meaningful, appropriate socioeconomic and equity measures must be included and it is critical that survey questions are formulated to take account of women's own perspectives and interpretations. Health and economic data should be longitudinal and integrated, and data sets should contain contextual legal, political, and health services variables at country, regional, and local levels. Supporting the data gathering, analytic and reporting capacity of nations is an important goal. United Nations statistics provide an example of how gender equity and economic equality can be monitored simultaneously at the country level, resulting in useful equity and empowerment indices that facilitate international comparisons (UNDP, 1999).

Why propose a unified framework of women's health?

Research is costly, but so is the failure to understand. It would be nearly impossible to test the entire model proposed in this paper. Yet, advances in our understanding of women's health have come through multi-disciplinary work that expands paradigms: an example is the burgeoning literature describing the physical and mental health effects of gender, labor market, and household roles. These studies take a large step forward in integrating gender equity (fairness in resource distribution) with socioeconomic position and rewards. Contextualizing studies in historical and geopolitical frameworks is a next big step, along with deepened exploration of how patterns may vary across different points in the lifecourse and for different birth cohorts. An advantage of this combined framework is its applicability to health outcomes across nations and cultures. It allows us to understand what in the patterning of women's health is universal and what is unique, and to develop humane and effective policies that promote equity, equality, and well-being.

Acknowledgements

The leadership of Sara Arber, Myriam Khlat, and CICRED in organizing the seminar on "Social and economic patterning of health among women" (Tunis, January 2000) is gratefully acknowledged, as are the insights, warmth and stimulation of colleagues who attended the meeting.

Notes

1. The United Nations uses two indices to capture gender related development and gender empowerment, the gender development index (GDI) and the gender empowerment measure (GEM) (UNDP, 1999, pp. 160–162). The GDI measures results for 143 countries in three key indicators of human development: life expectancy, educational attainment, and income, and adjusts those results for gender inequality. For every country, the GDI is lower than the UN's human development index (HDI), showing that gender inequality is universal. But in some cases, the GDI ranks higher than the HDI, suggesting that gender equality does not depend upon a country's income level or stage of development. There are developing countries that do better than richer industrialized nations in promoting women's participation in political and professional activities, as measured by the GEM (UNDP, 1999, p. 133). There are also differences among regions within countries.
2. This is quite different from organized religions as legal or political state-sanctioned authorities, which have often been associated with the oppression of women.
3. Information about the Demographic and Health Surveys, including the MEASURE project, is available at http://www.measuredhs.com.

References

Arber, S. (1991). Class, paid employment and family roles: Making sense of structural disadvantage, gender and health status. *Social Science & Medicine, 32*, 425–436.

Arber, S., & Cooper, K. (2000). In L. Annandale, & K. Hunt (Eds.), *Gender Inequalities in health*. Milton Keynes: Open University Press.

Barrett, H. (1995). Women in Africa: The neglected dimension in development. *Geography, 80*, 215–224.

Bassett, M. T., & Mhloyi, M. (1991). Women and AIDS in Zimbabwe: The making of an epidemic. *International Journal of Health Services, 21*, 143–156.

Bledsoe, C. H., Hill, A. G., Langerock, P., & D'Alessandro, U. (1994). Constructing natural fertility: The use of Western contraceptive technologies in rural Gambia. *Population and Development Review*, 20, 81–113.

Braveman, P. (1996). *Equity in health and health care: A WHO SIDA initiative*. Geneva: World Health Organization.

Brewster, K. L. (1994). Neighborhood context and the transition to sexual activity among young black women. *Demography, 21*, 603–614.

Brill, B., & Kobre, K. (1999). The power of small change. *San Francisco Examiner*, May 2–6. Http://www.examiner.com/microloans.

Clancy, C. M. (2000). Gender issues in womens health care. In M. B. Goldman, & M. C. Hatch (Eds.), *Women and health* (pp. 50–54). San Diego: Academic Press.

Coleman, J. S. (1988). Social capital in the creation of human capital. *American Journal of Sociology, 94*(Suppl.), S95–S120.

Dahlgren, G. (1990). Strategies for health financing in Kenya—the difficult birth of a new policy. *Scandinavian Journal of Social Medicine, 46*(Suppl.), 67–81.

Diez-Roux, A. V. (1998). Bringing context back into epidemiology: Variables and fallacies in multilevel analysis. *American Journal of Public Health, 88*, 216–222.

Dollar, D., & Gatti, R. (1999). Gender inequality, income and growth: Are good times good for women? World Bank, Development Economics Research Gronp, Poverty Reduction and Management Network, Working paper series, no. 1, 1999.

Frank, R. H. (1999). *Luxury fever: Why money fails to satisfy in an era of excess*. New York: The Free Press.

Geronimus, A. T. (1992). The weathering hypothesis and the health of African–American women and infants: Evidence and speculations. *Ethnicity and Disease, 2*, 207–221.

Geronimus, A. T., Anderson, H. F., & Bound, J. (1991). Differences in hypertension prevalence among US black and white women of childbearing age. *Public Health Reports, 106*, 393–399.

Geronimus, A. T., & Hillemeier, M. M. (1992). Patterns of blood lead level in US black and white women of childbearing age. *Ethnicity and Disease, 2*, 222–231.

Gielen, A., Ocampo, P., Faden, R., Kass, N., & Xue, N. (1994). Determinants of interpersonal violence during the childbearing year. *Social Science & Medicine, 39*, 781–781.

Gilligan, Carol. (1982). *In a different voice: Psychological theory and women's development*. Cambridge, MA: Harvard University Press.

Gottschalk, P., & Smeeding, T. (1997). Cross-national comparisons of earnings and income inequality. *Journal of Economic Literature, 35*(2), 633–687.

Graham, H. (1984). *Women, health and the family* (pp. 58–59). Brighton: Harvester Press/Wheatsheaf Books.

Graham, H. (1994). Gender and class as dimensions of smoking behavior in Britain: Insights from a survey of mothers. *Social Science & Medicine, 38*, 691–698.

Granovetter, M. S. (1973). The strength of weak ties. *American Journal of Sociology*, 78, 1360–1380.

Haan, M. N., Kaplan, G. A., & Syme, S. L. (1989). Socioeconomic status and health: Old observations and new thoughts. In J. P. Bunker, J. P. D. Gomby, & B. H. Kehrer (Eds.), *Pathways to health: The role of social factors* (pp. 76–135). Menlo Park, CA: The Henry J. Kaiser Family Foundation.

Hammel, E. A. (1990). A theory of culture for demography. *Population and Development Review*, 16, 455–485.

Hochschild Arlie, R. (1997a). *The time bind: When work becomes home and home becomes work*. New York: Henry Holt and Co..

Hochschild Arlie, R. (1997b). *The second shift*. New York: Avon Books.

Hogue, C. J. R. (2000). Gender, race and class: From epidemiologic association to etiologic hypotheses. In M. B. Goldman, & M. C. Hatch (Eds.), *Women and health* (pp. 15–23). San Diego: Academic Press.

Jarvis, G. K., & Northcott, H. C. (1987). Religion and differences in morbidity and mortality. *Social Science & Medicine*, 25, 813–824.

Jaspard, M., & Saurel-Cubizolles, M.-J. (2000). Violence envers les femmes et effets sur la santé. *Paper presented at the CICRED seminar on "Social and Economic Patterning of Health Among Women"*, January, Tunis.

Kaplan, G. A., Pamuk, E. R., Lynch, J. W., Cohen, R. D., & Balfour, J. L. (1996). Inequality in income and mortality in the United States: Analysis of mortality and potential pathways. *British Medical Journal*, 312, 999–1005.

Karoly, L. A. (1996). Anatomy of the US income distribution. *Oxford Review of Economic Policy*, 12, 77–96.

Karoly, L. A., & Burtless, G. (1995). Demographic change, rising earnings inequality, and the distribution of personal well-being, 1959–1989. *Demography*, 32, 379–405.

Kawachi, I. (1999). Social capital and community effects on population and individual health. *Annals of the New York Academy of Sciences*, 896, 120–130.

Kawachi, I., Kennedy, B. P., & Glass, R. (1999). Social capital and self-rated health: A contextual analysis. *American Journal of Public Health*, 89, 1187–1193.

Kennedy, B. P., Kawachi, I., & Prothrow-Stith, D. (1996). Income distribution and mortality: Test of the Robin Hood index in the United States. *British Medical Journal*, 312, 1004–1007.

Khlat, M., Sermet, C., & Le Pape, A. (2000). Women's health in relation with their family and work roles: France in the early 1990s. *Social Science & Medicine*, 50, 1807–1825.

Krieger, N., Rowley, D. L., Herman, A. A., Avery, B., & Phillips, M. T. (1993). Racism, sexism and social class: Implications for studies of health, disease, and well-being. *American Journal of Preventive Medicine*, 9, 82–122.

Lahelma, E., Arber, S., Kivelä, K., & Roos, E. (2001). Marriage, motherhood and work among British and Finnish women: Multiple health burden or multiple buffer? *Social Science & Medicine*, 54, 727–740.

Levin, J. S., & Vanderpool, H. Y. (1989). Is religion therapeutically significant in hypertension? *Social Science & Medicine*, 29, 69–78.

Lewis, P. (1999). World Bank says poverty is increasing. *New York Times*, June 3, C1.

Link, B. G., & Phelan, J. (1995). Social conditions as fundamental causes of disease. *Journal of Health and Social Behavior*, extra issue, 80–94.

Mason, K. O., & Smith, H. L. (2000). Husbands' versus wives' fertility goals and use of contraception: The influence of gender context in five Asian countries. *Demography, 37*, 299–311.

Mason, W. M., Wong, G. Y., & Entwisle, B. (1983). Contextual analysis through the multilevel linear model. In S. Leinhardt (Ed.), *Sociological methodology 1983–1984* (pp. 72–103). San Francisco: Jossey-Bass.

Matthews, S., & Power, C. (2001). Socioeconomic gradients in psychological distress: A focus on women, social roles and work-home characteristics. *Social Science & Medicine, 54*, 799–810.

McDonough, P., Walters, V., & Strohschein, L. (2001). Chronic stress and the social patterning of women's health in Canada. *Social Science & Medicine, 54*, 767–782.

McGuire, G. M., & Reskin, B. F. (1993). Authority hierarchies at work: The impacts of race and sex. *Gender and Society, 7*, 487–506.

Miller, M. A. (1995). Culture, spirituality and women's health [Review]. *Journal of Obstetrics Gynecologic and Neonatal Nursing, 24*, 257–263.

Nanda, A. K. (2000). Socio-economic determinants of health among women: Some evidence from a poor society. *Paper presented at the CICRED seminar on "Social and Economic Patterning of Health Among Women"*, January, Tunis.

Nathanson, C. (1980). Social roles and health status among women: The significance of employment. *Social Science & Medicine, 14A*, 463–471.

National Center for Health Statistics. (1998). *Health United States with socioeconomic status and health chartbook*. Hyattsville, MD.

Ocampo, P., Gielen, A. C., & Faden, R. (1995). Violence by male partner against women during the childbearing year: A contextual analysis. *American Journal of Public Health, 85*, 1092–1097.

Östlin, P., Sen, G., & George, A. (2001). Gender, health and equity. In T. Evans, M. Whitehead, F. Didenchsen, & A. Bhuiya (Eds.), *Challenging inequities in health: From ethics to action*. Oxford: Oxford University Press, Chapter 13.

Pappas, G., Queen, S., Hadden, W., & Fisher, G. (1993). The increasing disparity between socioeconomic groups in the United States, 1960 and 1986. *New England Journal of Medicine, 329*, 103–109.

Plata, M. I., & Calderon, M. C. (1995). Legal services: Putting rights into action—Profamilia—Colombia. *The American University Law Review, 44*, 1105–1111.

Power, C., Matthews, S., & Manor, O. (1998). Inequalities in self-rated health: Explanations from different stages of life. *Lancet, 351*, 1009–1014.

Razavi, S. (1997). Fitting gender into development institutions. *World Development, 25*, 1111–1125.

Rich, F. (1999). Who doesn't want to be a millionaire? *New York Times*, op-ed, November 20, A27.

Ruiz, V. L. (1987). *Cannery women, cannery lives. Mexican women, unionization and the California food processing industry, 1930–1950*. Albuquerque: University of New Mexico Press.

Scheper-Hughes, N. (1992). *Death without weeping: The violence of everyday life in Brazil*. Berkeley: University of California Press.

Scheper-Hughes, N. (1996). Small wars, invisible genocides. *Social Science & Medicine, 43*, 889–899.

Schultz, T. P. (1997). Inequality in the distribution of personal income in the world: How it is changing and why. *Paper presented at the annual meeting of the Population Association of America*, March 27–29, Washington, DC.

Science and technology (1995). Good intentions, road to hell? The World Bank's ideas for better health care in poor countries have not always worked out in practice. *The Economist*, October 7, 121–122.

Seeman, M. V. (2000). Mental illness in women. In M. B. Goldman, & M. C. Hatch (Eds.), *Women and health* (pp. 989–996). San Diego: Academic Press.

Seeman, T., Singer, B., Rowe, J., Horwitz, R., & McEwen, B. (1997). Price of adaptation-allostatic load and its health consequences. *Archives of Internal Medicine, 157*, 2259–2268.

Segura, D. (1989). Chicana and Mexican immigrant women at work: The impact of class, race, and gender on occupational mobility. *Gender and Society, 3*, 37–52.

Sen, A. (1984). Family and food: Sex bias in poverty. In A. Sen (Ed.), *Resources, values and development*. Cambridge, MA: Harvard University Press.

Sharma, M. (1995). What role can rights play in the work of international agencies? *The American University Law Review, 44*, 1097–1103.

Smeeding, T. M. & Gottschalk, P. (1995). The international evidence on income distribution in modern economies: Where do we stand? Invited paper for "Income distribution: Theory and evidence" session. International Economic Association World Congress, Tunis, December 1995. *Luxembourg income study working paper #137*, Maxwell School of Public Affairs, Syracuse University, Syracuse, NY.

Smith, K. R., & Waitzman, N. J. (1994). Women, work, and whether occupation matters: Differences in mortality by occupation in the US. 1971–1987. *Paper presented at the annual meeting of the Population Association of America*, Miami, FL.

Sowers, M. F. (2000). Menopause: Its epidemiology. In M. B. Goldman, & M. C. Hatch (Eds.), *Women and health* (pp. 1155–1168). San Diego: Academic Press.

Sullivan, D. (1995). Introduction. Conference on international protection of reproductive rights. *The American University Law Review, 44*, 969–973.

Thomas, D. (1990). Intra-household resource allocation: An inferential approach. *Journal of Human Resources, 25*, 635–664.

United Nations Development Program (UNDP). (1999). *Human development report 1999*. New York: United Nations.

United Nations Population Fund (UNFPA). (1999). *Women and health: Mainstreaming the gender perspective into the health sector*. Report of the expert group meeting 28 September–2 October, 1998, Tunis. United Nations, New York.

Von Korff, M., Koepsell, T., Curry, S., & Diehr, P. (1992). Multi-level analysis in epidemiological research on health behaviors and outcomes. *American Journal of Epidemiology, 135*, 1077–1082.

Wadsworth, M. E. J., & Kuh, D. J. L. (1997). Childhood influences on adult health: A review of recent work from the British 1946 National Birth Cohort Study, the MRC National Survey of Health and Development. *Pediatric and Perinatal Epidemiology, 11*, 2–20.

Walters, V., McDonough, P., & Strohschein, L. (2001). The influence of work, household structure, and social, personal and material resources on gender differences in health: An analysis of the 1994 Canadian National Population Health Survey. *Social Science & Medicine, 54*, 677–692.

Watkins, S. C., Goldstein, A., & Spector, A. R. (1992). Family planning patterns among Jewish and Italian women in the United States, 1900–1940. Unpublished paper.

Weisman, C. S. (1998). *Women's health care: Activist traditions and institutional change*. Baltimore: Johns Hopkins University Press.

Wiggins, R. D., Joshi, H., Bartley, M., Gleave, S., & Lynch, K. (2001). Geographical variation in women's health. A multilevel analysis of long-term illness among women in the ONS Longitudinal Study of England and Wales. *Social Science & Medicine, 54*, 827–838.

Wilkinson, R. G. (1992). Income distribution and life expectancy. *British Medical Journal, 304*, 165–168.

Wilkinson, R. G. (1996). *Unhealthy societies: The afflictions of inequality*. London: Routledge.

Williams, D. R. (1997). Race and health: Basic questions, emerging directions. *Annals of Epidemiology, 7*, 322–333.

Williams, D. R., & Collins, C. (1995). US socioeconomic and racial differences in health: Patterns and explanations. *Annual Review of Sociology, 21*, 349–386.

Williams, K., & Umberson, D. (2000). Women stress, and health. In M. B. Goldman, & M. C. Hatch (Eds.), *Women and health* (pp. 553–562). San Diego: Academic Press.

Wolff, E. (1995). *Top heavy: A study of the increasing inequality of wealth in America*. New York: The Twentieth Century Fund Press.

Wolf, W. C., & Fligstein, N. (1979). Sex and authority in the workplace: The causes of sexual inequality. *American Sociological Review, 44*, 235–252.

Wong, G. Y., & Mason, W. M. (1991). Contextually specific effects and other generalizations of the hierarchical linear model for comparative analysis. *Journal of the American Statistical Association, 86*, 487–503.

World Bank. (1994). *Population and development: Implications for the World Bank*. Washington, DC (p. 75).

World Bank. (1998). *Engendering development: Enhancing development through attention to gender*. Draft report and commentary.

World Bank. (2000). *World development report 2000/1, consultation draft*, January.

Zavella, P. (1987). *Women's work and Chicano families: Cannery workers of the Santa Clara valley*. Ithaca, NY: Cornell University Press.

17
HEALTHY BODIES, SOCIAL BODIES
Men's and women's concepts and practices of health in everyday life

Robin Saltonstall

Source: *Social Science & Medicine*, 36:1 (1993), 7–14.

Abstract

Using interview data from white, middle-class men and women, ages 35–55, the research explores the phenomenological, embodied aspects of health. Health is found to be grounded in a sense of self and a sense of body, both of which are tied to conceptions of past and future actions. Gender is a leitmotif. The body, as the focal point of self-construction as well as health construction, implicates gender in the everyday experience of health. The interplay between health, self, body, and gender at the individual level is linked to the creation of a sense of healthiness in the body politic of society. If social psychological theories of health are to reflect adequately the everyday experience of health, they must begin to take into account the body as individually and socially problematic.

Introduction

Sociologists and anthropologists of medicine have largely focused their research on sickness and illness, thus obscuring social scientific investigations of health and healthiness. Analyses which have taken health as their focus have examined the structural, cultural, and material aspects of health, and not the phenomenological elements, especially those related to the body [1].

The body as problematic is beginning to be more evident in some sociological investigations. Recent analyses of fitness have begun to address embodiment, health, and self [2]. Espeland [3] and Kotarba [4] examine the explicit role played by the body in the construction of self in their studies of giving blood and experiencing chronic pain. Olesen *et al.*, in their research on the mundane ailment, have proposed a new concept of self, "a physical self" [5]. This new perspective on the body is due in part to the recognition that sociological theory has tended to cast human beings as primarily cognitive and rational actors, while neglecting to account for nondeliberate actions (habits), for affective phenomena (emotions), and for the body as more than simply a surface upon which social and cultural meanings are bestowed [6–15].

I argue in this paper that the experience of 'being healthy' is another instance in which the phenomenological body is explicitly salient. No longer can the body be considered theoretically as an abstract universal concept, but must be considered in its concreteness as a lived experience of socially and historically situated men and women. This lived experience entails simultaneous processes of interpretation and communication: interpretation of one's own and other's particular bodies and communication of one's self as healthy and as member of a social group. Gender is an underlying theme.

I propose that social psychological theories of health need to take account of the body as personal and socially situated in the construction of self (and other selves) as healthy. This requires bringing into the theoretical foreground the processes and practices of everyday life through which the body is constructed and known in its concreteness and particularity.

Methodology

This research is based on open-ended, unstructured interviews with 9 white, middle-class men and 12 white, middle-class women, ages 35–55. The sample of convenience was limited in size due to financial considerations. None of the respondents had children and all had significant others. The selection of respondents for the research who were partnered and without children alleviated having to address the effects of parenthood and single-hood on health behavior. Interviewees were informed that the interview could be as long as necessary or convenient for them. Typical questions included: Do you consider yourself a healthy person? How do you account for your healthiness? What kinds of things do you do for the sake of health? How do you know if someone else is healthy? and so forth. To analyze interview data, I used the grounded theory method of iteratively coding and categorizing data to uncover thematic categories [16].

Findings related to respondents abstract concepts of health are presented first, followed by related findings concerning the body and self in health, the reflexivity of self and body in health, and gendered differences in the phenomenological experience of self and body. Findings related to health practices are then presented and include discussions of body maintenance, 'body insignia,' and the interplay between gender norms and health practices. The concluding section draws out implications of the research for social psychological theories of health.

Men's and women's concepts of health

In general, men and women shared similar ideas about what constitutes health. The cosmos of health depicted in definitions included most aspects of being human: physicality, consciousness, emotions, spirituality, and social situation (family, work, and income level). The idea of health was closely associated with the idea of 'well being;' that is, abstract notions of health and healthiness were identified with the positive aspects of 'being' in the world and were grounded in lived experience. Some definitions were so encompassing that they approached amorphousness, but their grandness indicated the degree to which contemporary men's and women's ideas of 'health' have become synonymous with a particular condition or state of 'life' itself. As is discussed below, the homogeneity between men's and women's abstract conceptions of health dissipated into gender specific forms when everyday actions were considered.

Many men and women defined 'health' comprehensively, referring to it as a state or condition of being, and often relating this condition to capacity, performance, and function:

> My definition of health would be physical, mental and emotional well being (male).

> (Health is) being balanced in the things you do (female).

One striking variation was that women frequently alluded to friends or family in their definitions of health (while men rarely did so):

> A really healthy person is a well person, they take care of themselves and their family and friends, . . .

> Its also being loved and being able to love.

Body and self in health

Without exception, men and women cited the actuality of being bodied in their concepts of health. Some references to the body were explicit, as in:

> I'm a healthy person because I'm in shape physically, I'm not overweight, . . . I have good muscle tone, . . . (male).

> (Health is) . . . when I'm in shape, I feel energetic, and I've got good color in my cheeks (female).

Others were implicit:

> ... The bottom line is that I am able to go through my day and accomplish what I have to do without any physical or mental encumbrances (male).

Both men and women conceptualized healthiness as flickering in nature, and health as a transitory state and a process related to the lived body. As one man phrased it:

> Health is living. You're alive and you're healthy or you're not healthy as you go along. It's like a living through.

The body's history was also seen as contributing to the temporality and transiency of health [17–20]:

> ... I guess health is a relative term anyway. I don't exercise that much... I want to but its a time problem and I have allergies. They're only slightly debilitating, but I have them... (male).

Definitions of health often referred to deliberate, intentional action involving the body. Each person was seen as having a biological base, a body, and what one did with that body resulted in various states of health. Both men and women mentioned body-oriented protocols such as avoiding smoking, abstaining from drinking, eating 'good' foods, getting sleep, and exercising as being essential to health. In short, health was conceptualized as creation [22, 23] and accomplishment [24, 25] of a bodied, thinking individual.

The concept of self was implicit in concepts of health, either as the intentional actor making decisions about health actions, or as the consciousness interpreting bodily signs and signals, or as the being performing an action. The self as healthy had both physical and metaphysical dimensions. When asked to describe health and being healthy, respondents moved back and forth between references to themselves as physical bodies and as sentient beings. "I'm in good shape", "I have good muscle tone", "I've got good color", and "I feel energetic", "I feel good", "I feel challenged".

Respondents' catalogued a kind of 'health inventory' which encompassed internal and external, visible and invisible, physical and metaphysical dimensions of themselves. The health inventory included things one's self was believed to 'have' and things one's self was expected 'to do'. The former included one's own particular stock of corporeal and incorporeal health-related items such as body size and shape, strength, capacity to do, genetic endowment, and friends. The latter included one's health-related activities and practices, as in:

> I get enough sleep, I don't over exercise and I don't starve myself.

These 'haves' and 'doings' were often intermixed in responses:

> Health to me is the food you eat, how you carry yourself, from the clothes you wear, to the size you are, body fat, skin tone, and whether you're sick. I feel if you take care of yourself by working out and eating right, . . . you will be stronger and healthier (male).

> I know I'm healthy. I'm in good shape. I exercise regularly, I eat a very good diet. I know how to avoid getting colds and flus. I get enough sleep. I don't party and abuse my body. I guess, in a nutshell, I take care of myself (female).

As these remarks suggest, judging one's self as healthy involved a taking stock of one's health inventory—of one's self as both material body and conscious actor.

Respondents' regarded the balance of items in the health inventory as fluctuating with time and action. Individuals would refer to themselves as having been healthier at a former time, or as becoming healthier through certain activities. In sum, the sense of being healthy involved both a sense of self and a sense of body (a body self), both of which were tied to a conception of past and future actions.

The reflexivity of self and body

Berger and Luckmann refer to the 'eccentric' human relationship between organism and self in which the experience of self involves both being and having a body [26]. In this study, when interviewees took stock of themselves as healthy, body and self were not experienced as divided into two parts; that is, as dichotomous 'mind' and 'body' in the Cartesian positivist sense. Nor, as in the Cartesian fashion, was the body described as a vacuum which had been filled up with a mind and a soul [27]. Rather, body and self were described as reflexive aspects of one wholeness, one 'being'; neither complete without the other. The material, or somatic, and immaterial, or asomatic, represented different dimensions of the same self engaged in action in the world. I referred to this reflexive process as 'the self-soma process'.

The reflexivity of self and body could be heard in the alternating grammatical referents used by men and women to describe health. Due to the linearity of language, respondents had to separate references to bodied self and minded self grammatically into subject and direct object. However, the referent of the 'I' continually vacillated such that in one sentence the subject would be the bodied self, and in the next sentence, the subject would be the minded self. This reflected the disjuncture between lived experience and linguistic rules, for in lived experience body and self are related to and contingent on one another. The changing referent is evident in the following example:

when I wake up I reflect immediately on how I feel—whether I'm tight from the workout the day before and whether I feel like getting up at all . . . and whether I can't face the day and what I have to do . . . (female).

The relationship of self and body also had elements of contingency. That is, the state of one was seen as having the potential to affect the state of the other:

I know I'm healthy by the way I feel . . . when I go on a binge of junk food . . . I feel rotten as a person (male).

It's (being healthy) all those things I said. It's really a body feeling, but it's also my head. I can take on the world if my body feels good (female).

Healthiness was considered to be a product of a personal and particular self and body. That is, the experience of being bodied, of the intrasubjective pattern of interplay between self and body, was regarded as unique to the individual. This notion was reminiscent of Mead's theory of the self and social interaction, that each self is individual because of its unique sociality and complement of interactions [28].

I'd say it's a feeling. Either you feel it or you don't on any given day . . . for me it's how I feel and for someone else how they feel (female).

If a person feels that he or she has physical, mental and emotional well-being, then I would say that that person is healthy from that person's point of view. (Health is) very individual (male).

Respondents' characterizations of the reflexive, contingent, and unique nature of the experience of self and body in health dramatically demonstrates the integral nature of embodiment and self-hood. The experience of self as body and body as self constitutes the human experience, and as such, is saturated with notions of moral action and responsibility.

Gendered differences

While both women and men referred to the reflexiveness, contingentness, and uniqueness of self and body with respect to being healthy, there were nuances of difference between men and women in their descriptions of the interactive relationship between self and body. Men frequently referred to healthiness as 'keeping' or 'being in control' and 'minding' one's body. Men seemed to imagine themselves as having 'power over' relationship to their bodies.

> Taking control of your health . . . is the key to an overall sense of well-being (male).

Men spoke about their bodies as though they 'belonged' to them (in the same way that an object belongs to one). Women, on the other hand, generally did not use the language of ownership when talking about their bodies, but rather referred to their bodies as though their bodies had a momentum or subjectness of their own [29-31].

> A lot of times I keep on eating even though I know its not good for me . . . It's like my body just wants those things right then . . .

These gender differences became even more apparent when respondents described their health practices.

Men's and women's health practices in everyday life

The experience of being situated in a particular social and cultural circumstance was conspicuous when comparing men's and women's descriptions of their everyday health practices with their abstract definitions of heath and being healthy. The homogeneity between men's and women's abstract conceptions of health dissipated into gender specific forms when translated into action in the everyday world.

Men and women unanimously cited biological and physiological 'needs of the human body' for rest, exercise, and food in their definitions of health. The prevalence of references to food, rest, and exercise as being essential to being healthy suggested that these have become staples in the commonsense understanding of healthiness. There were degrees of difference, however, in ideas about how much and what type of exercise, food, and rest men and women 'needed'. In these cases, the ideas of the 'healthy' body as a social phenomenon infused with social meaning and of health practices as instances of the social construction of bodies as gendered, began to be evident in the data.

In my interviews, women usually listed food first in response to the question, 'What kinds of things do you do to be healthy?' They then mentioned exercise and rest. All of my male respondents mentioned exercise first, then sleep, and food usually tagged along as the last item of importance. When men did mention food, the nutrient quality was what was important. For women, the caloric value was also, if not equally, as important as the nutrient value. When I asked women about what men should do to be healthy, they still listed food as most important, sleep as next in importance, and exercise as least important (but not to be ignored by any means). When I asked men about what women should do to be healthy, most deferred, saying they didn't know or that the woman would have to decide for herself. One man responded with "the same thing (as I do), I guess, but less."

These responses referenced cultural notions of there being two kinds of human bodies, male and female [32]. Human bodies (one's own and other's) were seen as having similar needs, but different combinations and degrees of these needs depending upon whether they were male or female. These lay ideas about the healthy body are at odds with medical notions of a universal human body which only varies in its reproductive aspects. Furthermore, the conceptualization of the body in the commonsense world of my respondents as dichotomized into male body and female body (with further variations based on particular self as male body or female body within the gross categories of male and female) refutes the idea of a generic and universal body and underscores my theoretical contention that the body is continually and multiply differentiated in the process of constructing self as healthy.

Body maintenance

Respondents' comments showed that the production of health for the self involves 'body maintenance' [33]. This conceptualization refers to the contemporary notion that the body is like a machine and must be maintained because it is believed to be subject to aging, deterioration, disease, and abuse by oneself and others. Respondents' references to health practices were rife with mechanistic metaphors. For example, 'food' was referred to as 'fuel'; exercise concerned 'biomechanics' and 'improving the oxygen uptake' of the heart, the body's 'pump'; and being healthy was a matter of routinized 'workouts' designed to produce 'fitness'. These references reflected a mechanistic, industrial, work-oriented approach to being healthy.

Men and women often cited 'body maintenance' activities as essential to producing health for one's self. Body maintenance conceptions were undergirded by a notion of the body as protean, potentially vulnerable, and alterable [34].

> I exercise regularly. I eat a very good diet. I know how to avoid getting colds and flus. I get enough sleep. I don't party and abuse my body. I guess, in a nutshell, I take care of myself.

Men's and women's approaches to and notions of body maintenance were different, however. Men emphasized sports and outdoor activities—one specifically excluded aerobics because it was womanish, "for girls," as he put it. Eating well was also considered to be important, but was usually mentioned as a corollary to being able to do well in sports. Most men also mentioned tooth-brushing and flossing.

> ...A lot of days I don't feel like working out, but I do anyway. I push a little harder because I know that when I get through my workout, I'll feel better (male).

Women also mentioned physical activities, but the emphasis was not on sport activities but on exercise activities (many mentioned aerobics). Food consumption was important for women, but interestingly, they often referred to it using the verb "to diet" rather than, as did men, the verb "to eat well". (I read this as a linguistic reflection of men's and women's different relationship to food and the body.) Unlike men, most women mentioned caring for their skin, shaving their legs, getting their hair cut, and other appearance-related items as being basic to body maintenance.

> (To stay healthy) I try to keep things balanced. I don't over workout, I don't slug it; I try not to overeat, and I take care of all my personal needs . . . I use sunblock, shave my legs, keep my hair looking nice . . . (female).

These differences in emphasis and approach to body maintenance practices suggested that men were concerned with the body as the medium of action; function and capacity of the body were of paramount importance. Implicit in men's orientation was a concern with potentiality, with being able to act in the world. Women were also concerned with maintaining function and capacity, especially with respect to 'doing for others', but they were equally concerned with the appearance of their bodies and with keeping their bodies in a 'presentable' condition.

The concept of body maintenance reflects a conceptualization of the body as having 'inner' and 'outer' aspects [35, p. 18]. Inner aspects refer to optimal functioning, performance, capacity to do things, and the potential for breakdown (lack of capacity) while outer aspects refer to appearance, movement within social space, and the potential to be touched and heard.

Considering respondents' comments in light of the concept of the inner and outer body, men and women differed in their emphasis on inner and outer aspects of the body. Men tended to emphasize the inner body phenomena of function and capacity more than the outer body phenomena of appearance, while women focussed more or less equally on both inner and outer phenomena.

The concepts of the inner and outer body invoke phenomenological conceptualizations of 'my body' as a 'subject' (or 'agent' body) and as 'object' body. In her analysis of the effects on body identity of Cartesian dualism which divides the world into dichotomies of active/passive, subject/object, and mind/body, Young points out that body identities have been dichotomized into woman-body-as-passive/man-body-as-active [35–37]. Male interviewees comments more frequently referenced the subject body: "being able to go through my day and accomplish things", "being in shape physically so I can do things", and "having good muscle tone". Female respondents, on the other hand, more frequently referenced the object body, as in: "looking agile", "having good color and skin tone". This suggested that these men and women each maintained a unique phenomenological stance toward their bodies.

Estimating health in other selves: body insignia

Up to this point I have addressed men's and women's self-constructions of being healthy. The analysis now turns to the issue of the construction of others as healthy. As in the case of the construction of self as healthy, the perceived physical body and body practices play a prominent role in the construction of other selves as healthy.

Male and female interviewees used aspects of the body and body practices as indicators of the dimensions of another persons physical as well as ontological state of health. I referred to these cues as 'body insignia':

> If they have good skin color and glow, then I know they must know what they're doing with their life (female).
>
> Well, it's pretty easy. I just look at them, if they're not in shape, I say, 'Those people are not healthy' (male).

Even though, healthiness was not necessarily a point of observation for most respondents (as hair color or height would be), certain body insignia brought healthiness to the fore as an observation point. A person's skin color—either 'paleness' or 'glow' was referenced frequently as provoking questions about another's health. In addition, individuals associated certain body insignia with individuals, and if there were changes, the question of healthiness arose. For example:

> I can tell when J. (a dancer), has cramps—she doesn't move her usual way (female).

Gender norms

Gender norms often informed the interpreting of body insignia. Respondents used body insignia as indicators of the health of self's and other's state of womanhood or manhood, that is, as indicators of the degree to which self or other was 'correctly' gendered and followed gender norms.

> My mother always said you're a lazy person if you don't take care of your face and wear make-up . . . (female).
>
> I see a lot of girls in the weight room these days and it's too much. I mean I like how some of them look, but the real bulked up ones . . . that's not right (male).

Gender was also a recurrent theme in respondents' comments about their health practices. Even though they made similar general recommendations for themselves regarding what was required in order to be healthy (exercise, rest, 'good' food, and so forth), when they came to act on their recommendations in the everyday world, they were guided and constrained by social norms and situations. Some constraints related to 'appropriate' sites for health activities. As one man said regarding where he could exercise: "I can't do aerobics with all those girls." Or, as one woman remarked: "I can't run at night anymore now that we live in the city . . ."

The issue of public safety (and danger) and being femaled-bodied was a recurrent topic in women's narratives. Women often cited concern about being safe while exercising. Men did not cite public safety as a health-related issue for themselves personally or for men in general. When men and women who identified themselves as runners and cyclists were asked directly about safety and exercise, most responded that women risked bodily harm if they went out in the dark (unless accompanied by a man), and that men, too, were taking risks by exercising at night; however, the 'risks' for men referred to 'tripping and falling down' and/or 'hitting something' and not to personal bodily harm. In short, there were particular structural conditions related to female and male bodies; moreover, male and female bodies were each seen as having their own specific set of concerns regarding public safety and danger.

Other constraints related to norms of behavior for men and women. One man said:

> I'd do more (to be healthy), but I can't with my job hours. My boss at the lab would kill me.

The conflict between work and health activities was a common theme for men. Many mentioned time conflicts (between work and health activities) while others cited the 'unhealthiness' of 'normal' work-related practices such as frequent traveling, eating restaurant foods, and spending hours sitting in planes and meetings. A few men mentioned routines they followed in order to minimize the unhealthy aspects of their jobs, such as "walking around the building at least three times a day" or taking vitamins and sticking to their home time zone sleep and eating times when traveling. Despite acknowledgements of the 'unhealthiness' of occupational practices, work demands usually took precedence over health demands when making decisions about allocating one's time and efforts. For these respondents, the social norms of making a living and using ones body for economically productive (economic) labor were paramount, even if such activities meant not 'being healthy'.

One woman referenced norms of behavior for women when she said:

> My mother always said that women who eat small meals are more feminine.

Female respondents regularly linked healthiness, eating, exercise, and being thin in their responses. Three women stated directly that their exercise and eating activities were motivated as much by a desire to 'not be fat' as by a desire to be healthy. Another respondent, expressing a common view among women about health and 'not being fat', fortified her response with a comment that 'being thin really is healthier for you'. There were a number of references to ideas about amounts of food required by men and women; amounts required by women were generally considered to be smaller than those required by men, irrespective of what the man or the women did. Two women respondents said that they often ate less (for weight control purposes) even when they knew it might be healthier to eat more. In these cases, activities related to 'being healthy' were influenced by social norms related to gender and the body, which in American culture locate woman as object of the male gaze [38]. Moreover, that a culturally saturated health-seeking activity such as eating can verge into non-healthy behavior is exemplified by such states as anorexia and bulimia [39].

Some of my respondents were acutely aware of the relationship between healthiness, the body, and gender and regarded their health actions as challenges to existing gender norms:

> Masters (swimmers) women are special because they have instituted change into their lives and have been willing to be somewhat unconventional in doing it. (We) have had to unlearn that early socialization and grow comfortable with (our) physical selves... (we) open the door for other women.

In sum, gender was emergent in health doings in that specific ideas about what male and female healthy bodies 'do' were legitimated and reinforced through the taking of certain actions and not others by either men or women.

Implications of the research

This research suggests that the body is problematic in the lived experience of health. Selfhood, embodiment, and health are intertwined. If social psychological theories of health are to reflect this experience of health adequately, they must begin to take into account not only the body as individually and socially problematic, but also the practices and processes through which the body is constructed and known as personal, concrete, and particular.

In the commonsense world of my respondents, the body as concrete and particular was evident in respondents use of their own and other person's bodily signs and signals, or 'body insignia,' as indicators not only of physical health, but also of ontological health, or the healthiness of the self. Bodies were seen to bear personal and particular self-inflections.

Gender played a key role in interpreting and constructing one's own and other's bodies as concretely and particularly healthy. Respondents cited different bodily symbols of health for males and females, differentiating between male and female bodies and the needs and 'appropriate' health activities for each. The healthy body was rarely referenced in universal, non-gendered terms (except in comments referring to the human need for sleep, food, and rest); rather, the healthy body was considered in its context of who and where. That gender was a significant aspect of the lived experience of health follows from the view that gender is a fundamental social construction of self which has a biological base [30, p. 44]. The body, as the focal point of self-construction as well as health construction, implicates gender in the everyday lived experience of health.

As residents of a commonsense world, respondents health practices were instances in which self and body as gendered were constructed. The sense of self as healthy, as gendered, and as body, were intertwined, and were realized simultaneously in concrete habits and practices of daily life. Decisions about what actions to take to be healthy or 'health doings' were colored by ideas about appropriate masculine and feminine behavior. From a theoretical point of view, this suggests that the doing of health is a form of doing gender [40], This is not because there is an essential difference between male and female body healthiness, but because of social and cultural interpretations of masculine and feminine selves—selves which are attached to biological male and female bodies. Health activities can be seen as a form of practice which constructs the subject (the 'person') in the same way that other social and cultural activities do [41, 42]. Health actions are social acts, in interactionist terms, and the social objects pertinent to the experience of being healthy are the self and the body. Social order is negotiated, produced, and reproduced through interpretation and construction of selves as healthy and as bodies.

Health an the phenomenological body

Thus, health is not a universal fact, but is a constituted social reality, constructed through the medium of the body using the raw materials of social meaning and symbol. This contrasts with other views of health which regard health as a material issue [43], an objective state in policy analysis [44], or the absence of illness [45]. Even though health is seen as an organic and inherent reality independent of selves, it is a creation of those selves. It is one classificatory system for mapping self and others. Health actions are political actions enacted via the body which legitimate or challenge norms and ideas of the social body. Put differently, the interplay between health, self, body, and gender at the individual level is linked to the creation and recreation of a sense of healthiness in the social body, the body politic of society.

In sum, I have argued that health is a lived experience of being bodied which involves action (practical activity) in the world. Gender is an integral aspect of this process. With respect to social psychological theory development, this raises the body to a position of explicit saliency and refocuses analytic attention on the array of everyday ways and means that ideas are enacted and the social order is sustained by socially situated, bodied selves.

References

1. Currer C. and Stacey M. *Concepts of Health, Illness, and Disease*. Berg, Leamington Spa, 1986.
2. Glassner B. Fit for postmodern selfhood. In *Symbolic Interaction and Cultural Studies* (Edited by Becker H. S. and McCall M. M). University of Chicago Press, Chicago, 1990.
3. Espelande W. Blood and money: Exploiting the embodied self. In *The Existential Self in Society* (Edited by Kotarba J. and Fontana A.). University of Chicago Press, Chicago, 1984.
4. Kotarba J. The chronic pain experience. In *Existential Sociology* (Edited by Douglas J. and Johnson J.). Cambridge University Press, Cambridge, 1977.
5. Olesen V., Schatzman L., Droes N., Hatton D. and Chico N. The mundane ailment and the physical self: analysis of the social psychology of health and illness. *Soc. Sci. Med.* **30**, 449–455, 1990.
6. Wrong D. The oversocialized conception of man in modern society. *Am. Sociol. Rev.* **26**, 184–193, 1961.
7. Baldwin J. Habit, emotion, and self-concious action. *Sociol. Perspect.* **31**, 35–58, 1988.
8. Ferguson K. *Self, Society, and Womankind*. Greenwood Press, Westport, CT, 1980.
9. Kotarba J. A synthesis: The existential self in society. In *The Existential Self in Society* (Edited by Kotarba J. and Fontana A.). University of Chicago Press, Chicago, IL, 1984.
10. Hirst P. and Wooley P. *Social Relations and Human Attributes*. Tavistock, London, 1982.
11. Turner B. *The Body in Society*. Blackwell, London, 1984.
12. For a selection of femnist interpretations of the problematic of the body see: Hodge J. Subject, body, and the exclusion of women from philosophy. In *Feminist Perspectives in Philosophy* (Edited by Griffiths M. and Whitford M.). Indiana University Press, Indianapolis, IN, 1988; Gross E. Philosophy, subjectivity, and the body: Kristeva and Irigaray. In *Feminist Challenges: Social and Political Theory* (Edited by Pateman C. and Gross E.). Allen and Unwin, Sydney, 1986; Jagger A. and Bordo S. *Gender/Body/Knowledge*. Rutgers, New Brunswick, NJ, 1989; Riley D. *Am I That Name? Feminism and the Category of 'Women'*. University of Minnesota Press, Minneapolis, MN, 1988; Jacobus M., Keller E.

and Shuttleworth S. *Body/Politics: Women and the Discourses of Science*. Routledge, New York, 1990.
13. Freund P. Bringing society into the body. *Theory and Society* **17**, 839–864, 1988.
14. Lester M. Self: sociological portraits. In *The Existential Self in Society* (Edited by Kortarba J. and Fontana A.). University of Chicago Press, Chicago, IL, 1984.
15. Manning P. Existential sociology. *Sociol. Q.* **14**, 200–255, 1973.
16. Glaser B. and Strauss A. *The Discovery of Grounded Theory: Strategies for Qualitative Research*. Aldine, New York 1967.
17. See Herzlich's concept of the 'reserve of health.' Herzlich C. *Health and Illness*. Academic Press. London, 1973.
18. Pill R. and Stott N. Concepts of illness causation and responsibility: some preliminary data from a sample of working class mothers. *Soc. Sci. Med.* **16**, 43–52, 1982.
19. Blaxter M. The causes of disease: women talking. *Soc. Sci. Med.* **17**, 59–69, 1983.
20. Herzlich C. and Pierret J. *Illness and Self in Society*. Johns Hopkins Press, Baltimore, MD, 1984.
21. Blaxter M. *Health and Lifestyles*. Routledge, London, 1990.
22. Turner [6, p. 236] has suggested that each disease has an organic grammar, but the speech of the sick patient is "highly variable, creative, and idiosyncratic."
23. Sacks has noted a similar phenomenon with migraines: "If the foundations of migraine are based on universal adaptive reations, its superstructure may be constructed differently by every patient, in accordance with his needs and symbols. Migraine... starts as a reflex, but can become a creation." Sacks O. *Migraine*. Summit, New York, 1981.
24. The idea of health as an accomplishment leads to the notions that the responsibility for health resides with the individual and that the etiology of both health and illness can be traced to the habits and practives of the individual. See Crawford R. You are dangerous to your health: the ideology and politics of victim-blaming. *Int. J. Hlth Services* **7**, 663–680, 1978.
25. Crawford R. Healthism and the medicalization of everyday life. *Int. J. Hlth Services* **10**, 365–388, 1980.
26. Berger P. and Luckmann T. *The Social Construction of Reality*, p. 50. Anchor Doubleday, Garden City, NY, 1967.
27. Butler notes that in Cartesian, positivist thinking "The soul is what the body lacks; hence, the body presents itself as a signifying lack. That lack which is the body signifies the soul as that which it cannot show." Butler J. *Gender Trouble*, p. 135. Routledge, London, 1990.
28. Morris C. W. (Ed.) *Mind, Self, and Society, George Herbert Mead*. University of Chicago Press, Chicago, IL, 1967.
29. The concept of control and mastery which was prevalent in men's references to their bodies was less evident in the language of my female respondents. The relationship between self and body was experienced as more colateral than hierarchical. This mirrors some of the feminist theories that women's relationships are characterized more by affiliation and cooperation than are men's. See Gilligan C. *In a Different Voice*. Harvard University Press, Cambridge, MA, 1982; Jordan J., Kaplan A., Miller J., Stive I. and Surrey J. *Women's Growth in Connection*. Guilford, New York, 1991.

30. Dinnerstein D. *The Mermaid and the Minotaur: Sexual Arrangements and Human Malaise*. Harper, New York, 1976.
31. Diamond and Quinby have noted the prevalence of the language of 'control over one's body' in contemporary discourse, arguing that such language blinds us to other more nurturant and aesthetic conceptions of bodies. Diamond I. and Quinby L. American feminism in the age of the body. *Signs* **10**, 119–125, 1984.
32. Kessler S. and McKenna W. *Gender: An Ethnomethodological Approach*. University of Chicago Press, Chicago, IL, 1978.
33. Featherstone M. The body in consumer culture. *Theory Culture Society* **1**, 18–33, 1982.
34. Featherstone [31, p. 22] suggests that body maintenance is tied to a concept of plasticity of the body, such that, if we work hard enough we can alter our bodies.
35. Young I. The exclusion of women from sport: conceptual and existential dimensions. *Phil. Context* **9**, 44–53, 1979.
36. See Duquin M. Fashion and fitness: images in women's magazines advertisements. *Arena Rev.* **13**, 97–109, 1989, and [35] for discussions of women as body objects in the context of sport.
37. Rintala J. The gendered body: a synthesis and more paradox. *Arena Rev.* **13**, 134–145, 1989.
38. Young I. M. Breasted experience, the look and the feeling. In *Throwing Like A Girl and Other Essays in Feminist Philosophy and Social Theory* (Edited by Young I. M.). University of Indiana Press, Bloomington, IN, 1990.
39. Boskind-Lodahl M. Cindarellas stepsisters: A feminist perspective on anorexia nervosa and bulimia. *Signs* **2**, 342–356, 1976.
40. West C. and Zimmerman P. Doing Gender. *Gender Society* **1**, 125–151, 1988.
41. Blacking J. *The Anthropology of the Body*. Academic Press, London, 1977.
42. Douglas M. *Natural Symbols*. Vintage Press, New York, 1970.
43. Navarro V. *Crisis, Health, and Medicine, A Social Critique*. Tavistock-Metheun, London, 1986.
44. Spacapan S. and Oskamp S. *The Social Psychology of Health*. Sage, Newbury Park, CA, 1988.
45. Calnan M. *Health and Illness, The Lay Perspective*. Tavistock, London, 1987.

18

IDENTITY DILEMMAS OF CHRONICALLY ILL MEN

Kathy Charmaz

Source: *The Sociological Quarterly*, 35:2 (1994), pp. 269–88.

Consider this story. A 45-year-old man had had a serious heart attack 3 years before while cycling. Being a competitive cyclist had complemented and extended his identities as a hard-driving, no-nonsense businessman, a former military man, and the traditional breadwinner and head of his household. These masculine identities—male athlete, competitive businessman, Vietnam veteran, and breadwinner—formed the boundaries and content of his self-concept. A business failure just before his heart attack forced his wife to go to work. After his heart attack, his doctor prescribed a strenuous cardiac rehabilitation program. Without my asking, he stated, "I didn't know who I was for a while. I'd kind of [think], 'God, if I can do this exercise, I'll die again . . . [doing the exercise frightened him because having a heart attack while cycling vigorously almost killed him]. How to identify?'" I then asked, "How did you come to identify yourself?" He replied with the following:

> Well, what's the alternative? If death is on the one end, or do you want repeated heart attacks? We had one of our friends in the group [cardiac rehabilitation] who was in there for the second heart attack and he lasted 2½ years and he's my age but he let himself go—back to smoking and drinking and bad eating habits. So there is—I've heard this before—you get this invulnerable feeling—this invincible feeling and all of a sudden the hardest thing to accept is, "Hey, you are vulnerable. You can be hurt. You can die," you know, which you never thought of that before, or I never did. So that's still in the back of your mind.

Caught within the identity dilemma of forecasting himself as a potential dead man who had exercised hard or as a cardiac invalid who had not, this man had felt trapped in a web of uncertainty for months. However, like other men who participated in cardiac rehabilitation programs, this man eventually gained a sense of leaving death behind and regained a feeling of moving on with his life. But reminders of the fragility of life come more frequently and forcefully, as occurred with the sudden death of his friend. The earlier victory over death fades, the regained sense of invincibility crumbles, and the consciousness of uncertainty again heightens.

This story illustrates two essential properties of men's experience of chronic illness: (a) Illness can threaten masculine identities and lead to identity dilemmas, and (b) these dilemmas, like the illnesses themselves, can be recurrent and chronic.[1] Identity dilemmas for men revolve around the following oppositions: active versus passive, independent versus dependent, autonomy versus loss of control, public persona versus private self, and domination versus subordination.

Identity dilemmas ripple upon each other. Should the man above give up his exercise program, he would also relinquish his masculine identity as an athlete. He would face the identity dilemma of active athlete versus passive patient. Subsequently, if he adopted the identity of passive patient, he would also face identity dilemmas between having been the traditional breadwinner and decision maker and becoming the dependent partner in his marriage.

Chronic illness frequently comes to men suddenly with immediate intensity, severity, and uncertainty. Typically, men contract more serious and life-threatening chronic illnesses than women, who experience a higher incidence of degenerative diseases such as arthritis and multiple sclerosis (Conrad, 1987; Verbrugge, 1989; Verbrugge & Wingard, 1987). Therefore, men have more heart attacks and strokes earlier in life and die significantly more frequently and quickly than women (Verbrugge, 1985). Thus, the suddenness of illness, its intensity, and timing in the life course (usually middle age and older) pose special identity dilemmas for men.

Identities define, locate, characterize, categorize, and differentiate self from others. Identities develop both in stable roles and in emergent situations (Goffman, 1963; Weigert, 1986). Following Hewitt (1989), social identities derive from cultural meanings and community memberships that others confer upon the person. Personal identities define a sense of location, differentiation, continuity, and direction by and in relation to self. When identities of either type are internalized, they become part of the self-concept, what Turner (1976) defines as the relatively stable, coherent organization of characteristics, evaluations, and sentiments that a person holds about self (cf. Charmaz, 1991; Gecas, 1982). Identity dilemmas result from losing valued attributes, physical functions, social roles, and personal pursuits and their corresponding valued identities, that is, positive definitions of self, including socially conferred and personally defined positive identities. These dilemmas arise as people experience complicated problems, defined incapacities, and hard decisions that result from such identity losses.

Masculine identities reflect lifelong participation in the gender order (Connell, 1987) and are taken for granted by men when these identities remain stable. Chronic illness can undermine all the taken-for-granted identities that support and sustain a man's place in the gender order, including his place in the male dominance hierarchy among men (cf. Messner & Sabo, 1990; Sabo & Panepinto, 1990). To wit, chronic illness can alter or end men's participation in work, sports, leisure, and sexual activities. Hence, illness can reduce a man's status in masculine hierarchies, shift his power relations with women, and raise his self-doubts about masculinity. Consequently, chronic illness can relegate a man to a position of "marginalized" masculinity in the gender order (Connell, 1987; Messner & Sabo, 1990; Sabo & Gordon, 1992).

To date, the sociological literature has not addressed the circumstances that chronically ill men face. Nor have earlier researchers looked at these men's experience from the standpoint of gender-based conceptions of masculinity. Instead, the literature has largely remained gender-neutral and thus not only missed seeing the particular emergent structure of men's experience of chronic illness but also the identity dilemmas that they confront (see, e.g., Charmaz, 1987, 1991; Corbin & Strauss, 1988; Johnson, 1991; Kelleher, 1988; Kleinman, 1988; Strauss et al., 1984).

What is it like to be an active, productive man one moment and a patient who faces death the next? What is it like to change one's view of oneself accordingly? What identity dilemmas does living with continued uncertainty pose for men? How do they handle them? When do they make identity changes? When do they try to preserve a former self?

This chapter explores these questions by initiating the discussion of gender and male identity in chronic illness and by looking at four major processes that men with chronic illnesses experience: (a) awakening to death after a life-threatening crisis, (b) accommodating to uncertainty as men realize that the crisis has lasting consequences, (c) defining illness and disability, and (d) preserving self to maintain a sense of coherence while experiencing loss and change.² These categories build on each other, although accommodating to uncertainty, modes of defining illness, and ways of preserving self often reflect implicit meanings rather than explicit strategies. Here, uncertainty means awareness of imminent or eventual recurrence, degeneration, or death. Although uncertainty has long been a key theme in the chronic illness literature, the focus has been on uncontrollable embarrassing, incapacitating, or painful symptoms and further episodes (cf. Reif, 1975; Schneider & Conrad, 1983; Wiener, 1975). By also studying men who suffer potentially life-threatening conditions, uncertainty in relation to death in chronic illness becomes explicit.

Awakening to death

Death. The first identity dilemma comes when men realize that death could occur—now. Clinging to former identities in hope of minimizing the symbolic threat of death by defining illness as minor could risk their lives. Acknowledging the threat of death could cost them their most valued identities. When wholly unanticipated, the threat of death shakes men to their very core. Within moments or brief hours, the disruptive crisis removes them from familiar former identities to that of patient, possibly of dying patient. Crisis can overtake them without earlier warnings. Even illnesses such as diabetes or cancer may not become manifest until a crisis.[3] Occasionally, as the athlete above, another man's crisis awakens or reawakens a man to his own vulnerability, aging, and death (cf. Karp, 1988).

Some men invoke gender-based reasoning such as the male midlife crisis (Jaques, 1965; Levinson, Darrow, Klein, Levinson, & McKee, 1978; Sabo, 1990) to account for what happens to them even as illness develops. One man believed he was having a midlife crisis—that his life was falling apart, "There's a point I was thinking, 'This is a midlife crisis; this is just a state, or this is a stage you're going through.'" Later, his doctor told him that his aorta was literally ripping apart.

Awakening to death comes as an unbelievable shock when a man (a) sees himself as too young to die, (b) defines himself as exceptionally healthy, or (c) has had no earlier episodes or heralding symptoms. Young clinical psychologist Neil A. Fiore (1984) sought help for what he believed was an infection on his testicle only to find the physician talking "calcification," "surgery," "cancer," "death." When younger men have heart attacks, particularly the first one, they often do not know what is happening to them (cf. Cowie, 1976; Frank, 1991; Johnson, 1991). The athlete above recounted his heart attack at age 42:

> I was on my bicycle going on just a routine ride for me and . . . I just went down. I didn't know what happened. . . . So I had no indication that I [was having a heart attack]—no chest pains, no shortness of breath, no the typical [symptoms of] how you feel. I couldn't even tell you what it feels like.

He awoke in the hospital to find himself partly paralyzed, which did not faze him, but the news that he had had a heart attack infuriated him. When I asked him what raised his fury, he juxtaposed the finality of heart disease with the injustice of having paid his dues already by stopping smoking, limiting drinking, getting in shape, and losing weight. All this work and then, the biggest injustice, "It's just I'm too young. . . . Why me?"

Once men realize or are told what has happened, identity dilemmas emerge. When men believe that they have narrowly survived their crisis, at least at first they assume it means vulnerability, a greatly increased risk of dying, a radically altered life. A substantially foreshortened future? Death? Now real and perhaps soon. They now connect death with personal identity. Several men made statements such as the following: "I know that I am mortal."

"We all 'know' that we are going to die, but when you come close to death, you see it is true." "I am not immune to death."

The prospect of immediate death darkens the present and shades the future. While in crisis, men see living and dying as discrete categories. Their sense of betrayal by their bodies evokes anger, self-pity, and envy of the healthy. Once certain futures now look uncertain, even ended. Though premature death now seems possible, these men remain unaware of lasting illness and disability if they are unfamiliar with their diagnoses, their disease process, and other men who have the same condition (cf. Charmaz, 1991).

When men define awakening to death as only a discrete, immediate event, they limit the critical period to the initial crisis. As Speedling's (1982) men who had heart attacks, such men initially view getting through this crisis as the passage to an unchanged future. Several men who had had bypass surgery or other circulatory procedures questioned whether they were suitable subjects for a study of experiencing chronic illness. They believed their surgery had effected the necessary repairs. For them, not only the threat of death was over, but also the illness. A referral to my study, especially if by their nurse, undermined their construction of illness as an acute episode.

Eventually, men's routine interactions and unforeseen daily obstacles turn early glimmers of awareness into growing cognizance that illness remains. They learn lessons in chronicity during everyday routines that have become much more arduous and time-consuming than before. For example, buttoning a shirt or tying a shoe becomes a formidable task to a man whose stroke has affected his dominant side. Playing his usual round of golf becomes impossible for a man who had a recent serious heart attack. Lessons in chronicity can challenge men's assumptions about male mastery and competence, thereby leading them into depression (cf. Dahlberg & Jaffe, 1977; Hodgins, 1964). Treating illness and its consequences as problems to solve is consistent with men's gender-related behavior (Tannen, 1990). Inability to solve these problems erodes their personal identity. A 45-year-old man with heart disease disclosed that for 6 months, "I thought my life was over. Cardiac Cripple."

The identity issues emerging in awakening to death are not limited to men, but they are embedded in the medical diagnoses these men received and the social conditions they experienced. Women responded similarly when they found themselves facing unanticipated life-threatening crises. However, women, even heart patients, reported much more difficulty in getting physicians to view their symptoms as real. Subsequently, practitioners, relatives, and the women themselves wondered if they fabricated their symptoms. Hence, these women met serious diagnoses with relief (cf. Charmaz, 1991). In contrast, men who had crises acknowledged their symptoms but initially glossed over their present or potential seriousness. Further, they seldom had trouble in getting practitioners to attend to their developing symptoms.[4]

What mitigates the overwhelming implications of awakening to death for identity? When might a man gain through having a crisis?

Awakening to death can result in direct, positive consequences for identity. Not only do moments of crisis crystallize when defined and met with a spouse or partner, so also do identities. During crisis and its immediate aftermath, most married men felt tremendous affirmation of their valued identities in the family as they awakened to death (cf. Johnson, 1991; Speedling, 1982). They received an outpouring of care, comfort, and love from their wives and families. These men often bragged about how supportive and helpful their wives had been. Even men who had had troubled marriages felt that their wives affirmed, valued, and supported them. Statements such as, "Marge was right there every minute; she even stayed at the hospital those first few nights" were common ones. To these men, their wives had provided the essence of "being there" for them. They were vigilantly attentive, helpful advocates, and loving companions throughout the crisis. These women provided their husbands with a continuing link to both past and future identity through the intensity of their involvement in the present.

Thus, these men received identity validation that not only confirmed positive social identifications and private self-definitions but also implicitly affirmed their gender identities as men in the household. Paradoxically, that validation came when they were most physically dependent but derived from their central positions as husbands (which also validates the wife or partner's identity and role as helpmate and caregiver).

Identity supports to provide validation for unattached single men, however, usually were much less available. They weathered crises largely on their own. Here, their situations resembled those of single women who often had to fend for themselves during crises and within the health care system. Older widowed and divorced women, however, typically received more caring and comfort from adult children than their male counterparts. The occasional exception occurred when divorced men's first wives, or gay men's friends gave them care and support through their crises.[5] Generally, if single men had no caring children or close friends, they were particularly bereft. Thus, constructing a personally valued and socially validated identity became more problematic for them than for those who had ready access to families.

Accommodating to uncertainty

In which ways do men define and handle uncertainty? A casual observer might find that men often accommodate to uncertainty by ignoring, minimizing, or glossing over it. But what do such actions mean to men who do so? Their way of accommodating to uncertainty assumes "bracketing" (Husserl, 1970) the event that elicited it. Bracketing means setting this event apart by putting a frame around it and treating it as something separate and removed from the flow of life. The impact of the event upon identity lessens when this event is separated from social and personal identity. Through bracketing, men define uncertainty as having boundaries—those limited to flareups and crises.[6] To the extent that men bracket uncertainty, they avoid letting it permeate their thoughts and alter their identities. Thus, bracketing raises identity dilemmas because it poses maintaining past identity at cost to health against taking illness into account at risk to social and personal identity.

Bracketing reduces awareness of uncertainty. But why might men who remain at least partly aware of continued uncertainty not make prescribed lifestyle changes because of it? First, these men cannot envision themselves as dead and may see themselves as risk takers and winners. Second, their earlier habits merge with their conception of masculine identity. Third, they have lost hope of genuinely effecting change and decide to live on their own terms for whatever time they have left. In each case, they usually do not foresee the possible kind or degree of disability and debility. Rather, they see themselves as remaining the same or as dead. Yet men can use uncertainty to retain power and privilege in their homes. Then, wives who cajole and try to control them get responses such as, "Why should I care what I eat? I'm going to die anyway." Fertile grounds for marital strife develop in each case (cf. Peyrot, McMurray, & Hedges, 1988). Subsequently, identity dilemmas arise when spouses disagree on bracketing or acknowledging uncertainty.

Eventually most men realize that their bodies have changed. Subsequently, they become aware of uncertainty—uncertain episodes, uncertain treatment effects, uncertain complications—an uncertain life. Awakening to death and acknowledging continued uncertainty is sobering. Reappraisals follow. These reappraisals can lead to epiphanies marking major turning points for men and their families (cf. Charmaz, 1991; Denzin, 1989; Gordon, 1990). When men acknowledge continued uncertainty, their reappraisals bring reflection and self-appraisal. Men who had attended much more to their work than to their families decide to devote more time to the latter. Men who describe themselves as driven by their Type A behavior believe that they have to relinquish it before it kills them. The man above who had viewed himself as a cardiac cripple for 6 months saw his heart attack quite differently 2 years later:

> I would say, "Thank you, thank you," type of thing. But you know, had it not been for my heart attack—I'm grateful it happened now, 'cause it changed my life considerably and so [I] have a lack of words [to describe it]. Yeah, I thank my heart attack for that. In one way I'm grateful.

Reappraisals of productivity, achievement, relationships all alter what these men defined as valuable. Their forced reappraisals led to setting priorities, making decisions, and also, coming to terms with their pasts and presents. A middle-aged executive regretted his behavior in his first two marriages and resolved to maintain his third. These appraisals lead to assessments of self and identity. The middle-aged attorney reflected:

> When you are on the brink, so to speak, you begin to look at what things in your life are valuable and which aren't. And you begin to—and one of the things is real clear was I was glad that I did work where I tried to help other people rather than having a garage full of Mercedes. And it made me feel not like a saint, or anything, but it made me feel like not a bad person, not even like I was a good person. But I was all right; I was all right.

A resolve to live in the present frequently follows these initial reappraisals. The man above said, "I reflect on the past, leave the sadness and parts of myself that I don't consider functional anymore and try to live in the present." A young man believed that his earlier struggles to sift through and to sort out the past had kept him from attending to the immediate present and from knowing himself within it.

For young men, reappraisal can open paths to self-discovery. Getting a kidney transplant and being released from triweekly dialysis treatments resulted in reappraisal by the young man above. At that point, he suddenly had much more unstructured time. He reflected:

> And part of it is getting used to myself.... Getting used to my self, yeah, two words, because I didn't really have that much time to find out who I was before. I'd get glimpses now and again, and I'd go, "Oh, yuck," or "yeah, far out," you know, or "Maybe," you know. [I] caught a lot of those [glimpses].

Not uncommonly, men will be shaken by the initial crisis then gradually resume normal lives. Concurrently, they normalize their symptoms and regimens if they follow one. But before they resettle into a normal routine, they reappraise their lives and their actions.

After awakening to death and defining uncertainty, lifestyles, and also habits, rapidly change—at least for a while. Men quit working, change jobs, renegotiate their work assignments, or retire early. They follow a regimen, lose weight, stop smoking, and reduce drinking. Making permanent changes, however, means acknowledging uncertainty and treating its consequences as lasting. Several men with diabetes disclosed that they had not attended to their conditions until shocked by a diabetic crisis. One middle-aged manager previously had ignored his diet, his doctor's warnings, and his wife's nagging. After a harrowing struggle against death followed by loss of his foot, he not only acknowledged his own uncertain future but also tried to instruct unaware relatives and friends about the negative consequences of their lifestyles, "because, look what happened to me."

As young men grow older, their accommodations to uncertainty can form the foundation of their identities. As he looked back on having been a diabetic for more than two decades, a professor viewed his regimen as not only the means of reducing uncertainty by staving off further complications but also as the way he identified himself:

> I would not want to have to be preoccupied with it the way I was the first year or so. Ah, but at the same time, it is the ground of my life. *I have no idea who I would be, in a way, if I hadn't become diabetic*.... Just to have to internalize this regime must have made a great difference to my personality, I think ... I was a person who didn't eat unless someone sort of sat him down. And, I like to drink and drink and sometimes got quite intoxicated. Stay up all night, and not sleep, go days without sleeping. And I've now become the opposite of all that, like a field and ground thing [emphasis mine].

Defining illness and disability

As they accommodate to uncertainty, how do men define their conditions? How do these definitions affect their personal identity? These men viewed their conditions in four major ways: (a) an enemy, (b) an ally, (c) an intrusive presence, and (d) an opportunity. Definitions of illness as an enemy or an ally personify and make illness tangible. Definitions of it as an intrusive presence or an opportunity reveal the connectedness between body and self. At different points in time, a man may hold each definition. Similarly, different contexts that call forth different identities can elicit disparate, even paradoxical views of illness. Thus, a man can curse his illness as the enemy that ruined his life, but treat it as an ally deserving of respect when he attempts to obtain a disability benefit. Such seeming inconsistencies can reveal the extent to which illness has permeated a man's self-definition and self-concept. In any case, these definitions reflect and simultaneously shape narratives of knowing self through illness (Frank, 1993; Herzlich & Pierret, 1987) and, therefore, can result in raising or resolving identity dilemmas.

Definitions of enemies and allies both explicitly create personifications. However, viewing one's illness as an enemy objectifies and externalizes it and thus distances and separates it from at least personal, if not also, social identity (cf. Goffman 1961, 1963). Viewing illness as an ally emphasizes subjectivity and identification with it and thus integrates it with personal and, if disclosed, social identity. Illness as an intrusive presence brings it into the body as an unwelcome occupant that insidiously has become part of self rather than remaining external to it. Illness as an opportunity allows for revaluation, redirection, and reconstruction of self.

Changing definitions and revising the stories that frame them reveal new identifications. Yet these definitions are not always stories of self-change as

Frank (1993) describes. Rather, definitions of illness as an enemy typically testify to a man's continuity of self. Here, the narrative framing of the man's definition proclaims that he remains the same though his body and situation may have changed.

Definitions of the illness spread to specific symptoms, treatments, and even to the body itself. A young man who had defined the dialysis machine as an enemy tried to make an ally of his new kidney transplant, which his body began to reject. To him, the transplant meant a direct route to his preferred identity as an involved graduate student. He said:

> Rejection is a very scary time . . . a very scary time because you have all these hopes and then the kidney—your body is saying, "Well, I don't agree with you, you don't need—this isn't your kidney." And you're saying, "Well, agree with me, this is . . ." and you get into conversations, I got into conversations with my kidney and my body.

Images of enemies and allies are present, although sometimes implicit, in the competitive discourse of victories and losses that middle-aged and younger men frequently invoke when talking about their illnesses. Norman Cousins (1983) titles his chapter on dealing with his heart attack, "Counterattack." Lee Foster (1986) states, "The record for longevity on a kidney machine, the last time I checked, was fourteen years, and if I stay on dialysis I aim to break the record" (p. 526). Arnold R. Beisser (1989), a psychiatrist who became quadriplegic due to poliomyelitis, took a similar stance toward his disability:

> When I became disabled, I even tried to turn my disability into a competitive sport. I did everything possible to deny the cripple in me. I had no use for him, and no place in my concept of myself for disability. Much of what I have written here has been about my search to find something of worth in that image of the cripple, something with which I could identify without regret.
>
> (p. 80)

Beisser wrote his book at age 62; he became ill at 27. Visible disabilities, such as Beisser's wheelchair use, result in social identifications that cause or complicate problems in self-definition. If so, definitions of illness and disability as an intrusive presence are likely to follow. Anthropologist Robert F. Murphy had had a productive career before a benign tumor left him progressively paralyzed. He (1987) comments:

> [F]rom the time I first took to the wheelchair up to the present, the fact that I am physically disabled has been in the background of my

conscious thoughts. Busy though I might be with other matters and problems, it lingers as a shadow in the corner of my mind, waiting, ready to come out at any moment to fill my meditations. It is a Presence. I, too, had acquired an embattled identity, a sense of who and what I was that was no longer dominated by my past attributes, but rather by my physical defects.

(p. 104)

Murphy's wheelchair use permeated his consciousness of self, as well as others' consciousness of him, and symbolized his loss of power. Other meanings and symbols emerge when the context and situation are different. When first ill, Beisser (1989) laid flat on his back for a year. He recalled when he first sat in a wheelchair, "I felt as though my power had been restored. I had far greater difficulty in breathing, and it lasted only three or four minutes. But who cared! It was position that counted, and I associated this one with being able to take care of myself" (p. 24).

Later, Beisser's disability elicited rudeness, stigma, invaded space, and loss of privacy, which raised and reinforced identity dilemmas. Like Beisser, several of my middle-aged and younger interviewees took years to reconcile the identity dilemmas that illness thrust upon them. Older working-class men were resigned to their situations and built lives around illness. Middle-class men sought to make illness and disability meaningful, to recast them into something through which positive identification could be made. Their quest resembled that of the younger and middle-aged women respondents (both middle and working class), but these women ordinarily articulated their concerns more directly and arrived at positive conclusions more readily. Nonetheless, by seeking to make illness meaningful, these men changed their definition from illness as an enemy or an intrusive presence to an experience with positive consequences. The professor above first received his diagnosis while he had a diabetic crisis and nearly died. Afterward, he viewed both his body and his illness as enemies who were trying to kill him. But over the years, his definition changed:

> It's [his illness] an enemy that I've made an ally of. Really, I don't think I'd still be here, if I hadn't been diabetic. It's like the paradox of the return of the prodigal son. It kicked me out of Eden alright, having to, you know, be on my best behavior so much and think about when to shoot up and all that. But it was what I needed.

From this vantage point, this man learned how central being diabetic was to his sense of identity. He remarked, "Probably if I were less narcissistic and obsessive, I would be a poorer diabetic. It's sort of like diabetes and me, we were made for each other."

By making illness an ally, men can use it as an opportunity for reflection and change. Arthur Frank (1990) refers to illness explicitly as "an opportunity, though a dangerous one" (p. 1). He writes, "Illness takes away parts of your life, but in doing so it gives you the opportunity to choose the life you will lead, as opposed to living out the one you have simply accumulated over the years" (p. 1).

Whether men treat their conditions as enemies, allies, intrusions, or opportunities, their definitions are seldom mutually exclusive or static. That is, a man who sees illness as an ally because it led him to set priorities can still see it as an intrusive, even ominous presence in his life. Similarly, a man can treat his illness as an ally for a number of years only to redefine it as an increasingly intrusive presence if it steadily limits his activities. Which definition holds sway depends on the context and situation, the man's self-definition, and his responsibilities, actions, values, goals, and plans. As a result, many men appreciate what they learn while ill, but still struggle with preserving defining aspects of self from the past before illness.

Preserving self

Although certain major identities change, such as that of worker to part-time retiree, men with chronic illnesses try to lead normal lives. In doing so, they implicitly, and often explicitly, devote much effort to preserving self—aspects of a self known and valued in the past (see also, Charmaz, 1991; Johnson, 1991). Preserving self means maintaining essential qualities, attributes, and identities of this past self that fundamentally shape the self-concept. Thus, ill people relinquish some identities but retain others. By preserving self, men reconcile the identity dilemmas that chronic illness thrusts upon them. Johnson (1991) stresses roles and lifestyles in preserving self, but it means more than that. Rather, preserving self means maintaining a way of being in the world and a way of relating to and knowing self, others, and social worlds. Doing so reduces the marginalizing effects of illness. Through preserving self, men maintain continuity throughout the past, present, and future. Although he had to take a disability benefit, Ernest Hirsch (1977), a clinical psychologist with multiple sclerosis, still maintained identity continuity through remaining in the same organization, community, and close friendships. His former employer provided him with free office space and clerical help to enable him to do research and writing. Despite earlier worries about losing his masculinity and independence, he managed to preserve essential qualities of self although he endured profound physical and social losses. He writes:

> Whatever changes have occurred in me do not touch the core of my "self," which has remained pretty much the same. As far as other

people are concerned, I think I've remained much as always. Although I realize some changes have occurred, I feel a continuity with the past and have no difficulty recognizing myself as myself, and neither does anyone else.

(pp. 169–170)

As men come to terms with illness and disability, they preserve self by limiting encroachments from illness in their lives and controlling definitions of their illness and any disability, as suggested above. They also intensify control over their lives when they can and develop strategies that minimize the visibility and intrusiveness of illness, which I discuss briefly below. This reconciling of identity dilemmas takes illness into account, whether others believe that these men do it in a healthy way.

Recapturing the past self

Before men learn these new ways of preserving self, many of them assume that they will recapture the past self, or explicitly aim to do so. Here, they aim to reclaim the same identities, the same lives that they had before illness. Nothing less will do. For these men, their "real" selves are and must be only the past self (Charmaz, 1991; Turner, 1976). They lapse into invalidism and despondency if they cannot recapture their past selves. Jean B. Zink (1992), who has long been disabled and now suffers from postpoliomyelitis syndrome, compares herself with a male friend:

> Disability came to Bill in his mature life, which was full of fun and freedom, and he feels he was robbed of it. Bill's future is now in the past. Disability robbed me of a carefree youth but not of youth itself, which was full of innocence and idealism. My future was before me. Bill yearns for the past. I prayed for a future.... Bill lost the life that was precious to him, and now he ages with regret. I age with gratitude, regardless of the struggle, not because I am better than Bill but because my experience as I perceive it has demanded this of me. Bill seems to believe that the way things *were* should be pursued relentlessly. Bill uses his psychic energy to recapture the past. I use my psychic energy to maintain the present.
>
> (p. 60)

Except for women whose diseases caused severe mental impairment, women showed more resiliency and resourcefulness than men in preserving aspects of self, even though women were less likely to have spouses to bolster their efforts (see also, LeMaistre, 1985; Lewis, 1985; Pitzele, 1985; Register, 1987; Wulf, 1979). Women rarely persisted in tying their futures to recapturing their past selves when they defined physical changes as permanent. Quite possibly, women's earlier roles and identities fostered greater adaptability to illness.

Trying to recapture the past self does provide strong incentives to fight illness and to stave off death. When men believe in their doctors and in their treatment, their resolve to struggle maintains their hope. If so, then a man assumes that his past self will be preserved when his physician promises marked improvement. A middle-aged father of young sons commented about having cardiac bypass surgery:

> I felt—I was going to do everything I did before; otherwise, it wasn't worth having the surgery. . . . I wanted to be just the same as before. And, like for these children, it would be really devastating to them if I were to go ahead and say, "Well, I can't do this because of my heart; I can't do that," you know. You don't want to teach young children to be like that.

Attempting to recapture the past self has its pitfalls when all valued social and personal identities remain in an irretrievable past. Being unable to measure up to the past self results in further preoccupation with it, and heightens identity dilemmas. Arnold Beisser (1989) recalls how his desire to recapture his past self affected his courtship:

> [O]ne big thing separated us. I was in love with someone else. That someone else was me, or rather my image of what I used to be. My past was my standard and I carried it with me like a Pepsi generation commercial. And, of course, I assumed that everyone else, including Rita, was attracted to that same image.
>
> (p. 56)

Drastic lifestyle changes following illness such as reduced employment, forced retirement, rigid regimens, and broken marriages erode or collapse former identities entirely, one after another, like dominoes. Simultaneously, despondency about not recapturing the past self increases and renders preserving valued aspects of self more arduous. A middle-aged man with heart disease felt overwhelmed, immobile, and depressed when he compared his present precarious physical, financial, and marital statuses with his past fitness, financial security, and stable marriage. His fear of another heart attack combined with his lassitude led him to withdraw from everyone. He said, "I'd say I hit rock bottom about October, November last year. I got to where I don't care what happens to me, you know; I don't care what happens to anybody."

The distance increases between a man's past self, by now reconstructed in memory in idealized form, and present identities, as valued former identities collapse and new ones are viewed as negative. With each identity loss from chronic illness, preserving valued past "masculine" identities becomes more difficult. Not surprisingly then, Brooks and Matson (1982) found that the self-concepts of men with multiple sclerosis changed more negatively over time than those of women. Men draw upon the existing cultural logic that currently defines masculinity as they try to make sense of their altered selves and situations (cf. Denzin, 1991). When sexual performance forms the foundation of their conception of masculinity, impotency undermines their identities as men.

Preserving a past identity becomes particularly problematic when the basis for that identity is lost. After his heart attack, the man above was financially devastated. Both he and his wife valued traditional roles but he could no longer work full-time. Subsequent crises put more responsibility on his wife to get a full-time job, as his identity as the wage earner rapidly eroded. He said:

> She was fine throughout that [the financial crisis]—she didn't work [before then]; she worked part-time; now she's working full-time. So yeah, she blamed me for that, me being the provider and that type of thing. That hurts me too, you know.

Under these conditions, illness becomes the symbol of identities lost and the reason why attempts to preserve self flounder. This man explained, "This is the worst year of my life. In one month I lost health, a career. In a year I lost my capital; I almost lost my marriage—you could almost say that year I lost my marriage. My oldest daughter moved."

Problematic health strains an already strained marriage. It also strains a stable marriage when erosion of valued identities continues. As with retirement, chronic illness allows men who cut back or leave work to become new critics of their wives' and children's activities. Loss of control outside of the home leads to efforts to preserve self by exerting more control within it. To the extent that a man takes for granted that masculinity is embedded in power, the more likely he will tighten his control within the household as access to other arenas decreases. For example, as a retired bartender became housebound, his scrutiny of his wife's day increased and he became more critical and controlling. She could incur his wrath by failing to anticipate or to satisfy his dictates about the smallest household or personal care task.

Such men want to be in control. At this point, they implicitly realize that illness has marginalized their sense of masculinity (cf. Connell, 1987; Messner & Sabo, 1990). They cannot accept physical dependence, except, perhaps, upon wives. The demeaning nature of seeking help, being evaluated ("his doctor found out he was smoking again and read him the riot act"), of living on new, much less on someone else's, terms does not come easily. Rather than give up old habits, these men may flaunt them. If they cannot control their health, they may try to control someone else's response. To do this, they take risks—often many of them—and likely cast their wives and physicians as adversaries to outwit. In this way, they maintain their assumed status in the hierarchy of men and simultaneously exert dominance over women (cf. Sabo, 1990). At such a point, they also risk being identified as obstreperous, unmotivated, and mentally unstable by their practitioners (cf. Albrecht, 1992; Plough, 1986).

Dependency strains relationships and plays havoc with identity. But identity develops and is maintained through interaction. Partners often find themselves in an elaborate dance around dependency. Wives and partners may find themselves anxiously trying to protect shreds of their husbands' former identities while feeling overwhelmed by the escalating demands placed upon them (see, e.g., Lear, 1980; Strong, 1988).

These women provide pivotal identity supports for their partners that mute the identifying effects of dependency and loss. In contrast, dwindling identity supports accelerate dependency and loss in single men. Death, divorce, and distance left a 38-year-old man with advanced multiple sclerosis institutionalized and without family contact. After years of life-threatening crises, he felt disconnected from the world and from almost everyone. He said, "I don't think of death as gloomy; I see it as a release."

This man disdained the self he witnessed in illness. To him, it was not worth preserving. When talking about his teenaged years, his present immobility contrasted strikingly with his past activity. He said in wonder, "You know, I could do anything I needed to do. Like baseball, or football, or basketball. You know I did all those things—swimming. Now it's no more."

For him, the halcyon days of healthy youth remained in a faded past. But for others, the disparity between past and present identity enfolded the immediate present and foretold the future. A young man whose kidney transplant was failing questioned the value of living on the dialysis machine. The middle-aged attorney alluded to previously discovered that his condition was far more serious and complicated than he had initially thought and probably had resulted in minimal brain damage. Another surgery became necessary, but his health had deteriorated too much to risk doing it. Losses accrued. No stamina for backpacking. Memory losses canceled work. Social Security denied his disability claim. A legal victory against Social Security still did not force processing his claim. Pleas for more painkillers were refused. Increased blood pressure medications sapped his energy and drained his spirit. Despondent and unable to function as in the past, he said, "I don't do anything but sleep now." Six months later, he hanged himself in the room that had come to be his bedroom, office, and sanctuary.

These three men saw their lives shrinking and their chances for creating valued identities diminishing. Under these conditions, they each saw suicide as a reasonable way of resolving the identity dilemmas in which they found themselves.[7] In contrast, possibilities of expanding identities foster hope and desire to stave off disability and death. The self to be preserved is a developing self, ripe with potential for new, positive identities. For example, one man had recently won an award that brought him substantial recognition and travel, in addition to renewed friendships. The world was opening up to him, not closing down upon him. Quite spontaneously, he disclosed, "I don't want to die, I'm just a baby, a 52-year-old baby boy. I'm just starting; I don't want to die."

Preserving a public identity, changing a private identity

Some men claim public identities that reaffirm their pasts and demonstrate continuity with that past. They offer a public narrative of their lives in which chronic illness plays a minor or past role. In that way, they attempt to maintain their earlier position in the gender order. But to keep their public narrative creditable, they may have to devote vast amounts of energy to keeping illness contained and disability hidden or cloaked (cf. Charmaz, 1991). Their efforts are founded on assumptions of preserving masculinity. A man with diabetes could not manage both his wheelchair and a tray in the cafeteria. Because he could not bring himself to ask his coworkers for help, he skipped lunch and risked a coma rather than request help.

Simultaneously, men may maximize the significance of illness and disability in their private lives. At home, illness and disability engulf them and may engulf the entire household. Roger Ressmeyer (1983) found that he involved himself in unwise relationships because he needed a partner's support and backup work. Ironically, the independent public man can transform himself into a dependent patient at home. This stance allows the tyranny of the sickroom, promotes self-pity, and encourages physical dependence. Even when men do not become overly dependent, wives add hours to their day as they prepare special diets, assist in bathing, dressing, grooming, completing the daily medical regimen, and provide rides (cf. Corbin & Strauss, 1984; Gerhardt & Brieskorn-Zink, 1986).

Strategies for preserving self

Whether a complete disjuncture exists between the public and private identities, most men try to mute the effects of illness on socializing or working. They draw upon both taken-for-granted actions and explicit strategies to preserve their earlier selves and thus, maintain or re-create public and private identities. Their strategies involve careful timing, pacing, and staging to maintain appearances to others, and often, to self.

When they needed to keep working, men attended closely to ways they could quite literally preserve themselves to do so. These men planned and managed their appearance because looking sick could cost them their bosses' confidence, coworkers' support, or even their jobs. When they felt that they would be disadvantaged in their hierarchy of men, they told no one that they had a serious illness (see also Ressmeyer, 1983), avoided disclosing further episodes, or minimized their significance. One middle-aged man with renal failure discovered that his cronies of 30 years turned against him for receiving less strenuous tasks for a few months after he had a heart attack. This man decided not to be beaten by his coworkers' attitudes and kept his job. But he refused his supervisor's offers to reassign him to easier jobs to prove that he could still do the strenuous work.[8]

Being able to control the logistics for doing work, as well as the amount and type of work itself, allows men to preserve their work and themselves, including their assumptions about masculinity. Part of that control rests on also being able to control other people and the definition of the situation. An executive masked leaving the office early for his dialysis treatments by "attending meetings out of the office." Not even his secretary knew he was a dialysis patient. He believed that knowledge of his illness in the business community would reduce his stature as an aggressive competitor in the hierarchy of businessmen (cf. Sabo & Gordon, 1992). A salesman completed his sales calls in the morning when he felt and looked fresher, and did paperwork at home in the afternoons when he could take rest breaks. A professor referred questions to several bright students when he felt short of breath. An administrator moved his office to a wing closer to the parking lot. In all these cases, controlling time, pace, space, information, and people gave these men more control over ensuing interaction, impression-management, and identity.

How do men preserve self when they cannot exert this type of control? Their embarrassment about visible markers of illness resulted in avoiding encounters beyond their inner circles. The executive above maintained a policy of not socializing with business associates. By not attending cocktail or swim parties, he hid his restricted diet and his dialysis shunt. A craftsman with emphysema hid how hard walking had become. He lagged behind anyone who might observe him struggling to climb a few stairs. Later, as his coughing and spitting fractured ordinary conversation, he refused social invitations and reduced his work to a few projects that he could complete alone at home.

Not everyone assumes that illness and disability will become melded with identity. Some men remain strikingly resourceful in finding ways to remain vitally involved and simultaneously, to avoid having a stigmatized identity. Wheelchair use, for example, can give rise to developing a host of clever strategies for preserving self. One man arrived at social events early to position himself in an opportune location to see and greet friends. He found that people treated him as a commanding male when seated across from him but did not when they towered over him. When others were seated, he could position his body more forcefully in ways associated with manliness (Connell, 1983; Whitson, 1990). Such strategies preserve self as known in the past and, moreover, preserve assumptions about masculinity.

Discussion

Traditional assumptions of male identity, including an active, problem-solving stance, emphasis on personal power and autonomy, and bravery in the face of danger create a two-edged sword for men in chronic illness. On the one hand, these assumptions encourage men to take risks, to be active, and to try to recover, which certainly can prompt re-creating a valued life after serious episodes of illness and therefore bolster self-esteem. On the other hand, these assumptions narrow the range of credible male behaviors for those who subscribe to them. Hence, they foster rigidity in stance and set the conditions for slipping into depression. Men's assumed difference between masculine identity and the "lesser" identities of women and children shrink as they lose ordinary masculinizing practices (Connell, Ashenden, Kessler, & Dowsett, 1982; Whitson, 1990).

Thus, an uneasy tension exists between valued identities and disparaged, that is, denigrated or shameful, ones. A man can gain a strengthened or a diminished identity through experiencing illness. These are not mutually exclusive categories. Men often move back and forth depending on their situations and their perceptions of them. The grieving process in men may be negated or cause those who witness it such discomfort that they cannot give comfort. Men express their grieving in fear and rage as well as in tears and sorrow. But for many men who experience progressive illness and disability, grieving, instead of being a process, sinks into becoming a permanent depression. If so, they will likely abandon constraining medical regimens that erode their sense of mastery. Life becomes struggling to live on their own terms while waiting to die.

What are the conditions that shape whether a man will reconstruct a positive identity or sink into depression? Certainly, whether a man defines having future possibilities makes an enormous difference. The men in my study primarily founded their preferred identities in action. Subsequently, if they saw no valued realm of action available to them and no way to preserve a valued self, the likelihood increased that they would become despondent.

In summary, awakening to death causes men to face their mortality. Whether they view their illness as a discrete event or as causing continued uncertainty depends in part on whether their concepts of masculinity allow them to construct flexible roles and valued identities as men who have chronic illnesses. Otherwise, they accommodate to uncertainty by bracketing illness to acute episodes and crises, or they refuse to accommodate to it. In this sense, men take more individualistic stances toward their illnesses than do women, who are tied to a network of relationships that shape how they manage their illnesses. Acknowledging uncertainty as lasting, however, does prompt reappraisals and redirection for both men and women and shapes how they define illness and disability. Men more often view illness as an enemy to overcome or as an intrusive presence to control than do women.

Visible disability may reduce men's stature in the hierarchy of men more than its analogous consequences for women. If so, then men have greater incentives than women to try to recapture the past and their respective masculine identities in the past. Similarly, then, men have perhaps a greater stake in preserving self than women and the public identities that support this self.

A final point: A more exacting look at the differential experience of men and women who suffer from serious chronic illnesses will deepen sociological and professional understandings of how they make sense of their lives. As the research in chronic illness grows, studying men and women comparatively in conjunction with marital, age, and social class statuses, in addition to the type of illness, can substantially refine sociological interpretations of the narratives of chronically ill people.

Acknowledgements

Portions of this article appeared in a different form in *The Sociological Quarterly*, *35*(2), 269–288. © 1994 by the Midwest Sociological Society; permission granted. The paper was also presented at the annual meeting of the Society for the Study of Social Problems in Pittsburgh, August 18–20, 1992. I am indebted to Candee Nagle, Norman K. Denzin, David F. Gordon, Mark Mikkelson, Don Sabo, and three anonymous reviewers for their comments on an earlier draft. I thank David F. Gordon and Don Sabo for encouraging me to work in this area.

Notes

1 Chronic illness means experiencing ongoing or intermittent, recurrent, irreversible, and often, degenerative, symptoms of a disease process (cf. Freund & McGuire, 1991). I focus on what it means to have a disease, not on objectivist medical definitions, and address two of Conrad's (1987) subtypes of chronic illness: "lived-with-illnesses" (e.g., multiple sclerosis, chronic fatigue syndrome, renal failure, diabetes, post-poliomyelitis syndrome), which force adapting without immediate life threat, and those "mortal illnesses" (e.g., heart attack, stroke, cancer) that sufferers view as life-threatening and have lasting consequences whether or not they (a) know about these consequences and (b) experience immediate symptoms.

2 The data for this study are derived from 40 in-depth formal interviews of 20 men, 7 of whom were interviewed more than once, informal interviews, and a collection of personal accounts. Comparisons were made with 80 interviews with chronically ill women. The criteria for being interviewed included (a) adult status (over 21 years of age), (b) a diagnosis of a serious but not terminal chronic illness, (c) a disease with an uncertain course, and (d) effects of illness on daily life. When I first met the men, their ages ranged as follows: three under 40; six between 40 and 50; four between 50 and 60; five between 60 and 70, and the remaining two men were 73 and 85. Ten men worked at least part-time; others had retired or were too ill to work. In social class, they ranged as follows: eight men were working class or poor; six were middle class, and four were upper-middle class. Ten men were married.

Status attributes of the one half of the sample with whom I kept in touch (5 to 8 years) changed slightly over time (e.g., financial and marital). All of the men were white.

Grounded theory methods were used to analyze the data (Charmaz, 1983, 1990; Corbin & Strauss, 1990; Glaser, 1978; Glaser & Strauss, 1967; Strauss, 1987). The steps included (a) examining the interviews for gender differences, (b) studying men's interviews and written accounts for themes, (c) building analytic categories from men's definitions of and taken-for-granted assumptions about their situations, (d) conducting further interviews to refine these categories, (e) rereading personal accounts from the vantage point of gender issues (e.g., Fiore, 1984; Hirsch, 1977; Hodgins, 1964; Kelly, 1977; Murphy, 1987; Zola, 1982), (f) studying a new set of personal accounts (e.g., Beisser, 1989; Frank, 1990; Zink, 1992), and (g) making comparisons with women on selected key points. The processes in the major themes served to integrate the analysis.

3 Also, men report fewer illnesses and doctors' visits than women; men may not seek early care or routine checks that might result in averting crises (Freund & McGuire, 1991; Nathanson, 1989; Verbrugge, 1989; Verbrugge & Wingard, 1987;Waldron, 1976). Some men disattend to conditions such as diabetes or high blood pressure until they become crises.

4 Note that I refer to *initial* crises here. A man who becomes identified as a troublemaker, crock, mental case, mental incompetent, or an alcoholic will be hard-pressed to have his symptoms and views of treatment taken seriously (cf. Albrecht, 1992; Leiderman & Grisso, 1985; Millman, 1976; Plough, 1986).

5 The few gay men with whom I talked did not currently have love relationships.

6 The disease process affects the kind of the uncertainty that people experience. Laura Nathan (1990) points out that initially cancer patients and their families focus on recovery, but they cannot be sure when and if that recovery has occurred; they face continued uncertainty.

7 Kotarba (1983) details the story of a man in chronic pain who suffers one loss after another and commits suicide. His story reveals parallel conditions to those these men faced.

8 Most working-class jobs permit little flexibility. Middle-class jobs, in contrast, allow men more control over timing, scheduling, pacing, and using space during work. Kotarba (1983) suggests that working-class laborers may be relatively unconcerned about staying on the job because they can net 80% of their pay if they can claim a job-related disability. Ten years later, many working-class jobs are without access to benefits and even if they are available, workers are hard-pressed to prove that their illnesses or disabilities are job related. Thus, workers try to remain in their jobs.

References

Albrecht, G. L. (1992). The social experience of disability. In C. Calhoun & G. Ritzer (Eds.), *Social problems* (pp. 1–18). New York: McGraw-Hill.

Beisser, A. R. (1989). *Flying without wings: Personal reflections on being disabled*. New York: Doubleday.

Brooks, N. A., & Matson, R. R. (1982). Social psychological adjustment to multiple sclerosis. *Social Science & Medicine, 16*, 2129–2135.

Charmaz, K. (1983). The grounded theory method: An explication and interpretation. In R. M. Emerson (Ed.), *Contemporary field research* (pp. 109–126). Boston: Little, Brown.

Charmaz, K. (1987). Struggling for a self: Identity levels of the chronically ill. In J. A. Roth & P. C. Conrad (Eds.), *Research in the sociology of health care: The experience and management of chronic illness* (pp. 283–321). Greenwich, CT: JAI.
Charmaz, K. (1990). Discovering chronic illness: Using grounded theory. *Social Science & Medicine, 30*, 1161–1172.
Charmaz, K. (1991). *Good days, bad days: The self in chronic illness and time.* New Brunswick, NJ: Rutgers University Press.
Connell, R. W. (1983). *Which way is up?: Essays on class, sex and culture.* Sydney, Australia: Allen and Unwin.
Connell, R. W. (1987). *Gender & power: Society, the person and sexual politics.* Stanford, CA: Stanford University Press.
Connell, R. W., Ashenden, D. J., Kessler, S., & Dowsett, G. W. (1982). *Making the difference: Schools, families and social division.* Sydney, Australia: Allen and Unwin.
Conrad, P. (1987). The experience of illness: Recent and new directions. In J. A. Roth & P. C. Conrad (Eds.), *Research in the sociology of health care: The experience and management of chronic illness* (Vol. 6, pp. 1–31). Greenwich, CT: JAI.
Corbin, J. M., & Strauss, A. L. (1984). Collaboration: Couples working together to manage chronic illness. *Image, 4*, 109–115.
Corbin, J. M., & Strauss, A. L. (1988). *Unending work and care: Managing chronic illness at home.* San Francisco: Jossey-Bass.
Corbin, J. M., & Strauss, A. L. (1990). *Basics of qualitative research.* Newbury Park, CA: Sage.
Cousins, N. (1983). *The healing heart: Antidotes to panic and helplessness.* New York: Avon.
Cowie, B. (1976). The patient's perception of his heart attack. *Social Science & Medicine, 10*, 87–96.
Dahlberg, C. C., & Jaffe, J. (1977). *Stroke: A doctor's personal story of his recovery.* New York: Norton.
Denzin, N. K. (1989). *Interpretive biography.* Newbury Park, CA: Sage.
Denzin, N. K. (1991). *Images of postmodern society.* Newbury Park, CA: Sage.
Fiore, N. A. (1984). *The road back to health.* New York: Bantam.
Foster, L. (1978). Man and machine: Life without kidneys. In H. D. Schwartz & C. F. Kart (Eds.), *Dominant issues in medical sociology* (pp. 522–526). Redding, MA: Addison-Wesley.
Frank, A. (1991). *At the will of the body.* New York: Houghlin Mifflin.
Frank, A. (1993). The rhetoric of self-change: Illness experience as narrative. *Sociological Quarterly, 34*, 39–52.
Freund, P. E. S., & McGuire, M. B. (1991). *Health, illness, and the social body.* Englewood Cliffs, NJ: Prentice Hall.
Gecas, V. (1982). The self-concept. *Annual Review of Sociology, 8*, 1–33.
Gerhardt, U., & Brieskom-Zink, M. (1986). The normalization of hemodialysis at home. In J. A. Roth & S. B. Ruzek (Eds.), *Research in the sociology of health care: The adoption and social consequences of medical technologies* (Vol. 5, pp. 271–317). Greenwich, CT: JAI.
Glaser, B. G. (1978). *Theoretical sensitivity.* Mill Valley, CA: Sociology Press.
Glaser, B. G., & Strauss, A. L. (1967). *The discovery of grounded theory.* Chicago: Aldine.
Goffman, E. (1961). *Encounters.* New York: Bobbs-Merrill.

Goffman, E. (1963). *Stigma*. Englewood Cliffs, NJ: Prentice Hall.
Gordon, D. (1990). Testicular cancer: Passage to new priorities. In E. J. Clark, J. M. Fritz, & P. P. Ricker (Eds.), *Clinical sociological perspectives on illness & loss* (pp. 234–247). Philadelphia: Charles Press.
Herzlich, C., & Pierret, J. (1987). Illness and self in society. Baltimore: Johns Hopkins University Press.
Hewitt, J. (1989). *Dilemmas of the American self*. Philadelphia: Temple University Press.
Hirsch, E. (1977). *Starting over*. Hanover, MA: Christopher.
Hodgins, E. (1964). *Episode: Report on the accident inside my skull*. New York: Athaneum.
Husserl, E. (1970). *The crisis of the European sciences and transcendental phenomenology*. Evanston, IL: Northwestern University Press.
Jaques, E. (1965). Death and the midlife crisis. *International Journal of Psychoanalysis*, 46, 502–514.
Johnson, J. L. (1991). Learning to live again: The process of adjustment following a heart attack. In J. M. Morse & J. L. Johnson (Eds.), *The illness experience* (pp. 13–88). Newbury Park, CA: Sage.
Karp, D. (1988). A decade of reminders: Changing age consciousness between fifty and sixty years old. *The Gerontologist*, 28, 727–738.
Kelleher, D. (1988). Coming to terms with diabetes: Coping strategies and non-compliance. In R. A. Anderson & M. Bury (Eds.), *Living with chronic illness* (pp. 155–187). London: Unwin Hyman.
Kelly, O. E. (1977). Make today count. In H. Fiefel (Ed.), *New meanings of death* (pp. 181–194). New York: McGraw-Hill.
Kleinman, A. (1988). *The illness narratives: Suffering, healing, & the human condition*. New York: Basic Books.
Kotarba, J. A. (1983). *Chronic pain: Its social dimensions*. Beverly Hills, CA: Sage.
Lear, M. (1980). *Heartsounds*. New York: Simon & Schuster.
Leiderman, D. B., & Grisso, J-A. (1985). The Gomer phenomenon. *Journal of Health and Social Behavior*, 26, 222–231.
LeMaistre, J. (1985). *Beyond rage: The emotional impact of chronic illness*. Oak Park, IL: Alpine Guild.
Levinson, D., Darrow, J. C., Klein, E., Levinson, M., & McKee, B. (1978). *The seasons of a man's life*. New York: Knopf.
Lewis, K. (1985). *Successful living with chronic illness*. Wayne, NJ: Avery.
Messner, M. A., & Sabo, D. F. (1990). Toward a critical feminist reappraisal of sport, men and the gender order. In M. A. Messner & D. F. Sabo (Eds.), *Sport, men, and the gender order: Critical feminist perspective* (pp. 1–15). Champaign, IL: Human Kinetics.
Millman, M. (1976). *The unkindest cut*. New York: William Morrow.
Murphy, R. F. (1987). *The body silent*. New York: Henry Holt.
Nathan, L. E. (1990). Coping with uncertainty: Family members' adaptations during cancer remission. In E. J. Clark, J. M. Fritz, & P. P. Rieker (Eds.), *Clinical sociological perspectives on illness & loss* (pp. 219–233). Philadephia: Charles Press.
Nathanson, C. (1989). Sex, illness, and medical care: A review of data, theory, and methods. In P. Brown (Ed.), *Perspectives in medical sociology* (pp. 46–70). Belmont, CA: Wadsworth.

Peyrot, M., McMurry, J. F., Jr., & Hedges, R. (1988). Marital adjustment to adult diabetes: Interpersonal congruence and spouse satisfaction. *Journal of Marriage and the Family, 50,* 363-376.
Pitzele, S. K. (1985). *We are not alone: Learning to live with chronic illness.* New York: Workman.
Plough, A. (1986). *Borrowed time: Artificial organs and the politics of extending lives.* Philadelphia: Temple University Press.
Register, C. (1987). *Living with chronic illness.* New York: Free Press.
Reif, L. (1975). Ulcerative colitis: Strategies for managing life. In A. L. Strauss (Ed.), *Chronic illness and the quality of life.* St. Louis, MO: C. V. Mosby.
Ressmeyer, R. (1983, July 10). A day to day struggle. *San Francisco Examiner and Chronicle,* pp. 1-5 [California Living Sec.].
Sabo, D. F. (1990). Men, death anxiety, and denial: Critical feminist interpretations of adjustment to mastectomy. In E. J. Clark, J. M. Fritz, & P. P. Rieker (Eds.), *Clinical sociological perspectives on illness & loss* (pp. 71-84). Philadelphia: Charles Press.
Sabo, D. F., & Gordon, D. (1992, August). *Rethinking men's health and illness: The relevance of gender studies.* Paper presented at the Society for the Study of Social Problems, Pittsburgh, PA.
Sabo, D. F., & Panepinto, J. (1990). Football ritual and the social reproduction of masculinity. In M. A. Messner & D. F. Sabo (Eds.), *Sport, men, and the gender order: Critical feminist perspectives* (pp. 115-126). Champaign, IL: Human Kinetics.
Schneider, J. W., & Conrad, P. (1983). *Having epilepsy.* Philadelphia: Temple University Press.
Speedling, E. J. (1982). *Heart attack: The family response at home and in the hospital.* New York: Tavistock.
Strauss, A. (1987). *Qualitative analysis for social scientists.* New York: Cambridge University Press.
Strauss, A., Corbin, J., Fagerhaugh, S., Glaser, B. G., Maines, D., Suczek, B., & Wiener, C. (1984). *Chronic illness and the quality of life* (2nd ed.). St. Louis, MO: C. V. Mosby.
Strong, M. (1988). *Mainstay.* Boston: Little, Brown.
Tannen, D. (1990). *You just don't understand: Women and men in conversation.* New York: Ballantine.
Turner, R. (1976). The real self: From institution to impulse. *American Journal of Sociology, 81,* 989-1016.
Verbrugge, L. M. (1985). Gender and health: An update on hypotheses and evidence. *Journal of Health and Social Behavior, 26,* 156-182.
Verbrugge, L. M. (1989). The twain meet: Empirical explanations of sex differences in health and mortality. *Journal of Health and Social Behavior, 30,* 282-304.
Verbrugge, L. M., & Wingard, D. L. (1987). Sex differentials in health and mortality. *Women and Health, 12,* 103-145.
Waldron, I. (1976). Why do women live longer than men? *Social Science & Medicine, 10,* 349-362.
Weigert, A. J. (1986). The social production of identity: Metatheoretical foundations. *Sociological Quarterly, 27,* 165-183.

Whitson, D. (1990). Sport in the social construction of masculinity. In M. A. Messner & D. F. Sabo (Eds.), *Sport, men, and the gender order: Critical feminist perspectives* (pp. 19–30). Champaign, IL: Human Kinetics.

Wiener, C. J. (1975). The burden of arthritis. In A. L. Strauss (Ed.), *Chronic illness and the quality of life* (pp. 71–80). St. Louis, MO: C. V. Mosby.

Wulf, H. H. (1979). *Aphasia, my world alone*. Detroit, MI: Wayne State University Press.

Zink, J. B. (1992). Adjusting to early and late-onset disability. *Generations, 16*, 59–60.

Zola, I. K. (1982). *Missing pieces: A chronicle of living with a disability*. Philadephia: Temple University Press.